Preventive Cardiology

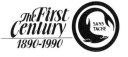

The First Century 1890-1990 SANS TACHE

Preventive Cardiology

Dennis M. Davidson, M.D.
Director, Preventive Cardiology Clinic
Stanford University School of Medicine
Stanford, California

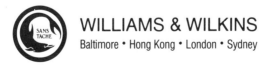

WILLIAMS & WILKINS
Baltimore • Hong Kong • London • Sydney

Editor: Jonathan W. Pine, Jr.
Associate Editor: Linda Napora
Copy Editor: Anne K. Schwartz
Designer: Wilma E. Rosenberger
Illustration Planner: Lorraine Wrzosek
Production Coordinator: Adèle Boyd

Copyright © 1991
Williams & Wilkins
428 East Preston Street
Baltimore, Maryland 21202, USA

Accurate indications, adverse reactions, and dosage schedules for drugs are provided
in this book, but it is possible that they may change. The reader is urged to review
the package information data of the manufacturers of the medications mentioned.

Printed in the United States of America

Library of Congress Cataloging-in-Publication Data

Davidson, Dennis.
   Preventive cardiology / Dennis M. Davidson.
      p.   cm.
   Includes index.
   ISBN 0-683-02350-0
   1. Heart—Diseases—Prevention. I. Title.
   [DNLM: 1. Coronary Disease—prevention & control. 2. Risk
Factors. WG 300 D252p]
RC682.D37 1991
616.1′205—dc20
DNLM/DLC
for Library of Congress   90-12455
                                                 CIP

90 91 92 93 94
1 2 3 4 5 6 7 8 9 10

To

Ralph and Amy Davidson

for a lifetime of love

preface

Despite the conventional wisdom of book publishing, this volume was written for a wide audience. It is my hope that it will serve as a readable introduction for health professionals and students to the exciting progress in preventive cardiology. Because clinicians from many specialties serve as primary caregivers, chapters on children, the elderly, and gender and hormonal considerations have been included, and interventions at the family and community level have been emphasized. I also intend to have the book serve as a reference for individuals working within the field; to that end, my source material has been cited extensively, particularly works published in the late 1980s in journals accessible through most medical libraries.

Coronary artery disease is a worldwide epidemic, well-established in industrialized countries, and soon to flourish in nations that are currently economically disadvantaged. To the extent that space allowed, I have attempted to reflect the many research endeavors and innovative community programs that are ongoing in various countries, while applauding the international cooperation that transcends ideology and is so characteristic of the preventive cardiology field.

Of particular interest to me have been the sociobehavioral and environmental factors, which have been less well studied to date than the physiologic indicators of risk. Early work indicates that there is a decided survival advantage at both the individual and the international levels to living under conditions of mutual trust and support, respect for our differences, and celebration of that which we hold in common. Toward that end, the international preventive cardiology and public health communities have been a constant source of inspiration for me. I am particularly grateful for the hospitality of colleagues during my visits and for the stimulation of our conversations at countless conferences.

I have been blessed with the example of many remarkable physicians in my professional growth, foremost of whom has been Dr. Paul Dudley White. A man who journeyed to equatorial Africa to meet Dr. Albert Schweitzer, who put to sea off Baja, California to record the electrocardiogram of a whale, and who walked from National Airport in Virginia to receive an award from the president of the United States at the White House, Dr. White continues to inspire me, years after his death.

Also of great importance to me have been cardiologists Evgueni Chazov and Bernard Lown, who have integrated their personal and professional concerns to lead us to a safer world. Cofounders of the International Physicians for the Prevention of Nuclear War, they continue to act as beacons for our journeys beyond national and cultural chauvinism to a future of hope for every child, woman, and man on this earth.

At the personal level, I am grateful to Doctors Richard D. Judge and Park W. Willis III, for their nurturance of my interest in cardiology during my early days in medical school. My divergence from traditional clinical and academic paths was stimulated and continues to be supported by my colleagues at Stanford University, Doctors Halsted R. Holman and John W. Farquhar. The Robert Wood Johnson Clinical Scholar Program and the National Heart, Lung, and Blood Institute Preventive Cardiology Academic Award gave me time to learn the principles and practice of preventive cardiology embodied herein, particularly through the opportunity to teach others.

For many of us, the heart has metaphorical meanings in emotional and spiritual spheres that extend far beyond its function as an electromechanical pump. It is my hope that the words that follow will touch you in many parts of your heart.

contents

Section I. Coronary Artery Disease

Section II. Indicators of Risk

Section III. Primary Prevention

Section IV. Prevention of CAD Events after Detection of Risk

Section V. Prevention of CAD Event Recurrence

Section VI. Dysrhythmias and Sudden Cardiac Death

Section VII. Cerebrovascular Disease

Section I

Coronary Artery Disease

1

epidemiology of coronary artery disease

During this century, coronary artery disease (CAD) emerged as the leading cause of death in industrialized countries (1, 2). In this book, *Hearts. Their Long Follow-up,* Dr. Paul Dudley White went back more than 50 years to review his cases as an intern at the Massachusetts General Hospital in 1912 and 1913. With characteristic precision, he noted several cases of atherosclerosis and angina pectoris, but noted confirmation by electrocardiogram was not possible "because such an instrument had not yet been installed in the hospital" (3).

Owing much to Dr. White and other pioneers in preventive cardiology, the epidemiology of CAD has been vigorously investigated during the last 50 years. During that time, the international cooperation of cardiovascular epidemiologists and other scientists first documented the rapid rise in mortality attributed to CAD and its sequelae in developed countries. More recently, decreases in CAD mortality rates have been noted in some economically advantaged countries (4), while lesser-developed nations continue to experience a rise (5).

Figure 1.1 illustrates the marked disparity in CAD mortality rates in women and men aged 30–69 from selected countries in 1985. The rates are adjusted for differences in age distribution among nations and are expressed in deaths per 100,000 persons.

For both women and men, rates in Northern Ireland are ten times higher than those in Japan. One may also note the remarkable similarity in rates in women from northern European countries, Canada, and the United States (6).

Although investigators have suggested that CAD may be associated with more than 200 indicators of risk (7), demonstration of cause and effect has been made in only a small percentage of these associations. Epidemiologic principles that strengthen a case for causality include strength and primacy of the relation, temporal sequence of presumed cause and effect, graded response of effect for a given "dose" of cause, independence of the presumed cause from other potential contributors to the effect, reproducibility of the effect when the cause is introduced in the original and other populations, and consistency with studies in vitro and in animals.

3

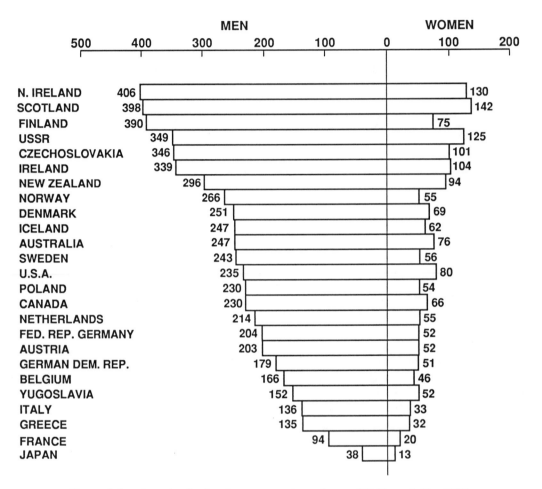

Figure 1.1. Age-standardized coronary artery disease (CAD) mortality, 1985.

Application of these criteria to the myriad of proposed indicators of CAD risk has yielded approximately ten categories of risk in addition to age. These factors are listed in Table 1.1 and form the basis for Chapters 3–12 of this volume. The presence and import of these indicators in childhood, in the early and middle adult years, and during the later years of life are then examined in Chapters 13–15.

INTERNATIONAL STUDIES

Regrettably, only a small number of the many exciting preventive cardiology studies and intervention programs can be covered in these pages. Further information is available in the published abstracts from the First and Second International Conferences on Preventive Cardiology held in Moscow (1985) and Washington (1989)

Table 1.1. Indicators of Coronary Artery Disease Risk

Lipids, lipoproteins, and nutritional intake
Blood pressure
Smoking
Family history
Diabetes mellitus
Physical activity
Obesity
Sociobehavioral and environmental factors
Gender and hormonal factors
Hematologic considerations

and in the CVD Epidemiology Newsletter distributed to members of the various national societies which comprise the International Federation and Society of Cardiology.

At the beginning of her book *On Call,* Jordan notes that "given that they were first to exist on the planet and currently make up the majority," she refers to the lesser-developed countries as "the First World" (8). Given the alarming increases in CAD risk indicator levels in those countries, the sequence of the global review below will follow her lead. After the poorer countries are discussed, the route will proceed by region, starting near the Greenwich meridian and circumnavigating eastward through representative countries.

Lesser-Developed Countries

In 1982, change in mortality from arterial diseases during the early 1970s was calculated. Of 28 developing countries, rates increased in 22 for men and 21 for women. Of eight countries with centrally planned economies, rates for men rose in seven; rates increased for women in six of the eight nations. As countries increased their per capita gross national product, the average annual rate of arterial disease mortality rose (9).

Rheumatic heart disease continues

to be the predominant cardiovascular disease throughout most of Africa, equatorial South and Central America, Egypt, Iran, Pakistan, Bangladesh, and other poor countries (5). However, the prevalence of smoking in many lesser developed countries is very high (10) (Table 5.1), and increases in other CAD risk indicators appear during transitions from rural to urban cultures within given countries.

For example, Kenyans who migrated from a rural area to Nairobi had significant elevations in blood pressure (11). Similarly, Asians moving to northwest London had high CAD mortality rates, but these were not entirely attributable to increased levels of risk indicators. Among Asians, the smoking rate remained low, and Hindus consumed less saturated fat and dietary cholesterol than the general British population (12). In contrast, for Muslims from Bangladesh living in east London, smoking rates were high, more saturated fat was consumed, and diabetes rates were higher than in the general population of London (13).

Among male Nigerian civil servants who had migrated from a rural area, the prevalence of hypertension increased to 35%; in women, it was 17%. Rates were higher among senior staff members; a majority over age 45 were hypertensive (14). Turks who migrated to the Federal Republic of Germany have higher levels of smoking and total blood cholesterol and have higher CAD mortality rates (15).

In Mexico, CAD rates increased nearly 40-fold from 1950 to 1983, particularly in the northern part of the country (16). A study in Ecuador documented dramatic rises in CAD rates, associated with migration to an urban area and increased consumption of saturated fat and salt (17). Stimulated by the International Teaching Seminars on Cardiovascular Epidemiology and Prevention, which have been held annually since 1968, a Latin American Working Group on Primary Prevention of Cardiovascular Disease and Epidemiology formed (18). Organizations such as these and the national heart associations encouraged by Dr. White and his successors will be necessary to combat the epidemic of CAD that will otherwise sweep these countries as their economies develop.

Northern and Western Europe

BELGIUM

Since 1970, CAD mortality has dropped significantly, probably due to reductions in cigarette use and consumption of saturated fats as well as a decrease of 50% in per capita salt use. Serum total cholesterol dropped significantly in the subsequent two decades (19), and stroke mortality in the elderly has decreased approximately 3% per year during that period (20). Investigators in the Belgian Heart Disease Prevention Project, a health education project, noted reductions in CAD mortality of more than 20% during its five-year span. The project was part of the World Health Organization European Collaborative Trial in the Multifactorial Prevention of Coronary Heart Disease (hereinafter "WHO Collaborative Trial") (21).

ENGLAND AND WALES

CAD rates in England and Wales continued to rise until the late 1970s (men) and early 1980s (women) (22). This may have resulted in part from little change in the past decade in blood cholesterol levels, despite dietary recommendations and health education efforts. In the mid-1980s, smoking prevalence in women and men varied by geographical area; approximately 23% of Oxford residents smoked compared with 40% of Londoners (23).

Differences in risk indicator levels have placed manual laborers at highest risk for CAD, despite a general trend toward lower rates throughout Great Britain (24); similar gradients were seen for the wives of laborers (25). Although manual workers smoked more than other men, differences in smoking rates between towns were higher than those between employment grades in a single town. Similarly, a wide range of mean blood pressures has been noted in towns participating in the British Regional Heart Study (26).

Dietary intake also varies considerably throughout England (27). Investigators found a close correlation between regions when infant mortality in 1921–1925 was compared with CAD mortality in 1968–1978. They concluded that poor nutrition in early life may increase susceptibility to the effects of an affluent diet later in life (28). They also noted a correlation between maternal mortality rates during 1911–1914 and stroke mortality in persons born during that period (29).

In the British portion of the WHO Collaborative Trial, the UK Heart Disease Prevention Project, self-reported cigarette smoking was reduced moderately, but changes in other risk indicators were small and not sustained. Fatal CAD events and nonfatal myocardial infarction incidence were not appreciably different in control and intervention groups after the 5–6 year surveillance (30). These findings stood in contrast to those in the Belgian trial reported above (21).

SCOTLAND

As shown in Figure 1.1, CAD rates in Scotland are second only to those in Northern Ireland. While most risk indicators in Scottish women and men are similar to those elsewhere in Europe, mean blood cholesterol levels exceed 250 mg/dl. Compared with persons living in Edinburgh, residents of North Glasgow are heavier smokers, have somewhat higher blood pressures, and have similar blood cholesterol levels (31). Social class and unemployment explain a considerable percentage of the geographical variability of CAD rates throughout Scotland (32).

FINLAND

During the 1950s and 1960s, a large increase in CAD mortality among Finnish women and men occurred, placing them among the highest in the world. Within the country, rates were much higher in the northern and eastern regions. Rates in men were approximately five times those in women. Since 1970, rates have declined (33), due in part to an intensive preventive cardiology program instituted in the North Karelia province in 1972 (34, 35).

These reductions were largely attributable to improvement in various CAD risk indicators (36). Smoking and high blood cholesterol, but not hypertension, were significant predictors of sudden cardiac death, while lipids and blood pressure were significantly related to nonsudden cardiac events (37).

GERMANY

After 1970, CAD mortality rates decreased significantly in the Federal Republic of Germany (FRG), while rates rose by at least 20% in both men and women in the German Democratic Republic (GDR) (6). GDR residents with the highest education level had better values for the major risk indicators than those with less schooling and were more interested in stopping smoking (38).

In the mid-1980s, approximately 40% of women and men in the FRG had blood cholesterol levels exceeding 250 mg/dl; a similar distribution was present in the GDR. Approximately 40% of men in the FRG and the GDR were smokers; prevalence of smoking among women was less in GDR (17% vs. 26%) (39, 40). In a 1988 FRG study in Essen, general practitioners and internists began dietary treatment at 240

mg/dl total cholesterol and drug therapy at 290 mg/dl (41).

A 1988 survey of health professionals in the GDR revealed that less than 10% of physicians smoked, while more than 30% of nurses and technicians did. Approximately one-third of both groups reported that they were never or seldom concerned about healthy diets (42). In a survey of physical activity and diet in the general population and in elite athlete groups, investigators expressed surprise at finding that a majority of GDR citizens were physically inactive. Elite athletes had diets more consistent with heart health than did the general public (43).

THE NETHERLANDS

Similar to what happened in other Western European nations, the onset of the CAD mortality decline in the Netherlands began around 1970 in the urbanized, western region of the country. Later in that decade, other regions experienced a downturn in CAD rates (44). In Zutphen, serum cholesterol determinations were done in 1960 in 829 middle-aged men. During 25 years of surveillance, these values were directly related to the incidence of myocardial infarction (MI) (45).

NORWAY

CAD rates in Norway rose through 1970, after which they have declined more than 30% in persons aged 40–49 and approximately 10% in persons aged 50–59 (46). In the Oslo Study, reduction of serum cholesterol (and to a lesser degree, reductions in smoking) produced a 47% lower rate of MI and sudden cardiac death in the intervention group, compared with the controls (47, 48). In the Tromsö Study, CAD mortality fell 40% in five years among men aged 39–49, compared with an 18% reduction in the entire country; the prevalence of smoking fell from 56% to 45%, and serum total cholesterol declined more than 10% between 1974 and 1987 (49).

SWEDEN

CAD mortality among Swedish men continued to increase until 1981, then began a slow decline. Nonfatal MI incidence also began to decrease at that time. Mortality rates in women declined slightly during the 1950s and 1960s, then began a steeper decline; however, nonfatal MIs in middle-aged Swedish women have increased. Serum cholesterol and blood pressure levels paralleled CAD mortality, while smoking prevalence was closely correlated with nonfatal MI rates (6, 50).

A series of comprehensive studies in Göteborg have added immeasurably to the epidemiology of CAD, particularly in women (51). In northern Sweden, residents have south Swedish, Finnish, and Lappish genetic backgrounds. Those in the latter two categories have higher rates of elevated cholesterol prevalence and CAD event incidence (52).

Eastern Europe

Throughout the 1980s, CAD incidence rates continued to rise among men and women in most Eastern European countries (6). This may have resulted in part from continued increases in consumption of animal fat while vegetable fat intake remained constant (53). As shown in Table 5.1, a majority of Eastern European men continued to smoke, compared with a lower prevalence of smoking among men in regions in the north and west of Europe. In women, these patterns were reversed (10).

CZECHOSLOVAKIA

From 1970 to 1985, CAD mortality rate increases in Czechoslovakia were among the lowest in Eastern Europe (10% in men, 2% in women) (6). From 1983 to 1987, however, women in North Bohemia

had a substantial increase in MI compared with the previous decade (54). Consumption of animal fat increased substantially during the 1980s, although smoking decreased somewhat among male industrial workers in one study (55).

POLAND

CAD mortality also continued to increase during the past two decades in Poland. Although CAD deaths are still higher in urban areas, mortality rates are increasing more rapidly in rural Poland. During this period, a decrease in the consumption of cereals, potatoes, fruit, and vegetables was matched by increases in consumption of meat (over 90% of fat in the diet was saturated animal fat). Mean blood pressure rose in both rural and urban areas, along with body weight, although cigarette smoking showed a modest decline in one study (56). From 1976 to 1986, the MI mortality rate decreased in Warsaw men, but it remained four times higher than for women in that city. In men, the prevalence of blood total cholesterol exceeding 270 mg/dl rose from 7% to 10%, while smoking prevalence was stable.

Elsewhere in Poland, CAD mortality rates continued to rise for both genders (57). Using guidelines from the European Atherosclerosis Society (58), investigators in the Poland-USA Collaborative Study on CVD Epidemiology estimated that approximately 45% of urban Polish women and men were hypertensive, compared with 31% of men and 43% of women in rural areas. While 56% of men smoked in both areas, fewer rural women were smokers (12% vs. 33%) (59).

SOVIET UNION

Throughout the Union of Soviet Socialist Republics (USSR), CAD mortality continued to increase from 1970 to 1985. The remarkable ethnic and racial diversity within the USSR has permitted comparisons among the various regions of the nation. For example, MI and stroke mortality rates are very high in Siberia along with high prevalence levels of hypertension and obesity. Hypertension is particularly high in the populations (largely Asian ethnicity) of southern Siberia, while it is lower (but increasing) among the natives of the Far North (60). In Moscow, MI mortality is increasing in both women and men aged 24–64 (61). Studies in Moscow children revealed that 26% of boys and girls had blood total cholesterol of 200 mg/dl or more; most had low levels of physical activity, but the prevalence of hypertension did not exceed 7% in either gender (62).

An active epidemiologic program in Lithuania has documented the importance of CAD risk indicators over a 15-year period (63). The prevalence of hypercholesterolemia was stable, but hypertension and hyperglycemia were diagnosed more frequently in the late 1980s (64). Investigators in Kiev have found similar prevalence and incidence rates for rural and urban residents of the Ukraine, although rural inhabitants have somewhat higher levels of CAD risk indicators (65). Two screenings of Leningrad men, eight years apart, revealed an increase in CAD prevalence from 13% to 19%. Improvement in blood lipid levels during the study period was associated with fewer CAD events (66). A majority of men throughout the nation continue to smoke (67).

Screening for CAD risk indicators in 15 Soviet cities revealed hypertension in 11 to 31% and smoking in 49 to 65%. Blood cholesterol levels of 200 mg/dl or more were present in 29% of girls and 15% of boys. Among adolescents aged 15 and 16, 32% of boys and 16% of girls smoked (68). As in other countries, smoking in this age group strongly correlates with smoking by other family members, so a strong national smoking prevention program has been instituted (69).

Mediterranean Countries

SPAIN

Although Spain ranks relatively low in CAD mortality, rates have continued to increase. Between 1970 and 1983, CAD mortality increased 49% in men and 25% in women aged 30 to 69 years. Rates in certain areas, such as the Canary and Balearic Islands, the agricultural areas of the south and southeast, and some industrial areas of the north, are more than two times higher than the lowest regions in Spain (70, 71). In a 20-year study of male industrial workers, three factors—smoking, systolic blood pressure, and hypercholesterolemia—were the best predictors of CAD mortality and total CAD events (72). In an urban (Madrid) population, CAD risk indicators in 2419 children were highly correlated with levels in their parents (73).

ITALY

Following World War II, consumption of animal fats rose in Italy; serum cholesterol rose along with CAD death rates until the late 1970s (74). After a brief plateau, mortality from cardiac causes began to decrease, attributable in part to continued treatment of high blood pressure in both genders, reduced smoking in men, and lower body weight in women (75). Several regions in Italy are served by intervention programs aimed at reducing CAD events (76), and school-based programs of cholesterol screening in children have begun. In one study, more than 12% of children aged 10 to 14 had blood cholesterol values exceeding 200 mg/dl (77).

LEBANON

Sibai and colleagues studied the effects of chronic stresses resulting from "war, a man-made disaster" in a case-control study of persons undergoing coronary angiography in Beirut during the preceding 14 years of war in their country. Factors such as the necessity to cross areas of sniping and random shellings were associated with twice the prevalence of CAD (78).

ISRAEL

Just south of Lebanon, Israel is also subject to the stresses engendered by conflicting ideologies. However, since 1970, Jews living there have experienced a dramatic decline in CAD mortality, although there has been no significant reduction in cigarette smoking or serum total cholesterol levels, and the percentage of calories coming from fat has increased. The investigators noted that this steep decline has not been shared by Arabs and Druse living there, although their rates were considerably lower than those for Jews in the mid-1970s (79). In a 23-year follow-up of more than 10,000 men who had immigrated to Israel from more than 20 countries, indicators of CAD risk were (in declining order of importance) diabetes, blood pressure, lipids, and smoking (80).

KUWAIT

From 1971 to 1986, CAD mortality and MI hospital admissions doubled. The government has initiated programs to reduce levels of smoking, blood cholesterol, and obesity, which have been important indicators of risk (81).

ASIA

PAKISTAN

A comparison of MI cases with a cross-sectional sample of persons from all four provinces of Pakistan revealed that the persons with CAD had higher prevalence levels of smoking, 16% of them were diabetic, and their mean blood cholesterol level was 230 mg/dl. A majority of smokers began before the age of 20 and attributed their adoption of smoking to parental models and cigarette advertisements. Use of hydrogenated oils, ghee, and butter is three times more likely than use of unsaturated oils (82).

INDIA

Several studies within India suggest that hypertension, diabetes, and smoking are the three major indicators of CAD risk (83). In Vellore, 45% of persons with angiographically documented CAD have total cholesterol levels under 200 mg/dl and triglycerides below 140 mg/dl; some persons with CAD had cholesterol levels below 150 mg/dl (84).

CHINA

The CAD crude death rate in the People's Republic of China (PRC) in 1984 was only one-tenth of that for Australia, Canada, and the USA, although stroke was five times more common than MI. The low mean serum total cholesterol values throughout the country may account for the low CAD rates (85).

In 1981, a joint research program in cardiovascular diseases was initiated by the PRC and the USA (86). From this collaboration, surveys have been done in several areas of the PRC. In the southern Chinese city of Guangzhou, mean total cholesterol levels in urban dwellers increased from 183 mg/dl to 204 mg/dl between 1983 and 1987. Rural men had values of 162 mg/dl and 181 mg/dl, respectively; rural women had levels 10 mg/dl lower in both surveys (87).

In other international joint studies, investigators demonstrated in Shanghai that, for serum total cholesterol levels above 135 mg/dl, there was a continuous increase in CAD mortality (no threshold) with increasing cholesterol levels (88). In Lhasa, Tibet, men and women have similar lipid and lipoprotein levels. Mean values were 166 mg/dl for total cholesterol, 55 mg/dl for HDL-cholesterol, and 94 mg/dl of LDL-cholesterol (89).

After a program of community and

physician education in rural China, sudden CAD deaths were markedly reduced and stroke mortality was more moderately decreased compared to a reference community. Values were also substantially lower in the intervention community than in a survey completed there 10 years earlier (90).

SINGAPORE

In 1988, the population of Singapore was 76% Chinese, 15% Malays, 7% Indians, and 2% from other ethnic groups. In both women and men, CAD death rates are approximately three times higher in Indians than in Chinese; Malays have rates nearly double those of the Chinese. Since 1980, CAD rates decreased in Chinese, but have been essentially unchanged in the other ethnic groups.

In men, smoking and hypertension were highest among the Malays, followed by Indians and Chinese. Diabetes was highest in Indians (29%) and was present in 20% of Malays but only 9% of Chinese. Blood mean total cholesterol levels were nearly identical in the three groups of men and women (220–231 mg/dl) (91).

JAPAN

Given the traditional Japanese diet high in sodium and low in saturated fat, epidemiologists have not been surprised to find stroke rates high and MIs low in number, with hypertension being the most important predictor of CAD events and stroke. Mean serum total cholesterol levels in 1980 were approximately 186 mg/dl in men over 30 and 191 mg/dl in women of the same age. Despite these relatively low figures, there is a direct linear relation between serum cholesterol and CAD events. Compared with persons having cholesterol levels below 180 mg/dl, the CAD relative risk of having a value of 240 mg/dl was 2.0 for men and 1.7 for women (92).

Smoking rates are particularly high in men, but low in women (93). While some studies have reported reductions in smoking (94), World Health Organization figures show a rise in adult per capita consumption (both genders) of 16% from 1970 to 1985 (10).

One study compared Japanese CAD mortality with that of Koreans, Chinese, and North Americans living in Japan. Men and women from the other countries were more likely to die from CAD than native Japanese: ratios for men and women were 1.11 and 1.12 for Koreans, 1.20 and 1.52 for Chinese, and 3.14 and 1.75 for North Americans (95).

Oceania

AUSTRALIA

CAD rates are highest in eastern Australia, among those born in Australia, and in lower socioeconomic groups. Rates peaked in Australia in the mid-1960s and have decreased more than 40% since, with the greatest reductions occurring on the east coast and among native-born Australians (96). The decrease has been attributed in part to less smoking and a preference for margarine over butter (97). In the Hunter region of New South Wales, CAD rates are among the highest in the country. Within that region, rates parallel differences in hypertension, cholesterol levels, smoking, and obesity, suggesting that preventive measures could modify the elevated rates (96). Rates in the southwestern city of Perth, already among the lowest in Australia, fell in all age-gender groups after 1968 (98).

In isolated Aboriginal communities in northern Australia, fasting cholesterol and glucose levels were quite low compared with those of urbanized Aboriginals and Australians of European background. However, their fasting insulin and triglyceride levels were uncommonly high for their low body mass and fasting glucose levels, suggesting to investigators that further urbanization might make them particularly susceptible to obesity and diabetes (99).

NEW ZEALAND

In 1980, CAD was the leading cause of death in New Zealand, accounting for 28% of mortality. MI rates were similar in Maori and non-Maori populations, but sudden cardiac death was three times more likely in Maoris (100). For persons of European ethnicity, CAD mortality decreased 22% and 13% (for men and women) between 1968 and 1981, due to a significant decline in sudden death rates. The CAD reductions were associated with reductions in dairy product consumption and cigarette smoking, reductions in serum cholesterol levels, improved control of hypertension, and increased habitual physical activity (101). Subsidies for dairy products were removed, and legislation was approved in 1972 allowing margarine to be made from polyunsaturated oils (102). Between 40 and 50% of the observed decline in CAD mortality could be attributed to changes in serum cholesterol and tobacco consumption (103).

During that period, however, CAD rates in New Zealand dropped more slowly than those in Australia. Observers in the two countries noted that New Zealand had a consistent decline in out-of-hospital mortality, but no reduction in nonfatal MIs. In the Australian cities Perth and Newcastle, both types of events declined.

North America

CANADA

In the early 1960s, CAD rates began to decline in Canadian women, followed by a decline in the rates for men a few years thereafter, but marked geographic differences in the onset of the decline and residual rates have been noted. Ontario has continued to exhibit the highest rates, although the decline in that province began early in both women and men. The Prairie region has continued to have the lowest rates; their decline, starting in the 1950s, was the first to become apparent. Pacific provinces have the second lowest rates for both genders, while Quebec has maintained its middle rank among the five regions. The Atlantic region has showed the slowest decline (104). Mortality from stroke in Canada has shown a consistent decline from as early as 1930 (105, 106).

The impact of various levels of risk indicators on CAD includes a 2.8-fold risk for smoking 20 cigarettes or more per day, 2.6 for a diagnosis of diabetes, 2.1 for total cholesterol of 280 mg/dl or greater, and 2.0 for hypertension. The percentage of CAD mortality attributable to various risk indicators has been estimated at 47% for smoking, 21% for hypertension, 8% for diabetes, and 7% for hypercholesterolemia (107).

In contrast to persons living in France, which has one of the lowest CAD rates in the world, French Canadians under the age of 65 have higher CAD mortality than do Canadians in English-speaking regions. Higher consumption of cigarettes and alcohol in French Canadian men produces strong but opposing effects on their HDL-cholesterol concentrations. Mean total cholesterol was 224 mg/dl, regardless of the alcohol use status (108).

UNITED STATES OF AMERICA

As has been noted for other countries discussed above, the CAD decline in the USA was not homogeneous. It apparently began in the 1950s in California and New York and did not occur in some regions of the mountainous west until after 1973 (109). The decline began earlier in women than in men. It was greater in men than in women of a given race (although men started at higher levels), was more pronounced in younger age groups, was more rapid in persons with professional standing than in manual laborers, and its rate was inversely related to socioeconomic status (110).

Medical care practices changed greatly in the USA during the past three decades; a smaller percentage of CAD deaths occurred outside the hospital. A nationwide hypertension detection and treatment campaign was carried out, and a similar effort is under way to reduce blood cholesterol levels through nutritional change. In addition, there were dramatic changes in the health habits of USA residents, particularly those who were more economically advantaged. Smoking declined steadily since the first Surgeon General's Report in 1964, vigorous physical activity became popular, and a desire for thinness has enabled many to reduce their weight closer to ideal levels. The latter two factors have coincided with a shift in eating habits toward lower fat and cholesterol consumption.

The CAD decline has been noted among the many ethnic groups in the country including men of Japanese ethnicity in Hawaii (111), native Americans residing in New Mexico (112), Texans of Mexican ethnicity (113), and blacks throughout the nation (114), although declines began later in poorer and less educated members of each ethnic group (115).

World Health Organization Studies

In keeping with the spirit of international cooperation that has characterized the preventive cardiology field since its inception, several major studies developed under the guidance of the World Health Organization (WHO) and its members

(116). Among these is the WHO Collaborative Trial in the Multifactoral Prevention of Coronary Heart Disease, which involved investigators from Belgium, Italy, Poland, Spain, and the United Kingdom (117).

To measure trends and determinants of cardiovascular mortality, CAD, and stroke morbidity, and the extent to which these changes result from risk modification efforts, the WHO Multinational **MONI**toring of Trends and Determinants in **CA**rdiovascular Disease (MONICA) project was begun (118). Table 1.2 lists participating nations.

The Countrywide Integrated Noncommunicable Disease Intervention (CINDI) Program seeks to develop an in-

Table 1.2. Countries Providing Collaborating Centers for WHO MONICA

Australia
Belgium
Canada
China
Czechoslovakia
Denmark
Finland
France
Germany
    Federal Republic of Germany
    German Democratic Republic
Hungary
Iceland
Israel
Italy
Japan
Malta
New Zealand
Northern Ireland
Poland
Romania
Scotland
Spain
Sweden
Switzerland
USA
USSR
Yugoslavia

Table 1.3.   Participating Countries in the WHO CINDI Project

Austria
Bulgaria
Canada
Czechoslovakia
Finland
Germany
  Federal Republic of Germany
  German Democratic Republic
Hungary
Iceland
Malta
Portugal
USSR
  Byelorussian SSR
  Estonian SSR
  Kharkov
  Khirgiz SSR
  Lithuanian SSR
  Moscow
Yugoslavia

tegrated approach to reducing those risk indicators that are common to more than one noncommunicable disease, such as smoking, unhealthy nutrition, physical inactivity, alcohol abuse, and psychosocial stress (119). Participating countries are listed in Table 1.3.

REFERENCES

1. White PD. Heart disease, 4th ed. New York: Macmillan, 1951.

2. Campbell M. The main cause of increased death rate from diseases of the heart: 1920 to 1959. Br Med J 1963;3:712–717.

3. White PD, Donovan H. Hearts. Their long follow-up. Philadelphia: Saunders, 1967.

4. Uemura K. International trends in cardiovascular diseases in the elderly. Eur Heart J 1988;9(suppl D):1–8.

5. Sindhvananda K. Problems of cardiovascular diseases and approaches to their solution in developing countries. In: Chazov EI, Oganov RG, Perova NV (eds): Preventive cardiology. London: Harwood Academic Publishers, 1985:313–322.

6. Uemura K, Pisa Z. Trends in cardiovascular disease mortality in industrialized countries since 1950. World Health Statistics Quarterly 1988;41:155–178.

7. Hopkins PN, Williams RR. A survey of 246 suggested coronary risk factors. Atherosclerosis 1981;40:1–52.

8. Jordan J. On call. Boston: South End Press, 1985.

9. Ioannidis PJ, Efthymiopoulou GD. International transeconomic trends of arterial disease in the mid-1970s. Am J Epidemiol 1982;115:278–297.

10. Masironi R, Rothwell K. Tendances et effets du tabagisme dans le monde. World Health Statistics Quarterly 1988;41:228–241.

11. Poulter N, Khaw KT, Mugambi M, Peart S, Sever P, Rose G. Longitudinal study of migrants from a "low-blood pressure population." Abstracts Second International Conference on Preventive Cardiology 1989;A102.

12. McKeigue PM, Marmot MG, Adelstein AM, et al. Diet and risk factors for coronary heart disease in Asians in northwest London. Lancet 1985;2:1086–1090.

13. McKeigue PM, Marmot MG, Syndercombe Court YD, Cottier DE, Rahman S, Riemersma RA. Diabetes, hyperinsulinemia, and coronary risk factors in Bangladeshis in east London. Br Heart J 1988;60:390–396.

14. Bunker CH, Ukoli FA, Omene JA, et al. Emergence of hypertension in a Nigerian population. Abstracts Second International Conference on Preventive Cardiology 1981;A3.

15. Bilgin Y, Doppl W, Klor HU, Ozal S, Federlin K. Comparison of coronary mortality in Turks living in Germany and in Turkey. Abstracts Second International Conference on Preventive Cardiology 1989;A62.

16. Chavez R, Escamilla A, Villa A, Lozano R, Escobedo J. Atherosclerosis: an outcome from epidemiologic polarization. Abstracts Second International Conference on Preventive Cardiology 1989;A60.

17. Zevallos JC, Torres FM, Ellison RC. Changes in dietary patterns among city migrants in the Andes of Ecuador. CVD Epidemiology Newsletter 1989;147–148.

18. Zevallos JC. The Latin American Working Group on Primary Prevention of Cardiovascular Disease and Epidemiology. CVD Epidemiology Newsletter 1989;144–146.

19. Kornitzer M. Evolution of coronary

heart disease mortality from 1958 in Belgium. Cardiology 1985;72:59–62.

20. Joossens JV. Trends in systolic blood pressure, 24h salt excretion and stroke mortality in elderly in Belgium. Abstracts Second International Conference on Preventive Cardiology 1989;A82.

21. Kornitzer M, DeBacker G, Dramaix M, et al. Belgian Heart Disease Prevention Project: incidence and mortality results. Lancet 1983;1:1066–1070.

22. Bowker T, Wilkinson P. A comparative cohort analysis of ischaemic heart disease mortality trends in the USA and England & Wales, 1954–1984. J Am Coll Cardiol 1990;15:183A.

23. Mann JI, Lewis B, Shepherd J, et al. Blood lipid concentrations and other cardiovascular risk factors: distribution, prevalence and detection in Britain. Br Med J 1988;296:1702–1706.

24. Marmot MG, McDowall ME. Mortality decline and widening social inequalities. Lancet 1986;1:394.

25. Marmot M. Socioeconomic determinants of CHD mortality. Int J Epidemiol 1989;18(suppl 1):S196–S202.

26. Shaper AG, Pocock, SJ. Risk factors for ischaemic heart disease in British men. Br Heart J 1987;57:11–16.

27. Cade JE, Barker DJ, Margetts BM, Morris JA. Diet and inequalities in health in three English towns. Br Med J 1988;296:1359–1362.

28. Barker DJ, Osmond C. Infant mortality, childhood nutrition, and ischaemic heart disease in England and Wales. Lancet 1986;1:1077–1081.

29. Barker DJ, Osmond C. Death rates from stroke in England and Wales predicted from past maternal mortality. Br Med J 1987;295:83–86.

30. Rose G, Tunstall-Pedoe HD, Heller RF. UK Heart Disease Prevention Project: incidence and mortality results. Lancet 1983;1:1062–1066.

31. Smith WC, Crombie IK, Tunstall-Pedoe HD, Tavendale R, Riemersma RA. Cardiovascular risk profile and mortality in two Scottish cities. Acta Med Scand 1988;suppl 728:113–118.

32. Crombie IK, Kenicer MB, Smith WC, Tunstall-Pedoe HD. Unemployment, socioenvironmental factors, and coronary heart disease in Scotland. Br Heart J 1989;61:172–177.

33. Tuomilehto J, Puska P, Korhonen H, et al. Trends and determinants of ischaemic heart disease mortality in Finland: with special reference to a possible leveling off in the early 1980's. Int J Epidemiol 1989;18(suppl 1):S109–S117.

34. Puska P, Tuomilehto J, Salonen J, et al. Changes in coronary risk factors during comprehensive five-year community programme to control cardiovascular diseases (North Karelia project). Br Med J 1979;2:1173–1178.

35. Puska P, Tuomilehto J, Salonen J, et al. Community control of cardiovascular diseases. Copenhagen: World Health Organization, 1981.

36. Salonen JT, Nissinen A, Tuomilehto J, Puska P. Contribution of risk factor changes to the decline in coronary incidence during the North Karelia Project: a within-community analysis. Abstracts Second International Conference on Preventive Cardiology 1989;A102.

37. Suhonen O, Reunanen A, Knekt P, Aromaa A. Risk factors for sudden and nonsudden coronary death. Acta Med Scand 1988;223:19–25.

38. Assmann A. Social gradient of coronary risk—everywhere?—Results from GDR. Abstracts Second International Conference on Preventive Cardiology 1989;A59.

39. Heinemann L, Heine H, Assmann A, et al. Risk factors in the population of the GDR-MONICA Study (1983/84). Acta Med Scand 1988;(suppl 728)144–149.

40. Greisler E, Joeckel KH, Gierspiepen K, Maschewsky-Schneider U, Zachcia M. Cardiovascular disease risk factors, CHD morbidity and mortality in the Federal Republic of Germany. Int J Epidemiol 1989;18(suppl 1):S118–S124.

41. Keil U, Doring A, Steinberg H. Awareness and treatment of hypercholesterolemia and physicians' attitude towards diagnosis and treatment of hypercholesterolemia: results from the F.R.G. Abstracts Second International Conference on Preventive Cardiology 1989;A13.

42. Mai C, Heinemann L, Barth W. Some aspects of health behaviour in health care per-

sonnel of the GDR. Preliminary results. CVD Epidemiology Newsletter 1989;88–89.

43. Heinemann L, Zerbes H, Thiel C, Barth W. Physical activity, diet, and cardiovascular risk in population versus elite athletes. CVD Epidemiology Newsletter 1989;105–107.

44. Mackenbach JP, Looman CW, Kunst AE. Geographic variation in the onset of decline of male ischemic heart disease mortality in the Netherlands. Am J Public Health 1989;79:1621–1627.

45. Kromhout D, Bosschieter EB, Drijver M, Coulander C. Serum cholesterol and 25-year incidence of and mortality from myocardial infarction and cancer. The Zutphen Study. Arch Intern Med 1988;148:1051–1055.

46. Thelle DS. Preventive cardiology in Norway: mortality trends and programmes. CVD Epidemiology Newsletter 1989;26–27.

47. Hjermann I, Velve Byre K, Holme I, Leren P. Effect of diet and smoking intervention on the incidence of coronary heart disease. Lancet 1981;2:1303–1310.

48. Holme I, Hjermann I, Helgeland A, Leren P. The Oslo Study: diet and antismoking advice. Prev Med 1985;14:279–292.

49. Bonaa KH, Thelle DS, Arnesen E, Forde OH. The Tromso Study. Trends in population coronary risk factors and ischemic disease mortality 1974–1987. CVD Epidemiology Newsletter 1989;27.

50. Wilhelmsen L, Johansson S, Ulvenstam G, et al. CHD in Sweden: mortality, incidence and risk factors over 20 years in Gothenburg. Int J Epidemiol 1989;18(suppl 1):S101–S108.

51. Bengtsson C, Lapidus L. The population study of women in Gothenburg, Sweden. CVD Epidemiology Newsletter 1989;23.

52. Stegmayr B, Nylander PO, Asplund K, Beckman L. Finnish and Lappish genetic influences on cardiovascular risk determinants and morbidity in Northern Sweden. CVD Epidemiology Newsletter 1989;21.

53. Epstein FH. The relationship of lifestyle to international trends in CHD. Int J Epidemiol 1989;18(suppl 1):S203–S209.

54. Bazika V, Tiserova J, Horakova D, Hrabovsky F. Fifteen-year register of myocardial infarction in the district of North Bohemia. CVD Epidemiology Newsletter 1989;83–85.

55. Simon J, Rosolova H, Buzkova J. Coronary risk factor changes in a middle-aged, male industrial population from 1976 to 1986. Abstracts Second International Conference on Preventive Cardiology 1989;A57.

56. Rywik S, Kupsc W. Coronary heart disease mortality trends and related factors in Poland. Cardiology 1985;72:81–87.

57. Rywik S, Wagrowska H, Broda G, et al. Epidemiology of cardiovascular diseases in Warsaw Pol-MONICA area. Int J Epidemiol 1989;18(suppl 1):S129–S136.

58. European Atherosclerosis Society Study Group. Strategies for the prevention of coronary heart disease: a policy statement of the European Atherosclerosis Society. Eur Heart J 1987;8:77–88.

59. Sznajd J, Rywik SL, Williams OD, et al. Poland-US Collaborative Study on CVD Epidemiology: CHD risk factor profiles for categories of European Atherosclerosis Society (EAS) guidelines. Abstracts Second International Conference on Preventive Cardiology 1989;A27.

60. Nikitin Y, Gafarov V, Feigin V, Astakhova T. CVD prevalence in west, south and north regions of Siberia. Abstracts Second International Conference on Preventive Cardiology 1989;A56.

61. Varlamova T, Zhukovski G, Naumova V. Changes in mortality and morbidity rates for myocardial infarction and stroke in Moscow male and female residents aged 25-64. Abstracts Second International Conference on Preventive Cardiology 1989;A60.

62. Alexandrov A, Issakova G, Demidova L, et al. Epidemiologic and preventive aspects of atherosclerosis precursors in Moscow schoolchildren. Abstracts Second International Conference on Preventive Cardiology 1989;A83.

63. Domarkiene S, Baubiniene A, Maceviciute N, Reklaitiene R, Sidlauskien D. Total and cardiovascular mortality in men aged 45–59 during fifteen year follow-up in Kaunas. Abstracts Second International Conference on Preventive Cardiology 1989;A65.

64. Domarkiene S, Tamosiunas A, Reklaitiene R, et al. Fifteen year trends of coronary heart disease and risk factors' prevalence among Kaunas men aged 45–59 years at entry. CVD Epidemiology Newsletter 1989;72–73.

65. Smirnova IP, Gorbas IM, Kvasha EA. Epidemiology of ischemic heart disease and its

risk factors in urban and rural populations of the Ukranian SSR. CVD Epidemiology Newsletter 1989;73–74.

66. Konstantinov VO, Lipovetsky BM, Ilyina GN, Plavinskaya SI. The time course of coronary heart disease and its main risk factors in a Leningrad male population. Abstracts Second International Conference on Preventive Cardiology 1989;A62.

67. Deev AD, Oganov RG. Trends and determinants of cardiovascular mortality in the Soviet Union. Int J Epidemiol 1989;18(suppl 1):S137–S144.

68. Oganov R, Chazova L, Alexandrov A, Britov A, Zhukovski G, Kalinina A. Prevention of cardiovascular diseases: USSR experience. Abstracts Second International Conference on Preventive Cardiology 1989;A62.

69. Chazova L, Prokhorov A, Alexandrov A, Prokhorova I, Sarsenova S. Smoking among adult and children populations and approaches to its prevention in the Soviet Union. Abstracts Second International Conference on Preventive Cardiology 1989;A23.

70. Balaguer-Vintro I, Sans S. Coronary heart disease mortality trends and related factors in Spain. Cardiology 1985;72:97–104.

71. Sans S, Tomas L, Balaguer-Vintro I. Consensus cholesterol conference in Spain. CVD Epidemiology Newsletter 1989;141.

72. Tomas-Abadal L, Varas C, Guiteras P, Balaguer-Vintro I. Coronary risk factors and survival probability in the Manresa Study (Spain). Abstracts Second International Conference on Preventive Cardiology 1989;A100.

73. Plaza I, Munoz T, Lopez D, et al. Fuenlabrada Study: familial associations of coronary risk factors. CVD Epidemiology Newsletter 1989;138.

74. Menotti A. Trends in CHD in Italy. Int J Epidemiol 1989;18(suppl 1):S125–S128.

75. Menotti A, Capocaccia R, Farchi F, Pasquali M. Recent trends in coronary heart disease and other cardiovascular diseases in Italy. Cardiology 1985;72:88–96.

76. Giamapoli S on behalf of the Di.S.Co. Project. Time trends of cardiovascular risk factors in the DISCO Project. Abstracts Second International Conference on Preventive Cardiology 1989;A62.

77. Montali A, Arca M, Antonini R, et al. Identification of high risk subjects through a cholesterol screening program carried out on school children and their families. Abstracts Second International Conference on Preventive Cardiology 1989;A66.

78. Sibai AM, Armenian HK, Alam S. Wartime determinants of arteriographically confirmed coronary artery disease in Beirut. Am J Epidemiol 1989;130:623–631.

79. Goldbourt U, Neufeld HN. Trends in coronary heart disease mortality and related factors in Israel. Cardiology 1985;72:63–74.

80. Goldbourt U, Yaari S. Coronary risk factors: their predictive value in a 23-year follow-up of CHD, stroke, cancer and all cause mortality. Abstracts Second International Conference on Preventive Cardiology 1989;A101.

81. Al-Owaish RA, Shah NM. Cardiovascular mortality and morbidity in Kuwait: trends, risk factors and prevention strategies. Abstracts Second International Conference on Preventive Cardiology 1989;A54.

82. Hussain A, Khan MZ, Tarar M, Mansoor MN. Cross-sectional survey of smoking pattern and use of hydrogenated oils in the Pakistani population. CVD Epidemiology Newsletter 1989;149–150.

83. Padmavati S, Kasliwal RR, Dhar A, et al. Epidemiology of coronary heart disease in India: a long term prospective study. In: Chazov EI, Oganov RG, Perova NV (eds). Preventive cardiology London: Harwood Academic Publishers, 1985;323–329.

84. Krishnaswami S, Prasad NK, Jose VJ. Lipid levels in Indian patients with coronary artery disease. Abstracts Second International Conference on Preventive Cardiology 1989;A9.

85. Tao S, Huang Z, Wu X, et al. CHD and its risk factors in the People's Republic of China. Int J Epidemiol 1989;18(suppl 1):S159–S163.

86. Data Preview from the People's Republic of China. Washington: U.S. Department of Health and Human Services, 1989.

87. Huang Z, Warnick R, Zhou Y, et al. Lipid trends in south China. Abstracts Second International Conference on Preventive Cardiology 1989;A52.

88. Chen Z, Peto R, Collins R, MacMahon S, Li W. Continuous positive relationship between serum cholesterol and coronary heart disease in a population with low mean

cholesterol. Abstracts Second International Conference on Preventive Cardiology 1989;A101.

89. Song A, Huang DX, Kesteloot H. Serum lipids in a Tibetan population sample. Abstracts Second International Conference on Preventive Cardiology. 1989;A7.

90. Zhang HX, Wang ZY. A 12-year community control of coronary sudden death and fatal stroke in a rural district in China. Abstracts Second International Conference on Preventive Cardiology 1989;A64.

91. Emmanuel SC. Trends in coronary heart disease mortality in Singapore. CVD Epidemiology Newsletter 1989;158–160.

92. Kodama K, Sasaki H, Shimizu Y, Kato H, Akahoshi M, Hosoda Y. Cholesterol and coronary heart disease in a Japanese population. A 26 year followup study. Abstracts Second International Conference on Preventive Cardiology 1989;A64.

93. Hatano S. Changing CHD mortality and its causes in Japan during 1955–1985. Int J Epidemiol 1989;18(suppl 1):S149–S158.

94. Ueshima H, Tatara K, Asakura S. Declining mortality from ischemic heart disease and changes in coronary risk factors in Japan, 1956–1980. Am J Epidemiol 1987;125:62–72.

95. Kono S, Isa AR, Ogimoto I, Yoshimura T. Cause-specific mortality among Koreans, Chinese and Americans in Japan, 1973–1982. Int J Epidemiol 1987;16:415–419.

96. Alexander HM, Balding DJ, Dobson AJ, Gibberd RW, Lloyd DM, Leeder SR. Risk factors and heart disease mortality. A regional perspective. Med J Aust 1986;144:20–22.

97. Hardey GR, Dobson AJ, Lloyd DM, Leeder SR. Coronary heart disease mortality trends and related factors in Australia. Cardiology 1985;72:23–28.

98. Martin CA, Hobbs MS, Armstrong BK, de Klerk NH. Trends in the incidence of myocardial infarction in Western Australia between 1971 and 1982. Am J Epidemiol 1989;129:655–668.

99. O'Dea K, White NG, Sinclair AJ. An investigation of nutrition-related risk factors in an isolated Aboriginal community in northern Australia: advantages of a traditionally-oriented life-style. Med J Aust 1988;148:177–180.

100. Beaglehole R, Stewart AW, Bonita R, Jackson RT, Sharpe DN. Myocardial infarction and sudden death in Auckland. NZ Med J 1984;97:715–718.

101. Beaglehole R, Jackson R. Coronary heart disease mortality, morbidity, and risk factor trends in New Zealand. Cardiology 1985;72:29–34.

102. Beaglehole R, Dobson A, Hobbs MS, Jackson R, Martin CA. CHD in Australia and New Zealand. Int J Epidemiol 1989;18(suppl 1):S145–S148.

103. Jackson R, Beaglehole R. Trends in dietary fat and cigarette smoking and the decline in coronary heart disease in New Zealand. Int J Epidemiol 1987;16:377–382.

104. Nicholls ES, Jung J, Davies JW. Cardiovascular disease mortality in Canada. Can Med Assoc J 1981;125:981–992.

105. Davies JW, Semenciw RM, Mao Y. Cardiovascular disease mortality trend and related risk factors in Canada. Can J Cardiol 1988;4(suppl A):16A–20A.

106. Nicholls E, Nair C, MacWilliam L, Moen J, Mao Y. Cardiovascular disease in Canada. Ottawa: Statistics Canada, 1986.

107. Semenciw RM, Morrison HI, Mao Y, Johansen H, Davies JW, Wigle DT. Major risk factors for cardiovascular disease mortality in adults: results from the Nutrition Canada survey cohort. Int J Epidemiol 1988;17:317–324.

108. Lupien PJ, Moorjani S, Jobin J, et al. Smoking, alcohol consumption, lipid and lipoprotein levels. Can J Cardiol 1988;4:102–107.

109. Wing S, Hayes C, Heiss G, et al. Geographic variation in the onset of decline of ischemic heart disease mortality in the United States. Am J Public Health 1986;76:1401–1408.

110. Higgins M, Thom T. Trends in CHD in the United States. Int J Epidemiol 1989;18(suppl 1):S58–S66.

111. Reed D, Maclean C. The nineteen-year trends in CHD in the Honolulu Heart Program. Int J Epidemiol 1989;18(suppl 1):S82–S87.

112. Becker TM, Wiggins C, Key CR, Samet JM. Ischemic heart disease mortality in Hispanics, American Indians, and non-Hispanic whites in New Mexico, 1958–1982. Circulation 1988;78:302–309.

113. Stern MP, Bradshaw BS, Eifler CW, Fong DS, Hazuda HP, Rosenthal M. Secular

decline in death rates due to ischemic heart disease in Mexican Americans and non-Hispanic whites in Texas, 1970–1980. Circulation 1987;76:1245–1250.

114. Gillum RF, Liu KC. Coronary heart disease mortality in United States Blacks, 1940–1978: trends and unanswered questions. Am Heart J 1984;108:728–732.

115. Secretary's Task Force on Black and Minority Health. Report of the Secretary's Task Force on Black and Minority Health. Volume IV: Cardiovascular and cerebrovascular disease. Washington: US Department of Health and Human Services, 1986.

116. Gyarfas I. The WHO Programme on Cardiovascular Diseases 1988–1989. CVD Epidemiology Newsletter 1989;1–4.

117. DeBacker G. WHO European Multifactorial Prevention Trial. In: Hofmann H (ed): Primary and Secondary Prevention of Coronary Heart Disease. Berlin: Springer-Verlag, 1985;1–7.

118. WHO MONICA Project Principal Investigators. The World Health Organization MONICA Project (Monitoring trends and determinants in cardiovascular disease): a major international collaboration. J Clin Epidemiol 1988;41:105–114.

119. Tsechkovski M, Shatchkute A, Svensson PG. Countrywide integrated noncommunicable diseases intervention (CINDI) programme. Abstracts Second International Conference on Preventive Cardiology 1989;A93.

2

pathophysiology of coronary artery disease

The consequences of coronary artery disease (CAD) in a given individual may be attributed to disparities in myocardial oxygen supply and demand. Determinants of demand include heart rate, blood pressure, myocardial contractility, and ventricular chamber size. During exercise, for example, increased myocardial oxygen demand results from increases in the first three factors. Disease states can also increase demand; thyrotoxicosis also elevates heart rate, blood pressure, and myocardial contractility until appropriately treated. Persons with dilated ventricles as a result of congestive heart failure will have an increased oxygen demand until therapeutic efforts to reduce ventricular size and restore normal hemodynamics are successful.

In persons with nondiseased coronary arteries, myocardial oxygen adjusts to meet oxygen demands, largely through arterial and arteriolar dilation, which provides a greater cross-sectional area and results in increased flow rates. This dilation results from neural and hormonal signals to the richly innervated muscular layers of the arterial wall. However, atherosclerotic involvement may decrease or prevent the ability of the affected arterial segment to dilate, limiting the maximal flow through the artery. In addition, dynamic obstruction of the artery through spasm or collapse may abruptly alter myocardial oxygen blood supply. Further, thrombosis at the site of such abnormalities or emboli originating at distal sites may also affect the delivery of oxygenated blood to myocardial cells.

In a recent review, Blankenhorn and Kramsch divide atherosclerosis into its two main components, atherosis and sclerosis. While the majority of research studies have focused on the former component, there is also active investigation into the pathophysiology and treatment of sclerosis of arteries (1).

In this chapter, the processes of coronary artery atherosis, sclerosis, spasm, and thrombosis are discussed in further detail.

ATHEROSCLEROSIS

Atheromas most commonly form in coronary, cerebral, carotid, iliac, and femoral arteries and in the aorta. The distribution of lesions among these sites may be determined by genetic as well as environmental conditions. In Europe and North America, dyslipidemias and coronary artery atherosclerosis are very prevalent, while persons in Japan are more likely to exhibit hypertension and cerebrovascular arterial involvement. Following the example of Ross (2), this chapter reviews evidence from human autopsy studies, investigations in nonhuman primates and other animals, and research at the cellular and molecular level. Prevailing models of atherosclerosis development incorporating these findings are then discussed.

Human Studies

The earliest indication of atherosclerosis is the fatty streak, a flat lesion composed of macrophages and smooth muscle cells that were filled with lipid. Above these elements are multiple layers of a smooth muscle cell type, which forms a fibrous cap. Deeper within the arterial wall is an area of necrotic debris, cholesterol crystals, and calcification. As lipid accumulates, the smooth muscle cells and macrophages become distorted, making accurate identification difficult. Rupture or roughening of the fibrous cap at the intimal surface can form a nidus from thrombus formation and further obstruction of the arterial lumen.

Although such streaks have been found in children from many countries (regardless of community prevalence of adult coronary artery disease), many investigators feel that this type of lesion is the earliest precursor of advanced arteriosclerotic plaques. Several investigators have noted that smooth muscle fibrous plaques develop later in life at the anatomic locations where fatty streaks are noted in children (2). By the third decade of life, proliferation of fatty streaks has peaked, and advanced fibrous plaques become more common in coronary arteries. Typically,

plaques in cerebral arteries appear in the following decade.

Sclerosis of atheromatous lesions may involve increased lesion collagen, destruction of medial elastin, and compositional changes in these fibrous proteins. These alterations can lead to reduced compliance, or elasticity, of vessel walls, particularly in persons with hypertension and diabetes mellitus. During aging, overall arterial compliance is reduced, particularly in the thoracic aorta and carotid arteries, which are the most compliant large vessels in adolescence (1).

Experimental Observations

Faggiotto and colleagues described month-by-month changes in the aorta and iliac arteries of nonhuman primates whose plasma cholesterol had been raised to the range of 500 to 1000 mg/dl by dietary means. After only 12 days of a high-fat, high-cholesterol diet in pigtail monkeys, they observed clusters of monocytes adhering to the endothelial surface at apparently random sites. At cell junctions, the monocytes migrated into the subendothelium, accumulated lipids, and appeared to be transformed into foam cells. This process resulted in fatty streaks similar to those found in human studies. The streaks expanded by continued migration of monocytes (which became macrophages) as well as through gradual accumulation of smooth muscle cells that accumulated lipid after their migration from the intima into the media.

After five months, the endothelial junctions over the fatty streaks appeared to widen, principally at arterial bifurcations and branches, where turbulent flow exists. Often, retraction was so pronounced that the fatty streak, its macrophages, and the underlying connective tissue were exposed to constituents of the blood stream, leading to platelet adherence, aggregation, and thrombosis. Subsequently, advanced smooth muscle proliferation was noted at these sites. A direct correlation was found between the blood cholesterol level, its rate of increase and duration, and the cellular and proliferative lesions (3, 4).

Endothelial cells can bind LDL-cholesterol through specific receptors and modify it to a form that can be recognized and ingested by macrophages that have specific receptors for native and modified LDL. This scavenger effect is part of normal function, but macrophages can injure the overlying endothelium, promoting the atherosclerotic process (2).

Platelet-derived growth factor (PDGF), a cationic protein that can be synthesized by endothelial and other cells and stored in platelets, is a chemotactic and mitogenic substance that can initiate and promote the expansion of smooth muscle migration and proliferation. This process, along with T lymphocytes, the connective tissue matrix, and lipid and lipoprotein accumulation, fosters the growth of the atherosclerotic plaque (5).

Smooth muscle cells also contain receptors for LDL and for growth factors other than PDGF, and they can synthesize prostacyclin (PGI_2) and other prostaglandin derivatives (2).

Endothelial cells are relatively impermeable to lipoproteins, and their normally smooth surface resists platelet adhesion. However, the endothelial lining may be altered through alterations in composition, by increased turnover or spreading of adjacent cells, or via denuding injury from mechanical or biochemical processes. Under such circumstances, platelets may be attracted to such sites, change their shape, and degranulate, releasing growth factors.

Pure atherosis, such as that seen in fatty streaks, may contribute to sclerosis through reductions in endothelium-derived relaxant factor (EDRF). In their studies of cynomolgus monkeys, Harrison and colleagues noted that intimal lesion formation reduces the production or delivery of EDRF, but the response of the media to its effects remains intact (6).

Autopsy studies have indicated that an adaptive phenomenon accompanies the progression of atherosclerotic plaque. Coronary arteries enlarge cross-sectionally, avoiding reduction in lumen stenosis, at least until plaque occupies 40% of the luminal area (7). Since angiographic evaluation has traditionally estimated lesions by the percentage decrease in lumen diameter, this compensatory arterial dilation may result in underestimation of the atherosclerotic process.

Response-to-Injury Hypothesis

These observations led Ross to formulate (and later revise) the hypothesis that interactions among endothelial cells, monocytes, macrophages, smooth muscle cells, platelets, and other bloodborne factors act to repair the wound through stimulation of smooth muscle cells and fibrous elements. If cellular migration and proliferation continue after healing has occurred, the lesions described above form in the intima, eventually leading to obstruction of the coronary artery lumen.

Figure 2.1 illustrates the current version of this hypothesis. The large clockwise cycle (**ABCDF**) represents the interaction of endothelium, macrophages, and platelets, as noted in experimentally induced hypercholesterolemia. Endothelial injury (**A**) results in growth factor secretion, to which monocytes are attracted (**B**). As the monocytes migrate into the subendothelium (**C**), they are transformed into macrophages, then into foam cells. Fatty streak formation results, with the release of other growth factors.

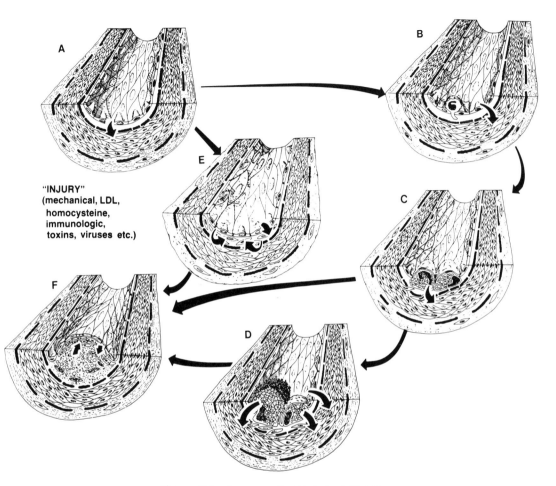

Figure 2.1 Response-to-injury hypothesis.

Fibrous plaques (**F**) may develop from fatty streaks (**C**), either through loss of the macrophages' overlying cover and subsequent platelet adhesion (**D**) or directly (**C–F**) through release of growth factors from macrophages or endothelial cells.

If the endothelium remains intact, increased turnover and growth factor formation by the endothelial cells may stimulate migration of smooth muscle cells from the media to the intima. Smooth muscle cell production of PDGF and growth factor secretion by the endothelial cells (**E**) can lead to plaque formation (**F**) (2).

CAD Risk Indicators and Atherosclerosis

The response-to-injury hypothesis should also be consistent with the epidemiologic evidence linking CAD to the risk indicators, described in the preceding chapter.

Chronic exposure to elevated LDL levels may alter the cholesterol: phospholipid ratio of the plasma membranes, leading to increased membrane viscosity and rigidity of endothelial cells, particularly at points of turbulent blood flow. Cellular retraction could then lead to injury of the denuded endothelium (2). Oxidative modification of LDL may also contribute to atherosclerosis, although this remains to be proven. Oxidated LDL may be toxic to the endothelium, initiating the injury sequence.

Several mechanisms have been proposed by which high blood pressure may lead to initiation or acceleration of atherosclerosis. These include shear stress of higher pressures on the endothelium and hormonal factors that may be toxic to endothelial integrity.

Among the many constituents of tobacco smoke, carbon monoxide (and resultant carboxyhemoglobin) and nicotine may disrupt endothelial integrity, increase platelet aggregation and adhesiveness, or induce the proliferation of smooth muscle cells.

In patients with diabetes mellitus, basement membrane abnormalities in smaller coronary vessels may account for the increased CAD risk. This process may result from injury by macrophages and their oxygen metabolites.

A relative lack of vigorous physical activity is associated with lower HDL-cholesterol levels, as is obesity. Reduction in the scavenger effect of this lipoprotein may enhance atherosclerosis.

Regression of Atheromatous Plaque

Because coronary artery blood flow is so critically dependent upon lumen patency, agents that can induce regression of plaque have been sought for many years. Experimental work in animals has encouraged investigators to seek similar results in humans.

As is explained in more detail in Chapter 3, CAD deaths decreased in the countries most affected by starvation during the First and Second World Wars (8). As Blankenhorn and Kramsch note, reversal of atherosis has been observed in rabbits, swine, dogs, chicks, pigeons, and subhuman primates such as rhesus and cynomolgus monkeys after hypercholesterolemic diets were withdrawn and plasma cholesterol levels were reduced. In early primate studies, removal of lesion collagen occurred slowly and only in the carotid and femoral arteries. Regression was achieved more readily in very early arterial lesions, with initial signs of reversibility noted as early as 4 weeks after serum cholesterol had returned to baseline. Both drug and exercise therapy has been demonstrated to reduce the rate of experimental lesion development (1). More recently, several studies have demonstrated regression in arterial lesions following reduction in serum total cholesterol and LDL-cholesterol levels (9). Quantitation of these studies has been facilitated by newer computer edge-detection algorithms.

Reversal of sclerosis after reduction of plasma cholesterol may allow for a reduction in myocardial ischemia even without a reduction in lesion size. Harrison et al. have suggested that increased ERDF production in coronary arteries after plasma cholesterol lowering may be responsible (6). Improved arterial compliance may also result from calcium channel blockade (1).

CORONARY ARTERY SPASM

Pioneers in cardiology such as Harvey and Heberden described chest pain at rest and noted its association with CAD; Osler suggested that angina pectoris is caused by a spasm of a large coronary artery (10). However, by the middle of the present century, coronary artery spasm was not considered to be significantly involved in myocardial ischemia (11). Prinzmetal et al. published their classic work in 1959, noting S-T segment elevation during patients' reports of chest pain at rest (12).

However, almost two decades elapsed before spasm was documented by hemodynamic monitoring, thallium scintigraphy, and angiography to be equivocably associated with angina pectoris and myocardial infarction. Further, episodes of asymptomatic ischemia were documented on continuous ambulatory electrocardiographic monitoring (13). It also became clear that the same patient could develop angina from increased demand, reduced supply, or both, leading to the term "mixed angina" (14). Ergonovine administration during coronary angiography showed that dynamic coronary constriction can occur in persons who have only exertional angina as well as those with rest pain (15).

Although work continues on the mechanisms of coronary artery spasm, it is reasonably clear that α-adrenergic blockade can reduce coronary vascular resistance, while β-adrenergic blockade may potentiate it. Active coronary vasoconstriction may be induced by cold, exercise, or cigarette smoking, limiting coronary artery flow in response to exercise or other stimuli that raise myocardial oxygen demand. Fortunately, nitrates and calcium-channel blockers can minimize or prevent such increases in coronary vascular tone (16). The prevalence of cigarette smoking in persons with vasospastic angina and no fixed coronary lesions is approximately double that in persons with only fixed lesions, and is nearly three times that of matched persons without CAD. Other CAD risk indicators are similar in the two groups with CAD, suggesting an etiologic role of smoking in coronary artery spasm (17).

The prevalence of smokers is also unusually high among cocaine users who experience myocardial infarction. In one series, eight of nine patients were smokers; the ninth subject had a family history of early CAD. Infarction development was unrelated to the route of cocaine administration. Recurrent ischemia was common among subjects who continued their cocaine use. The etiology of cocaine-induced ischemia is unclear, although several investigators have suggested norepinephrine-mediated α-adrenergic vasoconstriction. Other possibilities include increase platelet aggregability and thromboxane production and decreased endothelial prostacyclin release (18).

These new understandings, coupled with increased knowledge about the role of platelet aggregation and thrombosis in coronary artery obstruction (Chapters 12 and 16), have led to improved therapy for ischemic heart disease.

THROMBOSIS

It is now clear that thrombi play an important role in obstructive CAD, particularly at sites of atherosclerotic lesions (19). Apparent improvement in lumen narrowing may result from lysis or retraction of the clot, or through incorporation of the thrombus into the arterial wall with subsequent contraction. In unstable angina pectoris, eccentric stenoses are often associated with a ruptured atherosclerotic plaque and an associated thrombus (20). The association of these processes with prostaglandins and platelet aggregation continues to be an active focus for investigation (21). These topics are discussed further in Chapters 12 and 16.

REFERENCES

1. Blankenhorn DH, Kramsch DM. Reversal of atherosis and sclerosis. The two components of atherosclerosis. Circulation 1989;79:1–7.

2. Ross R. The pathogenesis of atherosclerosis—an update. N Engl J Med 1986;314:488–500.

3. Faggiotto A, Ross R, Harker L. Studies of hypercholesterolemia in the nonhuman primate. I. Changes that lead to fatty streak formation. Arteriosclerosis 1984;4:323–340.

4. Faggiotto A, Ross R. Studies of hypercholesterolemia in the nonhuman primate. II. Fatty streak conversion to fibrous plaque. Arteriosclerosis 1984;4:341–356.

5. Ross R. Platelet-derived growth factor. Lancet 1989;1:1179–1182.

6. Harrison DG, Armstrong ML, Freiman PC, Heistad DD. Restoration of endothelium-dependent relaxation by dietary treatment of atherosclerosis. J Clin Invest 1987;80:1808–1811.

7. Glagov S, Weisenberg E, Zarins CK, Stankunavicius, R, Kolettis GJ. Compensatory enlargement of human atherosclerotic coronary arteries. N Engl J Med 1987;316:1371–1375.

8. Schettler G. Atherosclerosis during periods of food deprivation following World Wars I and II. Prev Med 1983;13:75–83.

9. Blankenhorn DH, Nessim SA, Johnson RL, Sanmarco ME, Azen SP, Cashin-Hemphill L. Beneficial effects of combined colestipol-niacin therapy on coronary atherosclerosis and coronary venous bypass grafts. JAMA 1987;257:3233–3240.

10. MacAlpin RN. Coronary artery spasm: A historical perspective. J Hist Med Allied Sci 1980;35:288–311.

11. Braunwald E. Coronary artery spasm as a cause of myocardial ischemia. J Lab Clin Med 1981;97:299–312.

12. Prinzmetal M, Kennamer R, Merliss R, et al. Angina pectoris. I. A variant form of angina pectoris. Am J Med 1959;27:375–388.

13. Biagini A, Mazzei MG, Carpeggiani C, et al. Vasospastic ischemic mechanism of frequent asymptomatic transient ST-T changes during continuous electrocardiographic monitoring in selected unstable angina pectoris. Am Heart J 1982;103:13–20.

14. Maseri A, Chierchia S, Kaski JC. Mixed angina pectoris. Am J Cardiol 1985;56:30E–33E.

15. Crea F, Davies G, Romeo F, et al. Myocardial ischemia during ergonovine testing: different susceptibility to coronary vasoconstriction in patients with exertional and variant angina. Circulation 1984;69:690–695.

16. Winniford MD, Jansen DE, Reynolds GA, Apprill P, Black Hills LD. Cigarette smoking–induced coronary vasoconstriction in atherosclerotic coronary artery disease and prevention by calcium antagonists and nitroglycerin. Am J Cardiol 1987;59:203–207.

17. Scholl JM, Benacerraf A, Ducimetiere P, et al. Comparison of risk factors in vasospastic angina without significant fixed coronary artery narrowing to significant fixed coronary narrowing and no vasospastic angina. Am J Cardiol 1986;57:199–202.

18. Smith HW III, Liberman HA, Brody SL, Battey LL, Donohue BC, Morris DC. Acute myocardial infarction temporally related to cocaine use. Clinical, angiographic and pathophysiologic observations. Ann Intern Med 1987;107:13–18.

19. Fitzgerald, DJ, Rooy L, Catella F, FitzGerald GA. Platelet activation in unstable coronary disease. N Engl J Med 1986;315:983–989.

20. Fuster V, Chesebro JH. Mechanisms of unstable angina. N Engl J Med 1986;315:1023–1025.

21. Fuster V, Cohen M, Halperin J. Aspirin in the prevention of coronary artery disease. N Engl J Med 1989;321:183–185.

Section II

Indicators of Risk

3

lipids, lipoproteins, and nutrition

LIPID AND LIPOPROTEIN COMPONENTS

Lipids (cholesterol, triglycerides, and phospholipids) are transported in plasma in the form of large, macromolecular lipoprotein complexes. Cholesterol, the precursor of steroids, sex hormones, and bile acids, is also an important structural component of cellular membranes throughout the body. Brown and Goldstein have estimated that 93% of the body's cholesterol is located in cells, while only the 7% circulating in plasma predisposes to atherosclerotic disease (1). They also note that cholesterol is "the most highly decorated small molecule in biology," studies of which have resulted in thirteen Nobel Prizes (including their own) as of 1986 (2). It is transported largely as cholesterol esters, which are synthesized in cells or the plasma compartment. Triglycerides are an important source of energy, but are relatively insoluble in water, requiring their inclusion into lipoprotein form to reach various organs and tissues.

Lipoproteins are traditionally categorized by their density, composition, and electrophoretic mobility, which reflect the relative amounts of lipid and protein. Major classes include chylomicrons, very low density lipoproteins (VLDL), low-density lipoproteins (LDL), and high-density lipoproteins (HDL). In addition to a hydrophobic core, each has a surface of polar lipids and apolipoproteins of different types; composition varies considerably among the classes (Table 3.1) (3).

LDLs have been further fractionated by density into LDL_1 (also termed intermediate-density lipoproteins or IDL), LDL_2, and others. Similarly, ultracentrifugation of fasting plasma to isolate HDLs reveals predominantly HDL_2 and HDL_3 (4, 5).

Within each lipoprotein class, several apolipoproteins are found. To date, several families containing multiple individual apolipoproteins have been designated. Table 3.2 lists the location and some functions of the more important apolipoproteins.

Dietary fatty acids and cholesterol are esterified in the endoplasmic reticulum of intestinal mucosa cells, forming nonpolar triglycerides and cholesteryl esters. In the Golgi apparatus, they join various apolipoproteins and are secreted into the lym-

Table 3.1.   Lipoprotein Composition by Weight (a) (in Percentages)

Lipoprotein	Protein	Triglyceride	Cholesterol Free	Cholesterol Ester	Phospholipid
Chylomicrons	1–2	85–95	1–3	2–4	3–6
VLDL[b]	6–10	50–65	4–8	16–22	15–20
LDL	18–22	4–8	6–8	45–50	18–24
HDL	45–55	2–7	3–5	15–20	26–32

[a]Data from Schaefer EJ, Levy RI. Pathogenesis and management of lipoprotein disorders. N Engl J Med 1985;312:1300–1310.
[b]VLDL = very low density lipoprotein, LDL = low-density lipoprotein, HDL = high-density lipoprotein.

phatic and general circulations as nascent chylomicrons. There, the chylomicron matures by transferring apoA-I and apoA-II to HDL in exchange for apoC-II, apoC-III, and apoE. After migration to the surface of capillary endothelial cells, the apoC-II activates lipoprotein lipase (LPL) (found on the cell surface) to catabolize the core triglycerides of the mature chylomicron (6). Chylomicron remnants reenter the circulation and are taken up by apoB and apoE receptors in the liver. Receptor activity is influenced by dietary cholesterol and fat, as well as age. ApoC-III can inhibit the remnant uptake process.

Table 3.2.   Apolipoprotein Location and Function

ApoA-I	LCAT[a] activation; reverse cholesterol transport
ApoA-II	LCAT activation
Apo(a)	Covalently linked with ApoB-100 in LP(a)
ApoB-48	Chylomicron secretion
ApoB-100	LDL receptor recognition; VLDL secretion
ApoC-I	LCAT activation; inhibition of hepatic lipoprotein uptake
ApoC-II	LPL activation; inhibition of hepatic lipoprotein uptake
ApoC-III	LPL inhibition; inhibition of hepatic lipoprotein uptake
ApoE	LDL and remnant receptor recognition

[a]Abbreviations: HDL = high-density lipoprotein; LDL = low-density lipoprotein; LCAT = lecithin:cholesterol acyltransferase; LPL = lipoprotein lipase; VLDL = very low density lipoprotein.

VLDL is synthesized and secreted by the liver, and serves to transport endogenous triglyceride. After secretion into the circulation, it encounters LPL at the capillary wall surface. There VLDL is hydrolyzed, ultimately becoming LDL. This catabolism causes the release of free fatty acids and the formation of VLDL remnants that are metabolized in the liver through endocytosis involving LDL receptors on the surface of liver cells. If the number of these LDL receptors decreases, fewer remnants are metabolized in the liver, and more are available for hydrolysis to LDL (7).

In addition to catabolism from VLDL, some direct synthesis of LDL occurs, particularly in persons with homozygous familial hypercholesterolemia. LDL carries cholesterol throughout the body, where it is taken up by cellular endocytosis. Lysosomal acid lipases and proteases catabolize LDL through both receptor-dependent and receptor-independent mechanisms, releasing free cholesterol and amino acids. The number of available LDL receptors affects the plasma concentration by influencing both the rate of production (from VLDL) and the rate of clearance of circulating LDL; usually 60 to 80% of LDL is metabolized in the liver (7).

In addition to its other functions mentioned above, free cholesterol regulates the activity of LDL and HDL receptors, as well as the activity of 3-hydroxy-3-methylglutaryl coenzyme A (HMG-CoA) reductase, which is the rate-limiting enzyme of endogenous cholesterol synthesis. It also influences the activity of acylcoenzyme A:cholesterol acyltransferase (ACAT), the enzyme that esterifies free cholesterol within the cell. If the intracellular concentration of free cholesterol rises, LDL receptors are "down-regulated," and HMG-CoA reductase activity is decreased, while the activity of HDL receptors and ACAT are increased.

HDLs are produced directly in the liver and intestine as nascent HDL, but can also result from the catabolism of chylomicrons and VLDL. Using HDLs as substrate, lecithin:cholesterol acyltransferase (LCAT) catalyzes the conversion of free cholesterol to cholesterol ester. LCAT is activated by apoA-I and inhibited by apoC-II. During esterification, nascent (higher-density) HDLs are transformed into HDL_3. HDL_3 can scavenge cholesterol from peripheral cells that have apoA-I receptors. Depletion of intracellular free cholesterol results in an increase in LDL receptor activity and lower plasma LDL levels. The free cholesterol so sequestered is esterified by LCAT and transferred to the HDL core; during this reverse cholesterol transport process, HDL_3 becomes HDL_2. HDLs are catabolized in the liver and kidney (8).

Epidemiology

In 1950, Malmros reviewed studies of famine and arteriosclerosis, noting that Aschoff found less arteriosclerosis on autopsies done during the years of famine of World War I. Vartianinen and Kanerva made similar observations in Finland during World War II; Brozek, Wells, and Keys found fewer MIs among the starving population of Leningrad during those years. When German occupiers diverted dietary fat to munition production in Norway during World War II, coronary artery disease deaths fell (9). Schettler compared autopsy records from pathology institutes in Berlin, southern Germany, and Basel, Switzerland. Starving persons during World War II had markedly lower blood cholesterol levels, much less atherosclerosis, and lower heart disease rates (10).

Since the end of World War II, extensive investigations of the relationships of coronary artery disease (CAD), lipids/lipoproteins, and nutrition have been undertaken throughout the world, suggesting direct relationships between blood total cholesterol and CAD mortality (11, 12).

Total and LDL Cholesterol

In the Seven Countries Study, nutrition, lipids, and CAD were examined in 16 different population groups in Finland, Greece, Italy, Japan, the Netherlands, the United States, and Yugoslavia. Individual risk of CAD death during the first 10 years was directly related to baseline serum total cholesterol level (13).

In 1948, Framingham (Massachusetts) Heart Study investigators enrolled the first of their 5000 participants. After 14 years of surveillance of the women and men who were examined biannually, CAD morbidity and mortality was noted to correlate directly with baseline serum total cholesterol (14). Fractionation of total cholesterol samples and further surveillance confirmed that CAD mortality was directly related to LDL-cholesterol (15), which was estimated from the formula:

$$LDL\text{-}C = \text{Total cholesterol} - (HDL\text{-}C) - (VLDL\text{-}C)$$

where VLDL-cholesterol is estimated as ⅕ of serum triglycerides (16).

The Pooling Project investigators examined data from more than 12,000 men from eight studies in the United States. Men with baseline serum total cholesterol levels greater than the study mean of 235 mg/dl were significantly more likely to experience CAD events during follow-up (17).

In an attempt to control for heredity factors, investigators in the Ni-Hon-San study enrolled Japanese-American men in California, then matched the Japanese prefecture of their ancestors' origin with persons of Japanese ancestry living in Japan and Hawaii. Mean serum total cholesterol levels were highest in California men (226 mg/dl), intermediate in Hawaiian-Japanese subjects (219 mg/dl), and lowest in those residing in Japan (176 mg/dl) (18). MI incidence and CAD death rates paralleled the rank order of cholesterol values. Californians had a 50% greater incidence rate than Hawaiians, who had double the rate of the men living in Japan (19).

HDL Cholesterol

During the 1970s, several teams documented the inverse relationship of CAD and HDL-C (20–22), including the Framingham study, in which fractionation of total cholesterol began in the period 1969 to 1971 (15). These findings added to those of the Cooperative Lipoprotein Phenotyping Study, a case-control investigation of five populations totaling 6859 women and men of black, Japanese, and white ancestry in the United States. Investigators noted increased CAD risk in persons with HDL-C less than 45 mg/dl (23).

In a prospective Israeli study, the HDL-CAD relationship became even more pronounced in subjects above the age of 50 (24). Review of case-control studies reveals that HDL$_2$ levels are considerably different in MI survivors and control subjects (25).

In their examination of four major prospective studies in the United States,

Table 3.3. Conditions Affecting HDL-Cholesterol Levels

Higher HDL-C	Lower HDL-C
Female gender	Male gender
Estrogens	Progestins, androgens
Insulin	Diabetes (type I or II)
Alcohol	Smoking
Exercise	Diet high in carbohydrates or polyunsaturated fat
Weight reduction	Hypertriglyceridemia
Genetic hyperalphalipo-proteinemia	Genetic HDL-deficiency states

Gordon et al. estimated that a 1 mg/dl increment in HDL-C is associated with a CAD risk decrement of 2% in men and 3% in women (26).

HLD-C levels are higher in blacks and in women (27), as well as in persons with a lean body habitus and higher educational level, who are physically active, do not smoke, and consume a moderate amount of alcohol (28, 29). These, and other factors influencing HDL-C levels, are listed in Table 3.3.

For these reasons, the National Cholesterol Education Program Expert Panel recommends that low HDL-C be raised by hygienic means, such as smoking cessation, weight loss, and aerobic exercise.

Triglycerides

Whether triglycerides are an independent predictor of CAD remains controversial after more than three decades of research. Because of the interrelationships of lipid and lipoprotein variables (notably the inverse relation of HDL and triglycerides), multivariate analyses often result in the elimination of triglycerides from the final list of prognostic indicators. Age, obesity, fasting plasma glucose, and cigarette smoking are all positively associated with serum triglycerides, while physical activity is inversely related (30). These considerations led Hulley at al. to recommend abandonment of widespread screening and treatment of health persons for hypertriglyceridemia (31). However, triglycerides may be prognostically useful in women, and measurement of triglycerides is necessary to estimate LDL-C, so it is likely that they will continue to be a focus of clinical attention (32, 33).

Apolipoproteins

Although LDL-C and HDL-C have been documented as important prognostic factors, a number of investigators have suggested that apoB and apoA-I, respectively, are even more predictive. Maciejko and colleagues used stepwise discriminant and linear discriminant analyses to illustrate the superiority of apoA-I over HDL (34). Like HDL-C, apoA-I levels are positively related to alcohol intake, and are inversely related to body mass index and cigarette smoking (35).

ApoB, the principal protein of LDL-C, is associated with increased CAD risk (36). It is also elevated in men with a history of parental history of MI at an early age (37). Lipoprotein (a) and its apolipoprotein, (a), may prove to be equally useful in the prediction of CAD (38, 39).

ATHEROGENESIS

The epidemiologic studies stimulated in vitro research of the cellular and molecular mechanisms underlying the atherosclerotic process in man. Cultured macrophages have been used to understand a key component in atherosclerosis, the cholesteryl ester–filled macrophage (foam cell). In most types of macrophages, excess native cellular cholesterol leads to down-regulation of the LDL receptors on their surface, preventing a large influx of LDL-C into the cell. However, modified forms of LDL can lead to massive accumulation of cholesteryl ester in cultured macrophages; they enter via a receptor that is not subject to down-regulation (2). Another lipoprotein, β-VLDL, noted in familial dysbetalipoproteinemia, causes marked cholesteryl ester deposition in macrophages; it, too, is associated with a receptor not responsive to down-regulation (40).

Steinberg and colleagues postulate the following sequence: When plasma LDL levels are high, LDL is oxidized by the arterial endothelial cells. The modified LDL attracts monocytes that enter the subendothelial cells. The modified LDL also attracts monocytes that enter the subendothelial space, becoming macrophages. With their motility inhibited by the interaction, the macrophages accumulate the oxidized LDL and become foam cells (41).

Thus, the epidemiologic and pathophysiologic evidence linking LDL and atherogenesis is compelling. In contrast, the observed relation between low HDL and increased atherosclerosis is less well defined. The leading hypothesis is that HDL mediates reverse cholesterol transport, mobilizing cholesterol away from the arterial wall. Further laboratory work should illuminate the pathogenetic mechanisms involved (42).

Hereditary Aspects

Increased CAD rates have been associated with genetic disorders involving elevated LDL, triglycerides, and apoB, as well as decreased levels of HDL and associated apoproteins A-I and C-III (43–45).

Heterozygous familial hypercholesterolemia (FH) occurs in 1 in 500 persons: Those afflicted have only half the normal number of LDL receptors, and LDL is cleared from plasma at only two-thirds the normal rate (usually through receptor-independent pathways). LDL production is also increased in such individuals (46). Homozygous FH can occur when two heterozygotes mate (probability 1 in 250,000): One-fourth of their offspring will inherit the mutant LDL-receptor gene from both parents, resulting in a prevalence of 1 in a million persons. Because these individuals almost always develop symptomatic atherosclerosis (and often experience fatal MI) within their first two decades, plasmapheresis, portacaval shunt, and liver transplantation (to provide LDL receptors) have been used to reduce CAD risk (47–49).

Familial disorders in which persons display elevations of both LDL-cholesterol and triglycerides are termed familial combined hyperlipidemias. This usually results from an overproduction of apoB, and may respond to treatment with the major categories of lipid-lowering agents as discussed below (50).

Persons with low HDL levels may have one of several genetic diseases that have various degrees of association with CAD (51). Frequently, levels of apos A-I and C-III are reduced in persons with low HDL and early CAD. Familial hypoalphalipoproteinemia is the most common, being an autosomal dominant disorder. However, in Tangier disease, with low levels of apos A-I and A-II, the propensity toward early CAD may be mitigated by concomitant low LDL levels (43).

Black men living in the USA have higher HDL-C levels than white men. Studies to date have usually used ethnic self-identification rather than genetic markers, so the degree to which genetic mechanisms may account for this observed difference remains to be determined (52). Between 1960 and 1980, serum total cholesterol levels dropped in blacks only in men with 9 or more years of education; for other men and all women, there was no appreciable change in blacks, in contrast to the significant reductions in all categories of whites in the USA (53).

DEMOGRAPHIC CHARACTERISTICS

Age

Total and LDL cholesterol levels rise with age in both men and women (54). This may be due to decreased catabolism of LDL and apoB with increasing age, a condition that may be related to decreased LDL-receptor activity (55).

Recent studies indicate that both total cholesterol and its subfractions are predictive of future CAD events in the elderly. In the Framingham study, LDL-C and HDL-C were significant indicators of CAD incidence in women and men through the age of 82 (56). Similarly, men aged 60 to 79 in the Puerto Rico Heart Study who had baseline total cholesterol levels below 200 mg/dl had significantly fewer events during follow-up (57). In the Lipid Research Clinics Program Followup Study, total and LDL cholesterol were predictive of CAD events in men 65 and older during a follow-up period of eight and one-half years. Compared to those in the lowest quartiles, men in the highest quartiles for total and LDL cholesterol had relative risks of 3.2 and 4.8, respectively. After adjustment for other CAD risk indicators, both remained significantly predictive for CAD death (58).

There are few studies of intervention to lower lipid values in the elderly, but one study of institutionalized elders aged 60 to 93 demonstrated that diet can be safely altered to reduce fat and cholesterol without inducing deficiencies in protein, calcium, and the fat-soluble vitamins (59).

Gender

Lipid and lipoprotein levels are equal in boys and girls until puberty, after which

HDL-C levels in boys drops more dramatically. During young adulthood, LDL-C and VLDL-C are lower in women than in men, but this pattern reverses during the sixth decade. HDL values in women remain higher than in men until menopause, at which time the difference narrows (60, 61). In one study of premenopausal women, a 10 to 25% suppression of total and LDL cholesterol, as well as apoB, was observed during the luteal phase (62). In other studies, the differences have been smaller. In women taking oral contraceptives, LDL-C increases in direct proportion to the progestin content and inverse proportion to the estrogen strength. In addition, progestins decrease HDL-C. Unopposed replacement estrogens favorably influence LDL and HDL, while unopposed progestins have the opposite effect. The adverse effect on HDL is particularly noted with the 19-nor progestins (63).

DIETARY PATTERNS

In the USA, 35 to 37% of calories are taken from fat sources; there are virtually no differences with age and gender. Saturated fat consumption involves 12 to 15% of total calories: Values exceed 14% for boys and girls ages 2 to 11 (64). Table 3.4 lists the 10 most common sources in the USA diet for saturated fats and cholesterol according to the second National Health and Nutrition Examination Survey (NHANES II) (65).

Dietary Fat

Dietary saturated fatty acids vary in length from 4 to 18 carbon atoms. Often, they are all considered to have an adverse effect on blood lipids, but this effect is largely limited to fats high in lauric acid, myristic acid, or palmitic acid (12, 14, and 16 carbon atoms, respectively). Fatty acids with 4 to 10 carbon atoms do not increase

Table 3.4. Leading Sources of Dietary Saturated Fat and Cholesterol in USA Diets (Data from 11,658 Participants in the NHANES II Study)[a]

| Food | Rank | |
	Saturated Fat	Cholesterol
Hamburgers, cheeseburgers, meat loaf	1	3
Whole milk, whole milk products	2	4
Cheese, excluding cottage cheese	3	9
Beef steaks, roasts	4	2
Hot dogs, ham, luncheon meats	5	6
Donuts, cookies, cake	6	8
Eggs	7	1
Pork chops and roast	8	7
Butter	9	14
White bread, rolls, crackers	10	23
Liver	—	10
Chicken, including fried	16	5

[a]Adapted from Block G, Dresser CH, Hartman AM, Carroll MD. Nutrient sources in the American diet: quantitative data from the NHANES II survey. Am J Epidemiol 1985;122:27–40.

the cholesterol level, and stearic acid and oleic acids (18 bonds) can effectively lower blood cholesterol when either replaces palmitic acid in the diet (66). Since hydrogenation of vegetable oils containing oleic and linoleic acids yields stearic acid as an end product, the process of hydrogenation may not necessarily have an adverse effect on the lipoprotein profile. It appears that those saturated fatty acids that raise cholesterol do so by suppressing the synthesis of LDL receptors, among other possible mechanisms (67).

Polyunsaturated fatty acids appear to increase the clearance of LDL from plasma, through increased LDL-receptor activity. Linoleic acid, an omega-6 fatty acid, is the major polyunsaturated fatty acid in the diet. High doses of linoleic acid can reduce HDL-cholesterol (68), and apoA-I (69, 70), leading to recent moderation in offering diets with high polyunsaturated to saturated fat (P:S) ratios. Grundy has suggested that monounsaturated fats will not lower HDL (71), but Mensink and Katan had different findings in their study of persons who consumed either (*a*) an olive oil and sunflower oil diet (12.9% saturated fat, 15.1% monounsaturated fat, 7.9% polyunsaturated fat) and (*b*) a sunflower oil diet, containing 12.6% saturated fat, 10.8% monounsaturated fat, and 12.7% polyunsaturated fat. In men, HDL fell slightly in both groups; in women, HDL was unchanged (72).

Omega-3 polyunsaturated fatty acids, eicosapentanoic acid (EPA) and docosahexanoic acid (DHA), are found in cold-water fish (73). It has been suggested that low CAD rates in populations with high fish consumption may indicate a protective effect derived from these fatty acids (74). When taken in sufficiently large doses, omega-3 polyunsaturated fatty acids can markedly reduce triglycerides through inhibition of VLDL-triglyceride synthesis. This appears to be secondary to reduced incorporation of other fatty acids into triglycerides in the liver (75). However, LDL-cholesterol levels may rise as plasma triglycerides fall (76).

When the omega-3 polyunsaturated fatty acids replace saturated fats in the diet, LDL-cholesterol drops (77), but this does not occur if saturated fat intake remains constant (78). If the blood triglyceride level is normal, substitution of omega-3 or omega-6 fatty acids for saturated fats can cause a fall in HDL-C. When used for hypertriglyceridemia, however, HDL-C often rises as triglycerides fall (76).

Fish-oil capsules commonly available often contain as little as 180 mg of EPA and 120 mg of DHA. When only one or two capsules of this strength are taken by individuals with normal lipid values, no detectable changes occur in their lipid and lipoprotein profile (79).

In epidemiologic studies, population means for percentage of calories from saturated fats correlate directly with CAD rates. In the Seven Countries Study, saturated fat was less than 10% of calories in Greece, Italy, Japan, and Yugoslavia, where CAD rates were lowest. In contrast, Finland, the Netherlands, and the USA had the highest consumption of saturated fat (more than 15% of calories) accompanying their high CAD rates (13).

In prevalence studies, blood cholesterol levels and saturated fat intake correlated well. This was true in the Japan, Hawaii, and California cohorts in the Ni-Hon-San study (18), as well as in the Ireland-Boston Diet-Heart Study (80). Differences between groups often fitted changes in population mean serum cholesterol as derived from Keys' equation:

Serum cholesterol
$$= 164 + 1.3(2S\text{-}P) + 1.5\,(1000C/E)^{0.5}$$

where S and P are % calories from saturated and polyunsaturated fats, respectively; C is dietary cholesterol in mg/day; and E is total Kcal per day (81).

While animal products are the major source of saturated fat in the USA diet, some vegetable oils contain a very high percentage of saturated fat. Fortunately these "tropical" oils, coconut, palm, and palm kernel, represent less than 10% of the market.

Dietary Cholesterol

Metabolic ward studies confirm the hypothesized direct relationship between dietary cholesterol and blood cholesterol levels (82–84). At least three factors are involved in that relationship: composition of diet (proportions of saturated, polyunsaturated, and monounsaturated fats), baseline dietary cholesterol intake, and individual variability (85). It has been estimated that by decreasing dietary cholesterol from 750 mg to 250 mg, an individual consuming 2500 kcal would lower the blood cholesterol level by 8 to 15 mg/dl (86, 87). Other studies indicate that dietary cholesterol is related to CAD regardless of the blood cholesterol level (88).

The major effect of dietary cholesterol on LDL concentrations results from the suppression of LDL-receptor synthesis and the consequent delay in clearance of LDL and VLDL remnants.

By definition, all dietary cholesterol originates from animal sources. Accordingly, strict vegetarians are found to have substantially lower blood total and LDL cholesterol levels (89). When 250 mg of beef was added isocalorically to the diets of strict vegetarians, plasma total cholesterol rose by 19% within four weeks (90). Adding eggs (or increasing their use) in persons on a wide variety of diets usually increases the plasma total cholesterol levels significantly (91, 92).

For some years, physicians cautioned their patients to avoid shellfish because of increased cholesterol content. However, several species, such as oysters, clams, and scallops are relatively low in cholesterol, and all shellfish are very low in saturated fat, making them preferable to beef (93).

Dietary Fiber

Dietary fibers, those nondigestible remnants of plant cells, resistant to alimentary enzymes, can be subdivided by their water solubility. Most foods of plant origin contain both soluble and insoluble fibers, but they may be rich in one or the other. The natural gel-forming fibers (such as those abundant in oat bran, beans, fruit pectins, and guar gums) are water soluble, and they can be used to selectively lower LDL-C without detriment to HDL-C lev-

els. In contrast, wheat bran is rich in water-insoluble fibers and has no appreciable lipid-altering effects (94, 95). Population studies noting an inverse relation between dietary fiber and CAD have generally not distinguished between the two types (96). However, smaller studies of specific foods rich in the two types of dietary fiber have confirmed beneficial effects on several CAD risk indicators, including dyslipidemias, high blood pressure, obesity, and diabetes (97, 98).

Oat bran lowers LDL-C in a dose-response manner. In a double-blind study of low-dose consumption, Gold and Davidson investigated the effects of 34 g of oat bran daily in healthy medical students. Total cholesterol dropped from 178.8 to 169.3 mg/dl, and LDL-C was reduced from 108.4 to 99.0 mg/dl, but there were no significant changes in serum triglycerides or HDL-C (94).

Excess Calories

The Framingham investigators have noted correlations in adults of all ages between obesity and lipid and lipoprotein fractions. LDL-C levels and body weight were directly correlated in most age and gender subgroups, while HDL-C was inversely correlated to body weight in all subgroups (99).

The effect of excess calories (and consequent weight grain) on lipids and lipoproteins appears to have several determinants, including baseline weight and lipid levels, fatty acid composition of the diet, and concomitant physical activity. Contaldo et al. noted significant improvements in LDL-C, VLDL-C, and HDL-C after a mean weight loss of 21.7 kg in their obese subjects (100). In two other studies, HDL-C and VLDL-C improved after weight loss, but LDL-C did not. In the first, obese patients had no change in their diet composition during the study, which may have affected LDL-C concentrations (101). Wood et al. also failed to note significant LDL-C changes after weight loss induced by either increased physical activity or reduced caloric intake. Again, however, there was little change in dietary composition (102).

In the MRFIT study, decreases in total cholesterol, LDL-C, and triglycerides were directly related to weight loss, although those with the greatest weight loss had higher baseline lipid and lipoprotein values. In contrast, there was no significant difference in baseline HDL-C values among groups with different weight loss, yet those with the greatest weight loss had significantly greater changes in HDL-C (103).

In another study, spouse concordance of plasma cholesterol and triglyceride levels appeared to be mediated largely through relative body weight, rather than through similarity in diet composition and smoking habits. Since spouses were also concordant for hypertension, which is related to obesity, the investigators could not rule out the possibility that antihypertensive medications were responsible for the observed weight-lipid relationship (104).

Caffeine

In a study of 1130 male medical students in the USA followed for 19 to 35 years, a dose-responsive association of coffee consumption with clinically evident CAD was noted, with a relative risk of 2.49 among those consuming five or more cups per day (105). In a case-control study of women with nonfatal first MI before the age of 50, those consuming 10 or more cups of caffeinated coffee had a relative risk of MI of 2.0 compared to women who reported no coffee consumption (106). However, Framingham investigators found no association of coffee intake with CAD incidence in their participants, nor did they find a consistent relationship of blood total cholesterol to coffee consumption (107).

In contrast, investigators in the Tromsö (Norway) Heart Study concluded that coffee consumption is a major contributor to variation in levels in total cholesterol. Even after adjustment for other significant CAD risk indicators, mean serum total cholesterol levels in persons drinking less than one cup and those consuming 10 or more cups per day were 5.56 and 6.23 mmol/L (215 and 241 mg/dl), respectively (108). Another Norwegian study was designed to examine dietary habits, life-style, and coffee consumption; while associations were noted, they were too weak to account for the positive correlation between coffee drinking and serum cholesterol levels (109). In a Belgian study of more than 18,000 women and men, persons drinking three or more cups of coffee per day had higher serum total cholesterol and "non-HDL" cholesterol levels (110).

To distinguish between different sources of caffeine, Japanese men followed by the Honolulu Heart Program were examined. Their baseline coffee consumption was correlated with serum total cholesterol at baseline and six years later. Non–coffee drinkers had a mean cholesterol of 210 mg/dl, compared with 220 mg/dl in those consuming nine or more cups per day. There was no relation of cholesterol with tea or cola consumption (111). European studies have noted that boiled coffee raises serum cholesterol to a much greater extent than filtered coffee (112, 113).

Other acute effects of caffeine on the cardiovascular system include elevated blood pressure, catecholamine levels, plasma renin activity, and serum free fatty acid levels. However, tolerance develops quickly with chronic administration. It is also possible that the deleterious effects of coffee may be attributable to other constituents (114, 115). While some individuals with ventricular dysrhythmias may be sensitive to caffeine, a prospective trial of caffeinated and decaffeinated coffee showed no differences in total or repetitive ventricular dysrhythmias, despite increase in epinephrine and norepinephrine levels during caffeine consumption (116).

OTHER HEALTH HABITS

Alcohol Consumption

The relation of alcohol to lipid, lipoprotein, and apoprotein levels depends in part upon drinking and dietary patterns, as well as concomitant liver damage. Prospective studies have documented lower CAD rates in persons drinking up to five drinks per day than in nondrinkers or heavier drinkers. Such findings were consistent among studies in Japan and Hawaii (117), Massachusetts (118), Puerto Rico (57), London (119), Finland (120), and Yugoslavia (121). Among nondrinkers, some studies have not distinguished between never-drinkers and ex-drinkers. In the British Regional Heart Study, never-drinkers were at minimal risk (122). In the Tecumseh (Michigan) Study, ex-drinkers had a threefold greater risk of CAD than drinkers and never-drinkers (123). Persons consuming six or more drinks per day are at considerably greater risk for CAD and sudden cardiac death. Investigators in Chicago noted a persistence of this risk even beyond the first 10 years of surveillance (124).

Triglyceride levels are directly related to alcohol intake, even after adjustment for obesity and serum cholesterol level (123). Because diet is rarely assessed in studies of alcoholics, the independent effect of alcohol on LDL-C is not clear. Some have suggested that the apparent protective effect of alcohol on CAD applies only to those consuming high amounts of dietary cholesterol or saturated fat (125).

In contrast, HDL-C is usually increased with consumption in nonalcoholics. In alcoholics, Dai et al. noted increases in both HDL_2 and HDL_3 up to 450 ml of daily consumption, after which both total HDL and HDL_2 decreased. Alcoholic subjects with liver disease had higher HDL levels, and both subfractions decreased significantly during one month of abstinence (126).

Until recently, HDL_3 was not thought to exert a CAD protective effect (127). Possible pathways relating HDL-C and alcohol include: (*a*) mediation through sex hormones, reflected in increased HDL-C levels in women and decreased testosterone levels in alcoholic men; (*b*) increased degradation of VLDL; and (*c*) mediation through microsomal enzyme induction in the liver (126). In one study, cessation after long-term drinking resulted in decreases in HDL-C levels and lipoprotein lipase activity of approximately 40% (128).

Experimental studies of moderate alcohol consumption show a positive relation to apoA-I levels in doses as small as one drink per day (129, 130). Alcoholics with liver disease have reduced apoA-I levels (131); this is also noted during withdrawal (128, 132).

Given these findings, most clinicians recommend no change for persons drinking one or two drinks per day, but do not suggest that nondrinkers began alcohol consumption (133).

Smoking

Although many studies show no differences in LDL-C among persons of varying smoking status, one study of young women noted that nonsmoking oral contraceptive (OC) users had LDL levels 11.0 mg/dl lower than smoking OC users; among nonusers of OCs, the mean LDL level in nonsmokers was 5.1 mg/dl less (134).

The inverse relation between HDL-C and cigarette smoking is clearer. In the Lipid Research Clinics Program Prevalence Study, adjustment for age, gender, OC status, obesity, alcohol consumption, and regular aerobic exercise actually increased the difference in HDL-C between smokers and nonsmokers (135). HDL-C increases after smoking cessation; Stubbe et al. suggested that increases in dietary fat and carbohydrate might be related (136), and a later study in which diet was kept constant showed no differences in lipoprotein lipase, hepatic lipase, HDL-C, or other plasma lipid or lipoprotein concentrations (137).

Emotional Distress

While it is commonly perceived that emotional distress can adversely affect total blood cholesterol levels, there are few studies to document this belief. In a 1958 study, tax accountants were studied from January through June. Marked elevations of blood cholesterol were observed during the first two weeks of April, but levels returned to earlier values by June (138). When German manual laborers were exposed to job insecurity, increased shift work, and heavier work load, serum cholesterol levels increased (139). Taggart and Carruthers studied race car drivers, noting increased lipid levels during participation in their exciting sport (140).

Vigorous Physical Activity

Exercise effects on LDL-C have generally been small, both in cross-sectional comparisons of athletes and sedentary persons and in longitudinal training studies. Similarly LDL-C concentrations do not change appreciably with acute exercise in the absence of weight change or dietary modification (141).

In contrast, endurance athletes typically have higher HDL-C levels than sedentary individuals, probably secondary to reduced HDL catabolic rates (142). In training programs for nonathletes, HDL-C usually increases from 5% to 15%, although some studies report no change. Changes in HDL_2 and apo A-I parallel the changes in HDL-C concentration (141).

DISEASES AND DRUGS CAUSING DYSLIPIDEMIA

Several disease states or their treatment can cause abnormalities of lipid and lipoprotein levels. Such diseases include diabetes mellitus, hypothyroidism, liver disorders, dysglobulinemia, multiple myeloma, renal disorders, diseases of inflammation and infection, as well as myocardial infarction. Drugs associated with lipid and lipoprotein alterations include progestins, anabolic steroids, diuretics, β-adrenergic blockers, terbutaline, isotretinoin, cyclosporin, and corticosteroids.

In poorly controlled diabetes, LDL-C and VLDL-C increase, while HDL-C is lowered. In a study of 47 insulin-dependent diabetics, the 26 who chose to participate in an intensive treatment program (self-testing, self-adjustment of insulin delivered as continuous subcutaneous infusion) had a significant improvement in glycemic control. During the subsequent three years, all lipid and lipoprotein fractions were significantly better in the intensive control group than in those who continued their conventional diabetes control program (143). Treatment with weight reduction and a high fiber diet will also improve the lipid and lipoprotein profile. Hypothyroidism causes increased LDL-C and VLDL-C, but may also increase HDL-C. Hepatocellular dysfunction from a number of causes is associated with hypertriglyceridemia. Dysglobulinemias, resulting from chronic liver damage, multiple myeloma, and other causes, result in elevations of LDL-C and VLDL-C, as do the nephrotic syndrome and chronic renal failure (144).

Lipoprotein metabolism is altered in active rheumatoid arthritis and other chronic inflammatory arthritides; decreases in LDL-C, VLDL-C, and HDL-C are proportional to disease severity (145). Treatment of these disorders results in a variety of lipoprotein changes. Prednisolone and penicillamine improve the lipid profile, nonsteroidal antiinflammatory agents have no effect, and chloroquine worsens the lipoprotein disorders (146). The influence of infections on lipids depends on the causative agent; Gram-positive cocci and influenza appear to have little or no effect, while infection with Gram-negative bacilli markedly increases triglycerides, and hepatitis is accompanied by increases in both VLDL-C and LDL-C (147).

During the period from 24 to 72 hours after MI, serum total cholesterol levels drop, then gradually resume preinfarction levels after several weeks. However, measurements done within the first 24 hours after MI accurately reflect baseline conditions in both men and women, regardless of glucose tolerance (148, 149). Persons undergoing elective coronary angiography appear to have reduced levels of HDL-C for reasons not currently known (150).

While β-adrenergic blockers can lower HDL-C levels, terbutaline, a β-adrenergic agonist, raises HDL-C concentrations (151). In men and women treated with isotretinoin for acne, LDL-C and VLDL-C increased dramatically, while HDL-C levels dropped significantly. Within eight weeks of drug discontinuation, levels had been restored to pretreatment conditions (152). Cyclosporine significantly increases total and LDL-cholesterol levels, perhaps accounting for accelerated atherosclerosis in heart trans-plant survivors (153, 154). Anabolic steroids can reduce HDL-C levels (155), in some cases to less than half of their pretreatment level.

SAMPLING AND ANALYSIS

Although serum triglycerides will vary with time since the last meal, total cholesterol seems to be relatively independent of postprandial changes, allowing screening for total cholesterol throughout the day. Schilling and colleagues determined baseline total cholesterol values in normal volunteers, then fed them each of four isocaloric test meals varying in fat content. There were no appreciable differences in total cholesterol at fasting, two-hour, and four-hour sampling (156). Peric-Golia likewise found no differences between fasting and postprandial total cholesterol levels (157). Cholesterol measurements can vary as much as 15% depending on body position and consequent intravascular fluid shifts. Values obtained in winter are usually higher than those determined in summer months (158).

Strenuous efforts are being made to standardize laboratory methodology and improve its reliability and accuracy. The National Cholesterol Education Program in the USA has set a goal of ±3% for accuracy and reproducibility by 1992 (159). Three major desktop chemistry analyzers have been successfully tested against the College of American Pathologists standards (160), making them useful for office or community screening, if proper procedures for technique and materials are rigorously followed (161).

PUBLIC PERSPECTIVE AND POLICY

In 1983, the National Heart, Lung, and Blood Institute and the Food and Drug Administration in the United States sponsored two national probability telephone surveys; one sampled 4007 households and the other surveyed 1610 practicing physicians. While 64% of the public respondents thought reducing high blood cholesterol levels would have a large effect on heart disease, only 39% of the physicians so believed. Median range for physician initiation of diet therapy was 260 to 279 mg/dl; median for drug therapy commencement was 340 to 359 mg/dl. Physicians attributed considerably less preventive value to blood cholesterol reduction than to smoking cessation and blood pressure reduction.

In 1986, similar sampling was undertaken. The percentage of adults who considered that blood cholesterol reduction would have a large effect on heart diseases, rose to 72% (from 46% in 1983). The percentage who reported that they had their cholesterol checked rose from 35 to 46%; those who reported that they made dietary changes to lower their blood cholesterol rose from 14 to 23%. By the later study, physician attitudes had changed even more dramatically; 64% reported that they thought that reducing high blood cholesterol levels would have a large impact on heart disease, and their thresholds for dietary and drug treatment had dropped to 240 to 259 mg/dl and 300 to 319 mg/dl, respectively (162, 163). Many physicians attributed their change in attitude to the 1984 National Institutes of Health Consensus Conference on Lowering Blood Cholesterol (164).

In 1987, the European Atherosclerosis Society issued a policy statement formulated by scientists from 19 countries. They recommended an approach that combines population strategies and interventions with individual risk-reduction efforts. They recommended screening for blood cholesterol in all adults, with consideration of dietary therapy in individuals with values of total cholesterol exceeding 200 mg/dl and a goal of reducing individual levels to that value. They suggested that, for most persons with levels between 200 and 250 mg/dl, dietary advice and correction of other risk factors were most appropriate. Their report also summarized existing evidence about the importance of detection and treatment of the other major CAD risk indicators (165).

In January 1988, the report of the National Cholesterol Education Program (NCEP) Expert Panel on Detection, Evaluation, and Treatment of High Blood Cholesterol in Adults received widespread publication (166). This NCEP report recommended guidelines for all persons 20 years of age and older. Focusing on blood total cholesterol, the expert panel established three categories: values less than 200 mg/dl were termed "desirable," those from 200 to 239 mg/dl were designated as "borderline," and those 240 mg/dl and above were declared "high."

Individuals with values in the desirable range need only have their total cholesterol checked again within five years. Those in the high category should have lipoprotein analysis done, with further action dependent upon LDL level as described below. For those in the borderline category, recommended action depends upon other indicators of CAD risk or its established presence. If the individual has established CAD or two or more of the risk indicators listed in Table 3.5, then lipoprotein analysis should be done, with subsequent action dependent upon LDL level.

If definite CAD is present or if the individual has two or more other indicators of risk, then the goal is to reduce LDL below 130 mg/dl. If neither condition is true, but LDL remains above 160 mg/dl, the NCEP Expert Panel recommends the modest goal of reducing it below that level, while other clinicians strive for a lower level to minimize risk of CAD development.

Dietary treatment should be em-

Table 3.5. CAD Risk Indicators Other Than Dyslipidemia

- Male gender
- Family history of definite MI or sudden cardiac death (parent or sibling before age 55)
- Cigarette smoking (more than 10 cigarettes per day)
- Hypertension
- HDL-cholesterol less than 35 mg/dl on repeated measurement
- Diabetes mellitus
- History of definite cerebrovascular or occlusive peripheral vascular disease
- Severe obesity (30% or more over ideal weight)

ployed first, with drug therapy initiated only after an adequate trial of dietary modification.

DIETARY TREATMENT

The NCEP Adult Treatment Panel simplified earlier dietary recommendations; they suggest a two-step plan for dyslipidemias as shown in Table 3.6. Total caloric intake is adjusted to achieve and maintain desirable weight. Recommended intake of carbohydrates, protein, and the various forms of fatty acids is best expressed as percentage of total calories.

Table 3.6. NCEP Adult Treatment Panel

| Nutrient | Recommended Dietary Intake[a] (% of Total Calories) | |
	Step 1	Step 2
Total fat	<30%	<30%
Saturated fat	<10%	<7%
Polyunsaturated fat	Up to 10%	Up to 10%
Monounsaturated fat	10–15%	10–15%
Carbohydrates	50–60%	50–60%
Protein	10–20%	10–20%
Dietary cholesterol	<300 mg/day	<200 mg/day

[a]Adapted from the Expert Panel. Report of the National Cholesterol Education Program Expert Panel on detection, evaluation and treatment of high blood cholesterol in adults. Arch Intern Med 1988;148:36–69.

Given the number of grams of each nutrient in a serving, one can calculate calories using 9 calories/g for fats and 4 calories/g for carbohydrates and protein. Labeling information on breakfast cereals and some dairy products provides an excellent focus for teaching patients and their families to make these simple calculations as part of their food purchase and consumption habits.

It is also helpful to inquire about a typical day's food consumption pattern. After recording this information, substitutions can be recommended to reduce saturated fats and increase complex carbohydrates. For example, a breakfast of whole grain cereal, nonfat milk, whole wheat toast, and fruit spread would have less than 30% of its calories from fat sources, with no dietary cholesterol; its caloric intake would be approximately half that of a breakfast consisting of two eggs, bacon, toast with butter, and whole milk. The latter diet would have approximately half of its calories from fat (and the majority of those from saturated fat), and it would contain more than 600 mg dietary cholesterol. As indicated in Table 3.6, all individuals should strive for the step 1 diet with less than 30% of all calories coming from fat and 10% or less from saturated fat. Dietary cholesterol should be less than 300 mg/day.

The NCEP guidelines recommend a three-month trial period of the step 1 diet, with remeasurement of blood cholesterol at 4 to 6 weeks and at 3 months. If the minimal goals of LDL reduction have not been met after three months, then referral should be made to a registered dietitian. More vigorous efforts at the step 1 level may be encouraged, or further reduction of saturated fat intake (to less than 7% of total calories) and dietary cholesterol (less than 200 mg/day) may be indicated at that point. The panel recommended that a minimum of six months on dietary therapy alone transpire before consideration of drug therapy in persons without CAD or high LDL levels. However, in patients with LDL-C levels greater than 225 mg/dl or in persons with definite CAD, the practitioner may move to drug therapy earlier.

DRUG THERAPY

Several categories of drugs are now available for the treatment of dyslipidemias. Choice of medications for initial and subsequent therapy is largely predicated upon the lipid and lipoprotein abnormalities of the individual patient. Table 3.7 shows typical percentage changes with therapeutic levels of drugs from the bile acid sequestrant, nicotinic acid, HMG-CoA reductase inhibitor, and fibric acid groups. Summary figures in Table 7 have been derived from the major studies for cholestyramine (167–169), colestipol (170), niacin (171, 172), gemfibrozil (173–175), lovastatin (176), and combinations of these agents (177).

High LDL, Normal HDL and Triglycerides

Where a high LDL-C is the only abnormality, initial therapy with the bile acid sequestrants is a logical first step, given their performance in the large-scale intervention trials and their long record of safety. The primary action of these anion-exchange resins is binding bile acids in the intestinal lumen. The interruption of the enterohepatic circulation of bile acids leads to increased synthesis of bile acids

from cholesterol in the liver. This, in turn, stimulates hepatic LDL-receptor activity and removal of LDL from plasma. However, these changes may result in increased VLDL production and higher plasma concentrations of triglycerides.

Cholestyramine and colestipol are available in fine granular form in bulk cans or as individual packets (unit dose = 4g cholestyramine, 5g colestipol). Both must be mixed with water (or other substrates such as apple sauce or pineapple juice) and taken with meals. Cholestyramine is available in bar form, which is convenient when the patient is away from home. Because the bile acid sequestrants may interfere with absorption of other drugs if taken concurrently, it is advised that other medications be taken either more than one hour before or four hours after cholestyramine and colestipol administration. Interference has been reported with digitoxin, warfarin, thyroxine, thiazides, β-adrenergic blockers, fat-soluble vitamins, and folic acid.

Side effects include constipation, bloating, nausea, flatulence, and a sense of gastric fullness. Other agents would be preferable for persons with a history of peptic ulcer disease or hiatal hernia. Increasing dietary fiber intake will help constipation, as will concurrent administration of psyllium preparations, which will also serve to reduce LDL-C and apoB by 5 to 10% (178). Many patients experience a rise in serum triglycerides after bile acid sequestrant administration; in persons with triglyceride levels exceeding 500 mg/

Table 3.7. Typical Drug Effects on Lipids and Lipoproteins (% Change)

	TC	LDL	HDL	TG/VLDL
Bile acid sequestrants	(−)15–20	(−)20–30	(+)0–2	(+)0–5
Niacin	(−)10–15	(−)10–20	(+)10–20	(−)15–30
Gemfibrozil	(−)8–15	(−)8–15	(+)8–15	(−)35–45
Lovastatin	(−)20–35	(−)25–40	(+)5–10	(−)10–30

dl, these agents should not be used. Mild increases in alkaline phosphatase and transaminases may result from bile acid sequestrant therapy. These are usually transient, and they respond to dosage reduction or transfer to another type of agent. For this reason, liver function tests should be repeated within the first 3 months, and at 4- to 12-month intervals thereafter.

Average wholesale price to pharmacies in 1990 for these and other lipid-modifying agents are shown in Table 3.8 (179). On a yearly basis, costs for monotherapy of these agents at typical dosages are less than $200 for some brands of long-acting niacin, approximately $600 for gemfibrozil or probucol, approximately $900 for bulk bile acid sequestrant treatment, and approximately $600 to $1200 for lovastatin (20 mg vs. 40 mg daily). Given these considerations, some have suggested that drug treatment is most cost-effective for young persons with high LDL-C levels and other indicators of CAD risk, such as smoking or hypertension (180, 181).

High LDL and Triglycerides, Low HDL

High triglycerides are often accompanied by low HDL-C. When these abnormalities coexist with a high LDL-C, nicotinic acid (niacin) is a logical first choice. It decreases hepatic VLDL production and reduces LDL-C and triglyceride levels while raising HDL-C.

The major side effect, flushing, may be minimized by using sustained-release preparations. Flushing can also be reduced by taking niacin after meals. This prostaglandin-mediated effect can also be reduced by taking aspirin or nonsteroidal antiinflammatory drugs before the dose. Both forms are available at low cost, compared to other agents (182). Dosage is increased every 4 to 7 days until a daily dose of at least 1.5 g is reached; the dose may be

Table 3.8.   Average Wholesale Price to Pharmacies[a]

Medication Category	Unit Dose	Cost per Unit Dose (US $)	Typical Unit Doses per Day	Cost per Day
Bile acid sequestrants				
Cholestyramine	4 g		3–5	
Questran (bulk)		0.61		1.84–3.06
Questran (packets)		1.01		3.02–5.03
Choly-bar (bar)		1.08		3.24–5.40
Colestipol	5 g		3–5	
Colestid (bulk)		0.52		1.57–2.62
Colestid (packets)		0.73		2.19–3.65
Niacin (long-acting)	500 mg		3–6	
Slow niacin		0.07		0.21–0.42
Nicolar		0.42		1.25–2.08
Nico-Bid		0.60		1.80–3.00
Gemfibrozil				
Lopid	600 mg	0.47	2	0.94
Lovastatin				
Mevacor	20 mg	1.64	1–4	1.64–6.57
Probucol				
Lorelco	250 mg	0.49	4	1.95

[a]Data from Annual Pharmacists' Reference. Orodell, NJ: Medical Economics Inc., 1990.

raised to 3 g per day for further therapeutic effect. Occasionally, patients can tolerate doses up to 6 g per day, although a case of fulminant hepatic failure has been reported at that dose (183). Higher doses are more likely to result in elevations of hepatic enzymes, glucose, and uric acid. Other agents should be used for patients with a history of peptic ulcer, hepatic disease, hyperuricemia, or gouty arthritis. Blood glucose levels should be carefully monitored if niacin must be used in diabetics. Chemistry panel monitoring should take place every three to four months, with greater frequency at higher dosages.

Normal LDL, Low HDL, High Triglycerides

When high triglycerides and low HDL-C are the major abnormalities, either niacin or gemfibrozil represents a rational first choice. Gemfibrozil is a fibric acid derivative, but possesses properties different from clofibrate (which is no longer used to lower LDL-C due to toxicity) (184). Gemfibrozil increases lipolytic degradation of VLDL, reduces VLDL synthesis and secretion, and may lead to diminished cholesterol ester transfer from HDL to triglyceride-rich lipoproteins, thereby increasing HDL-C (175).

Gemfibrozil is available in 300 mg and 600 mg capsules; the usual dose is 600 mg twice daily with meals. Side effects are largely gastrointestinal, although blood glucose levels may rise slightly. Other agents should be used in persons with cholelithiasis or renal or hepatic disease. Prothrombin time should be carefully monitored during the early stages of therapy. Biochemical surveillance should also include periodic red and white blood cell counts.

Lovastatin

While cholestyramine, niacin, and gemfibrozil had all demonstrated reduced cardiovascular events in long-term trials by 1990, similar evidence was still not available for lovastatin, leading some to advocate caution in its use as a first-line drug. However, its powerful effects in lowering LDL-C (along with a modest HDL-C elevating effect) has led to its widespread use. It has also proved useful in maintaining adherence in individuals taking many medications.

Lovastatin inhibits HMG-CoA reductase production of LDL-C, while increasing LDL receptor activity and increasing the rate of receptor-mediated LDL removal from plasma. Dosage is usually started with a single 20 mg tablet with the evening meal and may be raised to 80 mg in a single or twice daily dose.

Myopathy (indicated by symptoms or asymptomatic elevation in creatinine kinase levels) occurs in a small percentage of patients; incidence is increased when lovastatin and gemfibrozil are used together (185), particularly in persons on prednisone or cyclosporine. Approximately 2% of treated patients have persistent increases in transaminase levels some 3 to 16 months after therapy commencement; these will revert to normal with discontinuation of therapy. Other reported side effects include gastrointestinal distress, skin rashes, fatigue, and insomnia. It does not appear that lens opacities are formed at a greater rate than normal aging suggests, but baseline and follow-up slit lamp examinations are still recommended. Lovastatin is contraindicated in persons with active liver disease and in women who are trying to become pregnant, are pregnant, or are nursing.

Probucol

Probucol lowers LDL-C slightly and HDL-C moderately, making it an unlikely candidate for therapy in most patients. However, it has been effective in reducing tendon xanthomas in persons with the

LDL-receptor absence or deficiency condition of familial hypercholesterolemia; the lower the HDL-C level drops, the greater the degree of xanthoma regression. It appears that probucol may modify HDL subspecies in a manner that facilitates reverse cholesterol transport and facilitates removal of cholesterol from peripheral tissues including diseased arterial walls. It also inhibits the oxidative modification of LDL, in addition to enhancement of bile acid secretion (186).

Side effects are largely gastrointestinal, particularly diarrhea. Tolerance to probucol in this regard usually occurs within several weeks. The long-term implications of probucol therapy are unknown.

Drug Combinations

Given the characteristics of individual lipid and lipoprotein disorders, and the specific biochemical actions of different drugs, certain combinations appear efficacious in treatment.

Bile acid sequestrants have been demonstrated to be effective with niacin in persons with heterozygous familial hypercholesterolemia (FH) (187) and in persons with all levels of blood cholesterol follow-ing coronary artery bypass surgery (177). Colestipol and lovastatin in combination increase the LDL fractional catabolic rate, and deplete cholesterol in LDL particles (188). The addition of gemfibrozil to lovastatin therapy does not appear to offer significant further LDL lowering and is associated with increased risk of myopathy (185). The magnitude of these changes are listed in Table 3.9.

LOW BLOOD CHOLESTEROL AND NONCARDIOVASCULAR DISEASE RISK

An inverse relationship between serum cholesterol and incidence of colon cancer was noticed in several large-scale cardiovascular disease trials in men (189–191). However, this association is strongest for deaths occuring within the first year after enrollment, suggesting that undetected cancer results in lowered total blood cholesterol values. Findings in several large-scale studies have been consistent with this hypothesis (192–194).

An association of low blood cholesterol and hemorrhagic stroke has been observed in persons of Japanese heritage living in Japan (195) and in Hawaii (196), as

Table 3.9. Percentage Change in Lipids and Lipoproteins

Drug	Daily Dose	Population	Total Chol[a]	LDL	HDL	Trig
Colestipol	30 mg	HeteroFH	−45%	−55%	+22%	−40%
Niacin[b]	6–7.5 g					
Colestipol	30 mg	CABS	−26%	−43%	+37%	−22%
Niacin[c]	3–12 g					
Colestipol	20 mg	Non FH	−36%	−48%	+17%	−8%
Lovastatin[d]	40 mg					

[a]Abbreviations: Chol = cholesterol; Trig = triglycerides; Hetero FH = heterozygous familial hypercholesterolemia; CABS = coronary artery bypass surgery; Non FH = elevated total and LDL cholesterol levels without familial hypercholesterolemia.
[b]Data from Kane JP, Malloy MJ, Tun P, et al. Normalization of low-density lipoprotein levels in heterozygous familial hypercholesterolemia with a combined drug regimen. N Engl J Med 1981;304:251–258.
[c]Data from Blaukenhorn DH, Nessim SA, Johnson RL, Sanmarco ME, Azen SP, Cashin-Hemphill L. Beneficial effects of combined colestipol-niacin therapy on coronary atherosclerosis and coronary venous bypass grafts. JAMA 1987;257:3233–3240.
[d]Data from Vega GL, Grundy SM. Treatment of primary moderate hypercholesterolemia with lovastatin (mevinolin) and colestipol. JAMA 1987;257:33–38.

well as in the Framingham (197) and MRFIT (198) studies. However, the risk for CAD and nonhemorrhagic stroke from aspirin, is positively related to blood cholesterol. Given the increased risk of hemorrhagic stroke, persons with a family history of hemorrhagic stroke without a high CAD risk profile may be well advised to avoid aspirin and be comfortable with a total cholesterol between 180 mg/dl and 199 mg/dl.

Multilevel Interventions

To achieve optimal reduction in CAD incidence, both individual and community interventions will be necessary. Targets for such efforts are listed in Table 3.10. Community-based studies have been successful in reducing blood cholesterol levels through intervention in several of the target groups. These include the Stanford Five-City Project (199), the Minnesota Heart Health Study (200), and the Pawtucket Heart Health Program (201), in the United States. In the North Karelia province of eastern Finland, a 10-year, community-based program of cardiovascular risk reduction resulted in a decrease in saturated fats of 20% in men and 14% in women, compared to a reference area elsewhere in Finland. Parallel changes in serum cholesterol levels were reported (202).

These efforts, along with secular changes in improved nutrition and orientation towards physical fitness, have resulted in significant decreases in mean serum cholesterol levels in the United States. Between 1960 and 1980, age-adjusted levels in women and men, 20 to 74 years of age, decreased from 217 mg/dl to 211 mg/dl in men and from 223 mg/dl to 215 mg/dl in women. Although decreases were significant in whites, this was not true in blacks or in persons with less than nine years of formal education. Changes in nutrition patterns during this period have undoubtedly contributed to the decline in CAD mortality, which began in some areas of the United States as early as 1960 (203). Reduction in total and saturated fat intake has also been associated with fewer new lesions in persons after CABS (204).

Table 3.10. Targets for CAD Reduction Efforts

Community
  Media
  Public opinion
  Legislators
  Food producers
Organizations
  Schools
  Worksites
  Grocery stores
  Restaurants
Specific groups
  Youth peer groups
  Families
  Low income and ethnic minority groups

REFERENCES

1. Brown MS, Goldstein JL. Lowering plasma cholesterol by raising LDL receptors. N Engl J Med 1981;305:515–517.

2. Brown MS, Goldstein JL. A receptor-mediated pathway for cholesterol homeostasis. Science 1986;232:34–47.

3. Schaefer EJ, Levy RI. Pathogenesis and management of lipoprotein disorders. N Engl J Med 1985;312:1300–1310.

4. Musliner TA, Krauss RM. Lipoprotein subspecies and risk of coronary disease. Clin Chem 1988;34(8(B)):B78–B83.

5. Small DM. HDL system: a short reveiw of structure and metabolism. In: Catapano AL (ed): Atherosclerosis reviews, vol. 16. New York: Raven Press, 1987:1–8.

6. Eckel RH. Lipoprotein lipase. A multifunctional enzyme relevant to common metabolic diseases. N Engl J Med 1989;320:1060–1068.

7. Grundy SM. HMG-CoA reductase inhibitors for treatment of hypercholesterolemia. N Engl J Med 1988;319:24–33.

8. Levy RI, Rifkind BM. The structure, function and metabolism of high-density lipoproteins: a status report. Circulation 1980;62(Suppl IV):IV4–IV8.

9. Malmros H. The relation of nutrition to health. A statistical study of the effect of the war-time on arteriosclerosis, cardiosclerosis, tuberculosis and diabetes. Acta Med Scand 1950;246(Suppl):137–153.

10. Schettler G. Atherosclerosis during periods of food deprivation following World Wars I and II. Prev Med 1983;12:75–83.

11. Keys A, Kimura N, Kusukawa A, (al. Lessons from serum cholesterol in Japan, Hawaii, and Los Angeles. Ann Intern Med 1958;48:83–94.

12. Pyorala K. Interpopulation correlations between serum cholesterol level and the occurrence of coronary heart disease. Eur Heart J 1987;8 (Suppl E):23–30.

13. Keys A. Seven countries: a multivariate analysis of death and coronary heart disease. Cambridge, MA: Harvard University Press, 1980.

14. Kannel WB, Castelli WP, Gordon T, McNamara PM. Serum cholesterol, lipoproteins, and the risk of coronary heart disease. The Framingham Study. Ann Intern Med 1971;74:1–12.

15. Gordon, T, Castelli WP, Hjortland MC, Kannel WB, Dawber TR. High density lipoprotein as a protective factor against coronary heart disease: the Framingham Study. Am J Med 1977;62:707–714.

16. Friedwald WT, Levy RI, Fredrickson DS. Estimation of the concentration of low-density lipoprotein cholesterol in plasma, without use of the preparative ultracentrifuge. Clin Chem 1972;18:499–502.

17. Pooling Project Research Group. Relationship of blood pressure, serum cholesterol, smoking habit, relative weight and ECG abnormalities to incidence of major coronary events: final report of the Pooling Project. J Chron Dis 1978;31:201–306.

18. Kagan A, Harris BR, Winkelstein W Jr, et al. Epidemiologic studies of coronary heart disease and stroke in Japanese men living in Japan, Hawaii and California: demographic, physical, dietary and biochemical characteristics. J Chron Dis 1974;27:345–364.

19. Robertson TL, Kato H, Rhoads GG, et al. Epidemiologic studies of coronary heart disease and stroke in Japanese men living in Japan, Hawaii and California. Incidence of myocardial infarction and death from coronary heart disease. Am J Cardiol 1977;39:239–243.

20. Miller GJ, Miller NE. Plasma-high-density lipoprotein concentration and development of ischemic heart disease. Lancet 1975;1:16–20.

21. Berg K, Borresen AL, Dahlen B. Serum-high-density-lipoprotein and atherosclerotic heart-disease. Lancet 1976;1:499–501.

22. Lewis, B. Relation of high-density lipoproteins to coronary artery disease. Am J Cardiol 1983;52:5B–8B.

23. Castelli WP, Doyle JT, Gordon T, et al. HDL cholesterol and other lipids in coronary heart disease. The Cooperative Lipoprotein Phenotyping Study. Circulation 1977;55:767–772.

24. Goldbourt U, Medalie JH. High density lipoprotein cholesterol and incidence of coronary heart disease—the Israeli Ischemic Heart Disease Study. Am J Epidemiol 1979;109:296–308.

25. Brugger P, Kostner GM, Kullich WC, Klein G. Plasma concentrations of high-density lipoprotein (HDL)-2 and HDL-3 in myocardial infarction survivors and control subjects. Clin Cardiol 1986;9:273–276.

26. Gordon DJ, Probstfield JL, Garrison RJ, et al. High-density lipoprotein cholesterol and cardiovascular disease. Four prospective American studies. Circulation 1989;79:8–15.

27. Linn S, Fulwood R, Rifkind B, et al. High density lipoprotein cholesterol levels among US adults by selected demographic and socioeconomic variables. The Second National Health and Nutrition Examination Survey, 1976–1980. Am J Epidemiol 1989;129:281–294.

28. Heiss G, Johnson NJ, Reiland S, Davis CE, Tyroler HA. The epidemiology of plasma high-density lipoprotein cholesterol levels. Lipid Research Clinics Program Prevalence Study. Summary. Circulation 1980;62 (Suppl IV):IV116–IV136.

29. Krauss RM. Regulation of high density lipoprotein levels. Med Clin North Amer 1982;66:403–430.

30. Cowan LD, Wilcosky T, Criqui MH, et al. Demographic, behavioral, biochemical, and dietary correlates of plasma triglycerides. Lipid Research Clinics Program Prevalence Study. Arteriosclerosis 1985;5:466–480.

31. Hulley SB, Rosenman RH, Bawol RD, Brand RJ. Epidemiology as a guide to clinical decisions. The association between triglyceride and coronary heart disease. N Engl J Med 1980;302:1383–1389.

32. Austin M. Plasma triglyceride as a risk factor for coronary heart disease. The epidemiologic evidence and beyond. Am J Epidemiol 1989;129:249–259.

33. Brunzell JD, Austin MA. Plasma trigylceride levels and coronary disease. N Engl J Med 1989;320:1273–1275.

34. Maciejko JJ, Holmes DR, Kottke BA, Zinsmeister AR, Dinh DM, Mao SJ. Apolipoprotein A-I as a marker of angiographically assessed coronary-artery disease. N Engl J Med 1983;309:385–389.

35. Meilahn EN, Kuller LH, Stein EA, Caggiula A, Matthews KA. Characteristics associated with apo- and lipo-protein levels in middle-aged women. Arteriosclerosis 1988;8:515–520.

36. Durrington PN, Ishola M, Hunt L, Arrol S, Bhatnagar D. Apolipoproteins (a), A1, B and parental history in men with early onset ischaemic heart disease. Lancet 1988;1:1070–1073.

37. Cambien F, Warnet JM, Jacqueson, A, Ducimetiere P, Richard JL, Claude JR. Relation of parental history of early myocardial infarction to the level of apolipoprotein B in men. Circulation 1987;76:266–271.

38. Rhoads GG, Dahlen G, Berg K, Morton NE, Dannenberg AL. LP(a) lipoprotein as a risk factor for myocardial infarction. JAMA 1986;256:2540–2544.

39. Anonymous. Apolipoprotein-B and atherogenesis. Lancet 1988;1:1141–1142.

40. Brown MS, Goldstein JL. Lipoprotein metabolism in the macrophage: implications for cholesterol deposition in atherosclerosis. Ann Rev Biochem 1983;52:233–261.

41. Steinberg D, Parthasarathy S, Carew TE, Khoo JC, Witztum JL. Beyond cholesterol. Modifications of low-density lipoprotein that increase its atherogenicity. N Engl J Med 1989;320:915–924.

42. Grundy SM, Goodman DS, Rifkind BM, Cleeman JJ. The place of HDL in cholesterol management. A perspective from the National Cholesterol Education Program. Arch Intern Med 1989;149:505–510.

43. Segal P, Rifkind BM, Schull WJ. Genetic factors in lipoprotein variation. Epidemiol Rev 1982;4:137–160.

44. Brunzell JD, Sniderman AD, Albers JJ, Kwiterovich PO Jr. Apoproteins B and A-1 and coronary artery disease in humans. Arteriosclerosis 1984;4:79–83.

45. Schaefer EJ. Clinical, biochemical and genetic features in familial disorders of high density lipoprotein deficiency. Arteriosclerosis 1984;4:303–322.

46. Goldstein JL, Kita T, Brown MS. Defective lipoprotein receptors and atherosclerosis. N Engl Med 1983;309:288–296.

47. Bilheimer DW, Goldstein JL, Grundy SM, Starzl TE, Brown MS. Liver transplantation to provide low-density-lipoprotein receptors and lower plasma cholesterol in a child with homozygous familial hypercholesterolemia. N Engl J Med 1984;31:1658–1664.

48. Thompson GR, Babir M, Okabayashi K, Trayner I, Larkin S. Plasmapheresis in familial hypercholesterolemia. Arteriosclerosis 1989;9(Suppl I):I152–I157.

49. Bilheimer DW. Portacaval shunt and liver transplantation in treatment of familial hypercholesterolemia. Arteriosclerosis 1989; 9(Suppl I):I158–I163.

50. Grundy SM, Chait A, Brunzell JD. Familial combined hyperlipidemia workshop. Arteriosclerosis 1987;7:203–207.

51. Lees RS, Lees AM. High-density lipoproteins and the risk of atherosclerosis. N Engl J Med 1982;306:1546–1548.

52. Watkins LO, Neaton JD, Kuller LH for the MRFIT Research Group. Racial differences in high-density lipoprotein cholesterol and coronary heart disease incidence in the usual-care group of the Multiple Risk Factor Intervention Trial. Am J Cardiol 1986;57:538–545.

53. National Center for Health Statistics-National Heart, Lung, and Blood Institute Col-

laborative Lipid Group. Trends in serum cholesterol levels among US adults aged 20 to 74 years. Data from the National Health and Nutrition Examination Surveys, 1960 to 1980. JAMA 1987;257:937–942.

54. National Heart, Lung, and Blood Institute. The Lipid Research Clinics Population Studies Data Book, vol 1: the prevalence Study. Washington DC: US Government Printing Office, 1980. NIH Publ. no. 80–1527.

55. Miller NE. Why does low density lipoprotein concentration in adults increase with age? Lancet 1984;1:263–267.

56. Kannel WB, Doyle JT, Shephard RJ. Prevention of cardiovascular disease in the elderly. J Am Coll Cardiol 1987;10:25A–28A.

57. Kittner SJ, Garcia-Palmieri MR, Costas R Jr, Cruz-Vidal M, Abbott RD, Havlik RJ. Alcohol and coronary heart disease in Puerto Rico. Am J Epidemiol 1983;117:538–550.

58. Bush T, Knoke J, Criqui M, Kritchevsky A. Total and LDL cholesterol as predictors of CHD death in elderly men: the Lipid Research Clinics' Program Follow-up Study. (abstr). CVD Epidemiol Newsletter 1988;43:22.

59. Goodwin, JS, Leonard AG, Hooper EM, et al. Concern about cholesterol and its association with diet in a group of healthy elderly. Nutr Rev 1985;5:141–148.

60. Rifkind BM, Segal P. Lipid Reserach Clinics reference values for hyperlipidemia and hypolipidemia. JAMA 1983;250:1869–1872.

61. Tell GS, Mittlemark MB, Vellar OD. Cholesterol, high density lipoprotein cholesterol and triglycerides during puberty: the Oslo Youth Study. Am J Epidemiol 1985;122:750–761.

62. Kim HJ, Kalkhoff RK. Changes in lipoprotein composition during the menstrual cycle. Metabolism 1979;28:663–668.

63. Bush TL, Fried LP, Barrett-Connor E. Cholesterol, lipoproteins, and coronary heart disease in women. Clin Chem 1988;34(8(B)):B60–B70.

64. Abraham S, Carroll MD. Fats, cholesterol, and sodium intake in the diet of persons 1–74 years: United States. Advance Data 1981;54:1–10.

65. Block G, Dresser CH, Hartman AM, Carroll MD. Nutrient sources in the American diet: quantitative data from the NHANES II Survey. Am J Epidemiol 1985;122:27–40.

66. Bonanome A, Grundy SM. Effect of dietary stearic acid on plasma cholesterol and lipoprotein levels. N Engl J Med 1988;318:1244–1248.

67. Spady DK, Dietschy J. Interaction of dietary cholesterol and triglycerides in the regulation of hepatic low density lipoprotein transport in the hamster. J Clin Invest 1988;81:300–309.

68. Mattson FH, Grundy SM. Comparison of effects of dietary saturated, monounsaturated, and polyunsaturated fatty acids on plasma lipids and lipoproteins in man. J Lipid Res 1985;26:194–202.

69. Shepherd J, Packard CJ, Patsch JR, Gotto AM Jr, Taunton OD. Effects of dietary polyunsaturated and saturated fat on the properties of high density lipoproteins and the metabolism of apolipoprotein A-I. J Clin Invest 1978;61:1582–1592.

70. Ehnholm C, Huttunen JK, Pietinen P, et al. Effect of a diet low in saturated fatty acids on plasma lipids, lipoproteins and HDL subfractions. Arteriosclerosis 1984;4:265–269.

71. Grundy SM. Comparison of monounsaturated fatty acids and carbohydrates for lowering plasma cholesterol. N Engl J Med 1986;314:745–748.

72. Mensink RP, Katan MB. Effect of a diet enriched with monounsaturated or polyunsaturated fatty acids on levels of low-density and high-density lipoprotein cholesterol in healthy women and men. N Engl J Med 1989;321:436–441.

73. Leaf A, Weber PC. Cardiovascular effects of n-3 fatty acids. N Engl J Med 1988;318:549–557.

74. Kromhout D, Bosschieter EB, Coulander C. The inverse relation between fish consumption and 20-year mortality from coronary heart disease. N Engl J Med 1985;312:1205–1209.

75. Nestel PJ, Connor WE, Reardon MF, Connor S, Wong S, Boston R. Suppression by diets rich in fish oil of very low density lipoprotein production in man. J Clin Invest 1984;74:82–89.

76. Connor WE. Hypolipidemic effects of dietary omega-3 fatty acids in normal and hyperlipidemic humans: effects and mechanisms. In: Simopoulos A, Kifer RR, Martin RE, (eds): Health effects of polyunsaturated fatty acids in seafoods. New York: Academic Press, 1986;173–210.

77. Illingworth DR, Harris WS, Connor WE. Inhibition of low density lipoprotein synthesis by dietary omega-3 fatty acids in humans. Arteriosclerosis 1984;4:270–275.

78. Rogers S, James KS, Butland BK, et al. Effects of a fish oil supplement on serum lipids, blood pressure, bleeding time, haemostatic and rheological variables: a double blind randomised controlled trial in healthy volunteers. Atherosclerosis 1987;63:137–143.

79. Davidson DM, Gold KV. n-3 fatty acids. N Engl J Med 1988;319:580–581.

80. Kushi LH, Lew RA, Stare FJ, et al. Diet and 20-year mortality from coronary heart disease. The Ireland-Boston Diet-Heart Study. N Engl J Med 1985;312:811–818.

81. Keys A, Anderson JT, Grande F. Prediction of serum-cholesterol responses of man to changes in fat in the diet. Lancet 1957;2:959–966.

82. Keys A, Anderson JT, Grande F. Serum cholesterol response to changes in the diet. II. The effect of cholesterol in the diet. Metabolism 1965;14:759–765.

83. Hegsted DM, McGandy RB, Myers ML, Stare FJ. Quantitative effects of dietary fat on serum cholesterol in man. Am J Clin Nutr 1965;17:281–295.

84. Mattson FH, Erickson BA, Kligman AM. Effect of dietary cholesterol on serum cholesterol in man. Am J Clin Nutr 1972;25:589–594.

85. Katan MB, Beynen AC. Characteristics of human hypo- and hyperresponders to dietary cholesterol. Am J Epidemiol 1987;125:387–399.

86. Hegsted DM. Serum cholesterol response to dietary cholesterol: a re-evaluation. Am J Clin Nutr 1986;44:299–305.

87. Stamler J, Shekelle R. Dietary cholesterol and human heart disease. The epidemiologic evidence. Arch Pathol Lab Med 1988;112:1032–1040.

88. Shekelle RB, Stamler J. Dietary cholesterol and ischaemic heart disease. Lancet 1989;1:1177–1179.

89. Sacks FM, Castelli WP, Donner A, Kass EH. Plasma lipids and lipoproteins in vegetarians and controls. N Engl J Med 1975;292:1148–1151.

90. Sacks FM, Donner A, Castelli WP, et al. Effect of ingestion of meat on plasma cholesterol of vegetarians. JAMA 1981;246:640–644.

91. Roberts SL, McMurry MP, Connor WE. Does egg feeding (i.e. dietary cholesterol) affect cholesterol levels in humans? The results of a double-blind study. Am J Clin Nutr 1981;34:2092–2099.

92. Edington J, Geekie M, Carter R, et al. Effect of dietary cholesterol on plasma cholesterol concentration in subjects following reduced fat, high fibre diet. Br Med J 1987;294:333–336.

93. Connor WE, Lin DS. The effect of shellfish in the diet upon the plasma lipid levels in humans. Metabolism 1982;31:1046–1051.

94. Gold KV, Davidson DM. Oat bran as a cholesterol-reducing dietary adjunct in a young, healthy population. West J Med 1988;148:299–302.

95. Council on Scientific Affairs. Dietary fiber and health. JAMA 1989;262:542–546.

96. Khaw KT, Barrett-Connor E. Dietary fiber and reduced ischemic heart disease mortality rates in men and women: a 12-year prospective study. Am J Epidemiol 1987;126:1092–1102.

97. Anderson JW, Tietyen-Clark J. Dietary fiber: hyperlipidemia, hypertension, and coronary heart disease. Am J Gastroenterol 1986;81:907–919.

98. Miranda PM, Horwitz DL. High-fiber diets in the treatment of diabetes mellitus. Ann Intern Med 1978;88:482–486.

99. Garrison RJ, Wilson PW, Castelli WP, Feinleib M, Kannel WB, McNamara PM. Obesity and lipoprotein cholesterol in the Framingham Offspring Study. Metabolism 1980;29:1053–1060.

100. Contaldo F, Strazzullo P, Postiglione A, et al. Plasma high density lipoprotein in severe obesity after stable weight loss. Atherosclerosis 1980;37:163–167.

101. Wolf RN, Grundy SM. Influence of weight reduction on plasma lipoproteins in obese patients. Arteriosclerosis 1983;3:160–169.

102. Wood PD, Stefanick ML, Dreon DS, et al. Changes in plasma lipids and lipoproteins in overweight men during weight loss through dieting as compared with exercise. N Engl J Med 1988;319:1173–1179.

103. Caggiula AW, Christakis G, Farrand M, et al. The Multiple Risk Factor Intervention Trial (MRFIT). IV. Intervention on blood lipids. Prev Med 1981;10:443–475.

104. Barrett-Connor E, Suarez L, Criqui MH. Spouse concordance of plasma cholesterol and triglyceride. J Chron Dis 1982;35:333–340.

105. LaCroix AZ, Mead LA, Liang KY, Thomas CB, Pearson TA. Coffee consumption and the incidence of coronary heart disease. N Engl J Med 1986;315:977–982.

106. Rosenberg L, Werler MM, Kaufman DW, Shapiro S. Coffee drinking and myocardial infarction in young women: an update. Am J Epidemiol 1987;126:147–149.

107. Wilson PW, Garrison RJ, Kannel WB, McGee DL, Castelli WP. Is coffee consumption a contributor to cardiovascular disease? Insights from the Framingham Study. Arch Intern Med 1989;149:1169–1172.

108. Thelle DS, Arnesen E, Forde OH. The Tromsö Heart Study. Does coffee raise serum cholesterol? N Engl J Med 1983;308:1454–1457.

109. Solvoll K, Selmer R, Loken EB, Foss OP, Trygg K. Coffee, dietary habits, and serum cholesterol among men and women 35–49 years of age. Am J Epidemiol 1989;129:1277–1288.

110. Pietinen P, Gebbers J, Kesteloot H. Coffee consumption and serum cholesterol: an epidemiological study in Belgium. Int J Epidemiol 1988;17:98–104.

111. Curb JD, Read DM, Kautz JA, Yano K. Coffee, caffeine, and serum cholesterol in Japanese men in Hawaii. Am J Epidemiol 1986;123:648–655.

112. Bak AA, Grobbee DE. The effect on serum cholesterol levels of coffee brewed by filtering or boiling. N Engl J Med 1989;321:1432–1437.

113. Stevsvold I, Tverdal A, Foss OP. The effect of boiled and filtered coffee on serum cholesterol and triglycerides in 5 counties in Norway. Eur Heart J 1988;9(Suppl A):87.

114. Curatolo PW. The health consequences of caffeine. Ann Intern Med 1983;98:641–653.

115. Myers MG. Effects of caffeine on blood pressure. Arch Intern Med 1988; 148:1189–1193.

116. Graboys TB, Blatt CM, Lown B. The effect of caffeine on ventricular ectopic activity in patients with malignant ventricular arrhythmia. Arch Intern Med 1989;149:637–639.

117. Yano K, MacLean CJ, Reed DM, et al. A comparison of the 12-year mortality and predictive factors of coronary heart disease among Japanese men in Japan and Hawaii. Am J Epidemiol 1988;127:476–487.

118. Gordon T, Kannel WB. Drinking habits and cardiovascular disease. The Framingham Study. Am Heart J 1983;105:667–673.

119. Marmot MG. Alcohol and coronary artery disease. Int J Epidemiol 1984;13:160–167.

120. Salonen JT, Puska P, Nissinen A. Intake of spirits and beer and risk of myocardial infarction and death—a longitudinal study in Eastern Finland. J Chron Dis 1983;36:533–543.

121. Kozararevic D, McGee D, Vojvodic N, et al. Frequency of alcohol consumption and morbidity and mortality. Lancet 1980;1:613–616.

122. Shaper AG, Wannamethee G, Walker M. Alcohol and mortality in British men: explaining the U-shaped curve. Lancet 1988;2:1267–1273.

123. Ostrander LD Jr, Lamphiear DE, Block WD, Johnson BC, Ravenscroft C, Epstein FH. Relationship of serum lipid concentrations to alcohol consumption. Arch Intern Med 1974;134:451–456.

124. Dyer AR, Stamler J, Paul O, et al. Alcohol consumption and 17-year mortality in the Chicago Western Electric Company Study. Prev Med 1980;9:78–90.

125. Ferrence RG, Truscott S, Whitehead PC. Drinking and the prevention of coronary heart disease: findings, issues and public health policy. J Stud Alcohol 1986;47:394–408.

126. Dai WS, LaPorte RE, Hom DL, et al. Alcohol consumption and high density lipoprotein in cholesterol concentration among alcoholics. Am J Epidemiol 1985;122:620–627.

127. Haskell WL, Camargo C Jr, Williams PT, et al. The effect of cessation and resumption of moderate alcohol intake on serum high-density-lipoprotein subfractions. A controlled study. N Engl J Med 1984;310:805–810.

128. Ekman R, Fex G, Johansson BG, Nilsson-Ehle P, Wadstein J. Changes in plasma high density lipoproteins and lipolytic enzymes after long term, heavy ethanol consumption. Scand J Clin Lab Invest 1981;41:709–715.

129. Camargo CA Jr, Williams PT, Vranizan KM, Albers JJ, Wood PD. The effect of moderate alcohol intake on serum apolipoproteins A-I and A-II. JAMA 1985;253:2854–2857.

130. Moore RD, Smith CR, Kwiterovich PO, Pearson TA. Effect of low-dose alcohol use versus abstention on lipoproteins A-I and B. Am J Med 1988;84:884–890.

131. Avogaro P, Cazzolato G, Bittolo Bon G. Lipids and apolipoproteins in heavy alcohol drinkers. In: Avogaro P, Sirtori CR, Tremoli E (eds): Metabolic effects of alcohol. Amsterdam: Elsevier/North Holland Medical Press, 1979;157–164.

132. Taskinen MR, Nikkila EA, Valimaki M, et al. Alcohol-induced changes in serum lipoproteins and in their metabolism. Am Heart J 1987;113:458–464.

133. Davidson DM. Cardiovascular effects of alcohol. West J Med 1989;151:430–439.

134. Willett W, Hennekens CH, Castelli W, et al. Effects of cigarette smoking on fasting triglyceride, total cholesterol, and HDL-cholesterol in women. Am Heart J 1983;105:417–421.

135. Criqui MH, Wallace RB, Heiss G, Mishkel M, Schonfeld G, Jones GT. Cigarette smoking and plasma high-density lipoprotein cholesterol. Circulation 1980;62(Suppl IV):IV70–IV76.

136. Stubbe I, Eskilsson J, Nilsson-Ehle P. High-density lipoprotein concentrations after stopping smoking. Br Med J 1982;284:1511–1513.

137. Quensel M, Soderstrom A, Agardh CD, Nilsson-Ehle P. High density lipoprotein concentrations after cessation of smoking: the importance of alterations in diet. Atherosclerosis 1989;75:189–193.

138. Friedman M, Rosenman RH, Carroll V. Changes in the serum cholesterol and blood clotting time in men subjected to cyclic variation of occupational stress. Circulation 1958;17:852–861.

139. Siegrist J, Matschinger H, Cremer P, Seidel D. Atherogenic risk in men suffering from occupational stress. Atherosclerosis 1988;69:211–218.

140. Taggart P, Carruthers M. Endogenous hyperlipidemia induced by emotional stress of racing driving. Lancet 1971;1:363–366.

141. Haskell WL. Exercise-induced changes in plasma lipids and lipoproteins. Prev Med 1984;13:23–36.

142. Thompson PD, Cullinane EM, Sady SP, et al. Modest changes in high-density lipoprotein concentration and metabolism with prolonged exercise training. Circulation 1988;78:25–34.

143. Rosenstock J, Strowig S, Cercone S, Raskin P. Reduction in cardiovascular risk factors with intensive diabetes treatment in insulin-dependent diabetes mellitus. Diabetes Care 1987;10:729–734.

144. Wallace RB, Pomrehn P, Heiss G, et al. Alterations in clinical chemistry levels associated with the dyslipoproteinemias. Circulation 1986;73(Suppl I):I62–I69.

145. Svenson KL, Lithell H, Hallgren R, Selinus I, Vessby B. Serum lipoprotein in active rheumatoid arthritis and other chronic inflammatory arthritides. I. Relativity to inflammatory activity. Arch Intern Med 1987;147:1912–1916.

146. Svenson KL, Lithell H, Hallgren R, Vessby B. Serum lipoprotein in active rheumatoid arthritis and other chronic inflammatory arthritides. II. Effects of anti-inflammatory and disease-modifying drug treatment. Arch Intern Med 1987;147:1917–1920.

147. Gallin JI, Kaye D, O'Leary WM. Serum lipids in infection. N Engl J Med 1969;281:1081–1086.

148. Gore JM, Goldberg RJ, Matsumoto AS, Castelli WP, McNamara PM, Dalen JE. Validity of serum total cholesterol level obtained within 24 hours of acute myocardial infarction. Am J Cardiol 1984;54:722–725.

149. Sewdarsen M, Vythilingum S, Jialal I, Nada R. Plasma lipids can be reliably assessed within 24 hours after acute myocardial infarction. Postgrad Med J 1988;64:352–356.

150. Genest JJ, Corbett HM, McNamara JR, Schaefer MM, Salem DN, Schaefer EJ. Effect of hospitalization on high-density lipoprotein cholesterol in patients undergoing elective coronary angiography. Am J Cardiol 1988;61:998–1000.

151. Hooper PL, Woo W, Visconti L, Pathak DR. Terbutaline raises high-density-lipoprotein-cholesterol levels. N Engl J Med 1981;305:1455–1457.

152. Bershad S, Rubinstein A, Paterniti JR, et al. Changes in plasma lipids and lipoproteins during isotretinoin therapy for acne. N Engl J Med 1985;313:981–985.

153. Gao SZ, Schroeder J, Alderman E, Hunt S, Valantine H, Wiederhold V. Incidence of accelerated coronary artery disease in heart transplant survivors: comparison of cyclosporin and azathioprine regimen. Circulation 1988;78(Suppl II):II-280.

154. Ballantyne CM, Podet EJ, Patsch WP, et al. Effect of cyclosporine therapy on plasma lipoprotein levels. JAMA 1989;262:53–56.

155. Crist DM, Peake GT, Stackpole PJ. Lipemic and lipoproteinemic effects of natural and synthetic androgens in humans. Clin Exp Pharmacol Physiol 1986;13:513–518.

156. Schilling FJ, Hashim SA, Leonardy JG. Effect of controlled breakfast on serum cholesterol and triglycerides. Am J Clin Nutr 1964;15:1–4.

157. Peric-Golia L. Postprandial serum-cholesterol. Lancet 1972;2:876.

158. Gordon DJ, Trost DC, Hyde J. Seasonal cholesterol cycles: the Lipid Research Clinics Coronary Primary Prevention Trial placebo group. Circulation 1987;76:1224–1231.

159. National Cholesterol Education Program. Recommendations regarding public screening for measuring blood cholesterol. Arch Intern Med 1989;149:2650–2654.

160. Burke JJ II, Fischer PM. A clinician's guide to the office measurement of cholesterol. JAMA 1988;259:3444–3448.

161. Naughton MJ, Luepker RV, Strickland D. The accuracy of portable cholesterol analyzers in public screening programs. JAMA 1990;263:1213–1217.

162. Schucker B, Bailey K, Heimbach JT, et al. Change in public perspective on cholesterol and heart disease. Results from two natural surveys. JAMA 1987;258:3527–3531.

163. Schucker B, Wittes JT, Cutler JA, et al. Change in physician perspective on cholesterol and heart disease. JAMA 1987;258:3521–3526.

164. Consensus Development Conference. Lowering blood cholesterol to prevent heart disease. JAMA 1985;253:2080–2086.

165. European Atherosclerosis Society Study Group. Strategies for the prevention of coronary heart disease: A policy statement of the European Atherosclerosis Society. Eur Heart J 1987;8:77–88.

166. The Expert Panel. Report of the National Cholesterol Education Program Expert Panel on detection, evaluation and treatment of high blood cholesterol in adults. Arch Intern Med 1988;148:36–69.

167. Lipid Research Clinics Program. The Lipid Research Clinics Coronary Primary Prevention Trial Results. I. Reduction in the incidence of coronary heart disease. JAMA 1984;251:351–364.

168. Lipid Research Clinics Program. The Lipid Research Clinics Coronary Primary Prevention Trial Results. II. The relationship of reduction in incidence of coronary heart disease to cholesterol lowering. JAMA 1984;251:365–374.

169. The Lovastatin Study Group. III. A multicenter comparison of lovastatin and cholestyramine therapy for severe primary hypercholesterolemia. JAMA 1988;260:359–366.

170. Nash DT, Gensini G, Esente P. Effect of lipid-lowering therapy on the progression of coronary atherosclerosis assessed by scheduled repetitive coronary angiography. Int J Cardiol 1982;2:43–55.

171. Knopp RH, Ginsberg J, Albers JJ, et al. Contrasting effects of unmodified and time-release forms of niacin on lipoproteins in hyperlipidemic subjects: Clues to mechanism of action of niacin. Metabolism 1985;34:642–650.

172. Canner PL, Berge KG, Wenger NK, et al. Fifteen-year mortality in coronary drug

project patients: Long-term benefit with niacin. J Am Coll Cardiol 1986;8:1245-1255.

173. Frick MH, Elo MO, Haapa K, et al. Helsinki Heart Study: Primary-prevention trial with gemfibrozil in middle-aged men with dyslipidemia. N Engl J Med 1987;317:1237-1245.

174. Mannien V, Elo MO, Frick MH, et al. Lipid alternations and decline in the incidence of coronary heart disease in the Helsinki Heart Study. JAMA 1988;260:641-651.

175. Tikkanen MJ, Helve E, Jaattela A, et al. Comparison between lovastatin and gemfibrozil in the treatment of primary hypercholesterolemia: the Finnish Multicenter Study. Am J Cardiol 1988;62:35J-43J.

176. Havel RJ, Hunninghake DB, Illingworth DR, et al. Lovastatin (mevinolin) in the treatment of heterozygous familial hypercholesterolemia. Ann Intern Med 1987;107:609-615.

177. Blankenhorn DH, Nessim SA, Johnson RL, Sanmarco ME, Azen SP, Cashin-Hemphill L. Beneficial effects of combined colestipol-niacin therapy on coronary atherosclerosis and coronary venous bypass grafts. JAMA 1987;257:3233-3240.

178. Bell LP, Hectorne K, Reynolds H, Balm TK, Hunninghake DB. Cholesterol-lowering effects of psyllium hydrophilic mucilloid. Adjunct therapy to a prudent diet for patients with mild to moderate hypercholesterolemia. JAMA 1989;261:3419-3423.

179. Annual Pharmacists' Reference. Orodell, NJ: Medical Economics Inc., 1990.

180. Oster G, Epstein AM. Cost-effectiveness of antihyperlipemic therapy in the prevention of coronary artery disease. JAMA 1987;258:2381-2387.

181. Kinosian BP, Eisenberg JM. Cutting into cholesterol. Cost-effective alternatives for treating hypercholesterolemia. JAMA 1988;259:2249-2254.

182. Alderman JD, Pasternak RC, Sacks RM, Smith HS, Monrad ES, Grossman W: Effect of a modified, well-tolerated niacin regimen on serum total cholesterol, high density lipoprotein cholesterol and the cholesterol to high density lipoprotein ratio. Am J Cardiol 1989;64:725-729.

183. Mullin GE, Greenson JK, Mitchell MC: Fulminant hepatic failure after ingestion of sustained-release nicotinic acid. Ann Intern Med 1989;111:253-255.

184. Oliver MF, Heady JA, Morris JN, Cooper J. A cooperative trial in the primary prevention of ischemic heart disease using clofibrate. Report from the Committee of Principal Investigators. Br Heart J 1978;40:1069-1118.

185. Illingworth DR, Bacon S. Influence of lovastatin plus gembrozil on plasma lipids and lipoproteins in patients with heterozygous familial hypercholesterolemia. Circulation 1989;79:590-596.

186. Yamamoto A, Matsuzawa Y, Yokoyama S, Funahashi T, Yamamura T, Kishino B. Effects of probucol on xanthomata regression in familial hypercholesterolemia. Am J Cardiol 1986;57:29H-35H.

187. Kane JP, Malloy MJ, Tun P, et al. Normalization of low-density lipoprotein levels in heterozygous familial hypercholesterolemia with a combined drug regimen. N Engl J Med 1981;304:251-258.

188. Vega GL, Grundy SM. Treatment of primary moderate hypercholesterolemia with lovastatin (mevinolin) and colestipol. JAMA 1987;257:33-38.

189. Williams RR, Sorlie PD, Feinleib M, McNamara PM, Kannel WB, Dawber TR. Cancer incidence by levels of cholesterol. JAMA 1981;245:247-252.

190. McMichael AJ, Jensen OM, Parkin DM, Zaridze DG. Dietary and endogenous cholesterol and human cancer. Epidemiol Rev 1984;6:192-216.

191. Schatzkin A, Hoover RN, Taylor PR, et al. Site-specific analysis of total serum cholesterol and incident cancer in the National Health and Nutrition Examination Survey. I. Epidemiologic follow-up study. Cancer Res 1988;48:452-458.

192. International Collaborative Group. Circulating cholesterol level and risk of death from cancer in men 40 to 69 years. JAMA 1982;248:2853-2859.

193. Sherwin RW, Wentworth DN, Cutler JA, Hulley SB, Kuller LH, Stamler J. Serum cholesterol levels and cancer mortality in 361,662 men screened for the Multiple Risk Factor Intervention Trial. JAMA 1987;257:943-948.

194. Knekt P, Reunanen A, Aromaa A, Heliovaara M, Hakulinen T, Hakama M. Serum cholesterol and risk of cancer in a cohort of 39,000 men and women. J Clin Epidemiol 1988;41:519–530.

195. Tanaka H, Ueda Y, Hayashi M, et al. Risk factors for cerebral hemorrhage and cerebal infarction in a Japanese rural community. Stroke 1982;13:62–73.

196. Kagan A, Popper JS, Rhoads GG, et al. Dietary and other risk factors for stroke in Hawaiian Japanese men. Stroke 1986;16:390–396.

197. Gordon T, Kagan A, Garcia-Palmieri M, et al. Diet and its relation to coronary heart diseases and death in three populations. Circulation 1981;63:500–515.

198. Iso H, Jacobs D, Wentworth D, Neaton JD, Cohen JD. Serum cholesterol levels and six-year mortality from stroke in 350,977 men screened for the Multiple Risk Factor Intervention Trial. N Engl J Med 1989;320:904–910.

199. Farquhar JW, Fortmann SP, Flora JA, et al. the Stanford Five-City Project: Effects of community-wide education on cardiovascular disease risk factors. JAMA 1990;264:359–365.

200. Mittlemark MB, Luepker RV, Grimm R Jr, Kottke TE, Blackburn H. The role of physicians in a community-wide program for prevention of cardiovascular disease: the Minnesota Heart Health Program. Publ Health Rep 1988;103:360–365.

201. Lefebvre RC, Lasater TM, Carleton RA, Peterson G. Theory and delivery of health programming in the community: the Pawtucket Heart Health Program. Prev Med 1987;16:80–95.

202. Pietinen P, Nissinen A, Vartiainen E, et al. Dietary changes in the North Karelia Project (1972–1982). Prev Med 1988;17:183–193.

203. Havlik RJ, Feinleib M, (eds): Proceedings of the Conference on the Decline in Coronary Heart Disease Mortality. Bethesda (MD): United States Department of Health, Education and Welfare; 1979. NIH Publ no. 79–1610.

204. Blankenhorn DH, Johnson RL, Mack WJ, Elzein HA, Vailas LI. The influence of diet on the appearance of new lesions in human coronary arteries. JAMA 1990;263:1646–1652.

4

hypertension

EPIDEMIOLOGY

More than 60 million persons in Canada and the United States have a systolic blood pressure (SBP) of 140 mm Hg or greater, a diastolic blood pressure (DBP) of 90 mm Hg or greater, or are taking blood pressure lowering medication (1–3). Similar prevalence rates have been documented in other Western countries. In Japan, the percentages of men and women with hypertension are even greater.

During the past two decades, however, many countries have engaged in widespread detection, evaluation, and treatment programs that contributed significantly to decreases in cardiovascular and cerebrovascular deaths. In the United States and Canada, expert panels issued reports in 1977, 1980, 1984, and 1988, providing guidelines for health professionals and community workers in their care of persons with high blood pressure (1–5). In the 1988 document, the panel recommended classification of blood pressure (BP) in persons aged 18 and older as shown in Table 4.1. Classifications are based on the average of two or more readings on each of two or more occasions (1).

Demographics

Changes in the prevalence of hypertension reflect several concurrent proc-

esses: continuation of persons previously diagnosed as hypertensives, the diagnosis of new cases, the death of hypertensive persons since the last enumeration, and the persistence of normal blood pressures in persons whose treatment has been discontinued. Most studies define a hypertensive person as one who is taking antihypertensive medication and/or has systolic or diastolic blood pressures exceeding predetermined levels after repeated measurements. Precise prevalence levels will depend on the threshold levels selected for diagnosis as well as the frequency and accuracy of the measurements.

AGE AND GENDER

Applegate has pointed out large differences in reports of hypertension prevalence in persons more than 65 years old. He attributes some of these differences to threshold value selection and others to frequency of measurement (6). In general, however, diastolic BP rises with age during adult life until approximately age 55, then is relatively constant. In contrast, systolic BP continues to rise with age (7). Isolated systolic hypertension (normal diastolic pressure) is present in approximately 10% of North Americans over age 70; the prevalence is doubled in women and men over 80 (8). Mean blood pressure values and prevalence of hypertension in women of a

Table 4.1. Blood Pressure Classification in Persons 18 Years and Older[a]

Blood Pressure (mm Hg)	Category
DBP	
<85	Normal BP
85–89	High normal BP
90–104	Hypertension (mild)
105–114	Hypertension (moderate)
>114	Hypertension (severe)
SBP (when DBP <90 mm Hg)	
<140	Normal BP
140–159	Isolated systolic hypertension (borderline)
>159	Isolated systolic hypertension

[a]Adapted from Joint National Committee. The 1988 report of the Joint National Committee on Detection, Evaluation, and Treatment of High Blood Pressure. Arch Int Med 1988;148:1023–1038.

given age, race, and culture are generally slightly lower than in men. In a prospective study of more than 119,000 US nurses, women with self-reported high BP had 3.5 times higher CAD incidence and a 2.6-fold stroke risk (9).

RACE AND ETHNICITY

Within a given country, marked BP differences may be observed in men and women of different racial and ethnic groups. Some of these differences may be attributed to differential access to health care and to disparities in socioeconomic conditions (10), as were particularly notable in the United States before enactment of civil rights legislation in the 1960s but are still present (11). However, black physicians also had a high incidence of hypertension during surveillance for an average of 22 years after their graduation from medical school (12). A marked difference in hypertension prevalence persists between black and white citizens of the USA who are 65 years and older; rates in black women are 50% higher than in their white contemporaries (13).

During the past two decades, widespread public education programs in the USA have dramatically reduced the number of persons whose hypertension is undiagnosed, untreated, or uncontrolled. This decline has been shared by blacks, in whom the prevalence of hypertension in the early 1960s was double that in whites (14, 15) (Table 4.2).

While the prevalence of hypertension in Mexican-American women and men is similar to that of non-Hispanic whites in the USA, the percentages of persons previously detected, treated, and controlled are lower (16). Hypertension prevalence in native Americans is lower than in whites, but it rises with migration to an urban environment (14).

Within the Japanese-American population, the prevalence of hypertension depends upon body weight and acculturation (17). It is slightly higher in Japanese-American men living in California than in their white counterparts, but is much lower in Japanese-American women at all ages. In Chinese-Americans living in Cal-

Table 4.2. Changes in Rates of Hypertension Prevalence, Awareness, Treatment, and Control in the USA from 1960–1962 to 1976–1980[a]

% Hypertensives	Women		Men	
	Black	White	Black	White
Previously undiagnosed	−20.6	−18.7	−34.8	−16.1
On medication	+12.5	+20.4	+22.4	+15.9
On medication under control	+18.3	+18.4	+11.1	+19.1

[a]Adapted from Rowland M, Roberts J (eds). Blood pressure levels and hypertension in persons ages 6–74 years. United States 1976–80. National Center for Health Statistics Advance Data, 1982.

ifornia, prevalence rates were similar to those of whites for men under 50 and for women of all ages. Older Chinese-Americans had slightly higher rates. Filipino-Americans of both genders have significantly higher rates of hypertension than whites or other Asian-Pacific Islanders (18).

The same California investigative team examined hypertension-related mortality in their state from 1969 to 1971 and from 1979 to 1981. During both periods, age-standardized rates were highest for blacks, followed by whites, and lowest for Asians and Pacific Islanders. Despite their high prevalence rates, Filipino-Americans had low mortality rates related to their disease. Rates among all groups declined more than 28% during that decade, but enumeration and continuing immigration limit more precise interpretation of those data. The authors note that recent immigrants remain closer to their homeland cultural habits and place more emphasis on group cohesion, social stability, and support from the family (19).

Family History

Familial tendencies to high blood pressure may result from genetic and environmental factors. Several investigators have compared relatives of persons with CAD at an early age with families with no evidence of CAD. Rissanen and Nikkila studied 211 men under the age of 56 residing in eastern Finland; 105 men had experienced MI, 53 had uncomplicated angina, and 53 were apparently free of CAD. Hypertension was three times more prevalent in the families of MI and angina patients than in control families (20). In a British study of 5362 subjects at age 36, deaths of fathers of subjects from hypertensive and coronary artery diseases were associated with significantly higher levels of both SBP and DBP (21).

Becker et al. studied siblings of 86 persons with CAD documented before age 60. Screening revealed that 48% of brothers and 41% of sisters were hypertensive; only 43% of these sibling were aware of their hypertension prior to screening (22). In one British study, however, first-degree relatives so identified were more likely to comply with a request to visit their physician than were relatives of normotensives (23).

Siblings of Johns Hopkins School of Medicine students who were hypertensive were three times more likely to have high blood pressure themselves (24). Investigators in the Tecumseh (MI) study found a strong correlation between parents' BPs and those of their children, particularly those offspring still living at home, suggesting the importance of shared environmental factors (25). In the Bogalusa (LA) study of school children, parents of those with blood pressures exceeding the 90th percentile were examined. Of these parents, 67% of blacks and 25% of whites were hypertensive (26). Connor et al. found a strong familial component for urinary sodium and for systolic BP, which may represent family similarities in sodium intake (27).

Twin studies have produced heritability estimates as high as 60 to 84% in males, but much lower values in women. Utah investigators concluded that genes contribute much more than shared environment to familial correlation of BPs (28).

PATHOPHYSIOLOGY OF HYPERTENSION AND CAD

Secondary Hypertension

Secondary hypertension is rare, and detailed screening for its causes in all newly diagnosed hypertensives is not considered cost-effective. An appropriate initial workup does include a routine biochemistry panel, urinalysis, determination of lipid and lipoprotein concentrations, and a resting electrocardiogram. Certain characteristics suggest an increased likelihood of secondary hypertension; these qualities include age less than 25, DBP above 120 mm Hg, sudden onset of high BP, bruits, or differential pulses (29). Other useful physical findings are abdominal or flank masses (polycystic kidneys), abdominal bruits (renovascular disease), and truncal obesity with pigmented striae (Cushing's syndrome) (1).

The American Heart Association offered guidelines for office evaluation of hypertension and its correctable causes. Pheochromocytomas can be detected by measurement of fasting plasma catecholamines or urinary metanephrine. A low serum potassium level may indicate primary aldosteronism. Renovascular hypertension before the age of 40 is more common in women and in the right renal artery; it is usually due to fibrous dysplasia. In later years, the etiology is more often atherosclerotic, and it is found more often in men. Screening for this disorder can be accomplished with a rapid-sequence intravenous urogram or a dynamic renal flow scan (30).

Primary Hypertension and CAD Risk Indicators

WEIGHT

Chiang and colleagues reviewed more than 20 population studies, finding in most linear associations of SBP and DBP with body weight (31). The Community Hypertension Evaluation Clinic program in the USA screened more than one million persons for hypertension between 1973 and 1975. Persons classifying themselves as overweight had hypertension prevalence rates 1.5 to 3 times higher than other screenees. The relative risk of hypertension among overweight persons aged 20 to 39 was 2 to 3; in individuals 40 to 64 years old, 1.5 to 2 (32). An Australian study produced similar results; in men under age 45, nearly two-thirds of cases of hypertension were attributable to obesity. In both women and men aged 25 to 64, approximately one-third of cases were related to overweight (33).

In the first National Health and Nutrition Survey (NHANES I) carried out in the USA between 1971 and 1974, triceps and subscapular skinfold measurements were employed to measure peripheral and centrally located body fat. Investigators concluded that high BP in middle-aged persons of both genders and different race groups is directly associated with centrally deposited body fat (34). Members of the Kaiser Permanente medical plan who had centrally deposited body fat were more likely to develop hypertension regardless of the initial level of obesity (35).

Meharry Medical College graduates were followed for an average of 22.5 years. The 433 black physicians (38 women, 395 men) were initially examined as medical students between 1958 and 1965; at that time none were hypertensive. At follow-up, 43.8% had developed high blood pressure. Those who were initially lean but became obese were the most likely to develop high BP. The risk ratio for those most obese at follow-up compared with the leanest group was 1.7 (36). In a study of Harvard University alumni, a relative risk of 1.6 of developing hypertension was noted in persons who gained 25 pounds or more since graduation (37).

PHYSICAL ACTIVITY

A study of Irish men found that leisure-time activity, but not exertion at work, was inversely correlated with SBP and DBP (38). In a California study, self-reported physical activity was inversely related to DBP (39). In a longitudinal study, low levels of self-reported physical activity predicted higher rates of hypertension development (40).

DIET

In the Honolulu Heart Study of men of Japanese descent, potassium and calcium intake was inversely correlated with blood pressure; their combined effect was greater than either alone(41).

In 1987, Pietinen and Huttunen reviewed studies relating dietary fat and BP. They concluded that evidence for the direct association is persuasive but not conclusive (42). Later, a study of Seventh-Day Adventists in the USA revealed that SBP was lower in black vegetarians, but not white vegetarians, than it was in persons not following a vegetarian diet (43).

ALCOHOL

In 1915, Lian noted a higher prevalence of hypertension in those French army officers with the greatest alcohol consumption (44). For several decades, this association was largely ignored. In recent years, however, considerable attention has been paid worldwide to alcohol-related hypertension. For comparison of the studies reviewed below, one drink of alcohol can be defined as 12 ounces of beer (3 to 5% ethanol), a 5-ounce glass of wine (12% ethanol), or a 1.5-ounce shot of spirits (80 proof = 40% ethanol). Each contains 0.6 ounces (17 ml = 13.6 g) of ethanol (45).

Acute Effects

In a British study of alcoholics, women and men (average age 44) with a mean daily alcohol intake of 196 g for many years had blood pressure monitoring before, during, and after detoxification. Initial BP was directly correlated to mean daily alcohol intake for the three months preceding admission; more than half of the subjects had initial BPs exceeding 140/90 mm Hg. Withdrawal symptoms were most pronounced in those with highest entry BPs. Blood pressures dropped during detoxification. Persistence of this effect depended upon abstention (46).

In a study of hypertensive men with high habitual alcohol intake, medications were continued during six weeks of usual drinking and a subsequent six weeks of consuming only a low-alcohol beer. Mean weekly alcohol intake decreased from 452 ml to 64 ml. Systolic and diastolic BP levels dropped 5.0 mm Hg and 3.0 mm Hg between the two periods (47). Earlier, the same investigative team found that, in normotensive men, decreasing intake from three drinkers per day to three drinks per week decreased systolic BP by 4 mm Hg but did not significantly change diastolic BP over a six-week period (48). Reductions of BP in normotensives who stop drinking may occur within one week. Howes asked subjects to drink 80 g of alcohol for four days, then stop. Four days later, their mean systolic and diastolic BPs had decreased by 8 and 6 mm Hg, respectively (49).

Chronic Effects

Klatsky and colleagues studied BP and usual drinking habits in 83,947 women and men who underwent a multiphasic health examination in the Kaiser Permanente system. Participants reported their consumption in one of three categories (in drinks per day): two or less, three to five, and six or more. In the lower category, men had similar BPs to controls; women had lower BPs. Both women and men reporting three or more drinks per day had higher systolic and diastolic BPs, and a higher prevalence of individuals with a BP of 160/95 or greater. Compared to nondrinkers, persons consuming six or more drinks daily had a prevalence of hypertension that was doubled in whites and 1.5 times in blacks.

The same investigators also reviewed

early Framingham Study data, noting that men who consumed 100 ounces or more per month had mean systolic BPs 7 mm Hg higher than lighter drinkers. Hypertension (>160/95) was twice as prevalent in persons who drank 60 ounces or more monthly compared with those drinking 10 to 29 ounces per month (50).

In Lipid Research Clinics Prevalence Study subjects, systolic and diastolic BPs were linearly correlated to alcohol intake; a daily consumption of 30 ml appeared to increase systolic BP by two to six mm Hg (51). In an Australian study, investigators noted a 1 mm Hg increment increase in systolic BP for every drink consumed daily by their male subjects. The half who drank most heavily were four times more likely to have systolic BP >140 mm Hg and were three times more likely to have a diastolic BP of 90 mm Hg or greater. Previous drinkers had BPs similar to nondrinkers (52).

However, investigators in approximately half of the reported studies have found a J-shaped relation between alcohol and BP (53). Analysis of the Tecumseh, Michigan study data revealed that minimal BP in subjects was associated with 1.5 drinks per week in men and approximately 4 drinks per week in women, independent of age and body weight (54).

Other investigations have found a threshold level above which BP rises. The Lipid Research Clinics study estimated this value to be 20 to 30 ml/day (51), as was true in 7011 men of Japanese descent in the Honolulu Heart Program (41). Initial data from the Kaiser study indicated a threshold of 90 ml daily. However, later studies from Kaiser revealed that the threshold effect was present only in women (55).

It is unclear whether the type of alcohol consumed is important. In two North American studies, greater pressor effects were noted in beer and liquor drinkers than in wine consumers (55, 56). However, Italian wine drinkers had a higher prevalence of hypertension than did nondrinkers of both genders (57).

Prospective studies have demonstrated greater increases in BP among heavy drinkers than nondrinkers, including the Peoples Gas and Western Electric studies in Chicago (58), the Framingham Offspring Study (59), and the Zutphen Study in the Netherlands (60).

PSYCHOSOCIAL AND ENVIRONMENTAL STRESSORS

Many studies in recent decades have focused on the relation of hypertension to psychosocial and environmental stressors. Table 4.3 contains a partial list of factors that may be related to the development of high blood pressure.

Observations that changes in autonomic and neurohumoral activity are elicited when persons are exposed to mental challenges or emotionally arousing stimuli have led to the hypothesis that prolonged exposure to such stressors may contribute

Table 4.3.   Psychosocial and Environmental Factors in Hypertension

Demographic, cultural, and community
1.   Education, social status, economic circumstances
2.   Ethnic and cultural considerations
3.   Modernization, crowding, migration
Interpersonal relationships
1.   Family and friends
2.   Workmates/colleagues
Self-appraisal
1.   Efficacy/esteem
2.   Health beliefs/perceptions
Personality factors
Psychosocial stressors
1.   Conflict/daily hassles
2.   Loss/bereavement/other major life events
Environmental stressors
1.   Occupational/worksite
2.   Noise/traffic
Behavioral responses
1.   Anxiety
2.   Anger/hostility

to hypertension. Persons with established high blood pressure have greater heart rate and BP responses when confronted with such stimuli. However, these associations do not establish cause and effect, so considerable experimental activity in animals and humans has been conducted in recent years. Because of the heterogeneity of hypertensives, it is expected that no single behavioral pattern will explain all cases of the disorder (61). There is increased confidence among clinical investigators that primary hypertension represents either a defect in neurocirculatory control or a relative predominance of neurogenic pressor mechanisms over depressor mechanisms (62).

Hypertension is more prevalent among persons with less education, lower social status, and poorer economic circumstances, even within racial and ethnic groups (63). These differentials may be related in part to higher levels of other risk indicators, such as smoking, obesity, and dietary habits (64), as well as less access to, or utilization of, medical care (65). Unfortunately, these inequalities are widening (66).

Ethnic and cultural factors may influence the appearance of hypertension and modify its treatment. Syme noted that hypertension is most prevalent in Western countries in situations where aspiration to upward mobility is thwarted and in which meaningful human intercourse is restricted (67). From this conceptualization, James and colleagues developed the notion of "John Henryism," in which a strong personality and determination to succeed coexist in an individual disadvantaged in other ways for dealing with one's environment. Syme's concept may also account for the higher prevalence of hypertension in persons whose primitive environment is exchanged for a modern one, either through migration or through modification of their home surroundings (68–70).

Harburg and colleagues found higher BP levels in city areas designated as high-stress by existing demographic, economic, and sociological conditions (71). The effects of such changes may be mitigated by the support of family and friends (72). For example, low levels of instrumental support among blacks in the southern USA were associated with a higher prevalence of high BP (73). In several countries, neighborhood clubs have formed for the purpose of enhancing hypertension treatment and other CAD risk modification (74).

Support from colleagues and workmates was found to be important in the same USA black community; both women and men were more likely to drop out from treatment if social support on the job was low (75). In the Netherlands, workers with supportive supervisors were less likely to become hypertensive than workers under similar stress without support (76).

Self-efficacy (77) and self-esteem (78) may contribute to improved adherence to blood-pressure–lowering interventions. One's perception of health has also been associated with actual health outcomes in prospective studies (79). Belief in the effectiveness of hypertension treatment correlates well with subsequent reduction in BP (80, 81).

Several studies have found support for the hypothesis that the coronary-prone (type A) behavior pattern is associated with hypertension, particularly the anger and hostility components of the behavior pattern (82–84).

Psychosocial stressors, such as widowhood and other major life events, might be expected to raise blood pressure, although direct measurement of BP is rarely reported under those circumstances. Environmental conditions, such as work circumstances, have been more clearly correlated with hypertension. Air traffic controllers and bus drivers have exhibited high prevalence rates of high BP (85), along with factory and construction workers (86, 87). Noise from industrial, residential, traffic, or airport exposure also leads to increase rates of hypertension (85).

Behavioral responses to stimuli may also engender elevated BP. While the influence of anxiety on BP is probably transient (88), persons with low assertiveness and low verbal and indirect-aggression patterns have higher blood pressure (89). Suppressed anger, accompanied by hypertension, predicted the highest mortality risk in a sample of the Tecumseh (Michigan) Community Health Study (90). In a study of prison inmates, the high level of suppressed hostility was not accompanied by a high prevalence of hypertension (91).

DIABETES

Diabetics often have concurrent hypertension; control of their high blood pressure is often more difficult than in nondiabetics (92). Several investigators have suggested that obesity, type II diabetes mellitus, and hypertension hold in common the characteristics of hyperinsulinemia, insulin resistance, or both, although direct proof is currently lacking (93).

Diuretic and β-blocker therapy can worsen both diabetic control and serum lipid/lipoprotein values (94). Because they have no adverse effects on these functions, α-adrenergic blockers, centrally acting agents, and converting enzyme inhibitors may be preferable for treating hypertension in the diabetic (95).

SMOKING

Cigarette smoking elevates SBP and DBP for at least 15 minutes; this effect is exacerbated and extended with concomitant caffeine intake (96). Further, cigarette smoking interferes with the pharmacologic treatment of hypertension, especially attempts at BP reduction in black patients using propranolol (97).

LEFT VENTRICULAR HYPERTROPHY

Hypertension is frequently accompanied by left ventricular mass increases and alterations in diastolic function (98). Some have suggested that the hypertrophy is more closely related to blood pressure during stressful situations than to basal blood pressure (99). Because it has also been associated with a limitation in coronary vasodilator reserve, hypertension-induced hypertrophy has been implicated in the development of angina. However, recent studies have documented angina in hypertensive patients due to microvascular disease in the absence of hypertrophic changes (100).

Echocardiography provides the most accurate assessment of left ventricular hypertrophy (LVH) as well as CAD incidence related thereto (101). Where echocardiographic studies are not available or affordable, electrocardiographic indices of LVH are available; efforts to improve their accuracy continue (102).

Regression of LVH after successful treatment of HBP has been documented by several investigative teams. Diuretics and nonspecific vasodilators appear to have little effect on regression, while the other major categories of blood-pressure-lowering drugs have demonstrated an ability to regress LVH (103). Weight reduction alone can decrease left ventricular mass in obese hypertensives (104).

SCREENING AND MEASUREMENT

The inherent variability of a person's blood pressure has long been recognized. While BP measurement is one of the most common procedures, it is often done incorrectly. In addition to the many procedural pitfalls, the emotional reactivity of the individual being checked adds to this variability. The "white-coat hypertension" phenomenon appears to be real, particularly when the white coat is worn by a physician and the subject is a woman (105). Investigations of myocardial function suggest that persons with BP elevations only in the physician's office have cardiac size and function similar to those of normotensive individuals (106). Given the high prevalence of hypertension and the costs and risks of various treatment modalities, accurate determination of blood pressure becomes paramount.

Measurement Techniques and Equipment

Persons should abstain from caffeine and smoking for at least 30 minutes prior to BP measurement. They should be seated, resting quietly for at least five minutes, with the arm at heart level. An appropriate size cuff should be used; the rubber bladder should encircle at least two-thirds (ideally 80%) of the arm circumference (107, 108). A mercury sphygmomanometer, a calibrated aneroid manometer, or a validated electronic device should be employed, recording both SBP and DBP, using Korotkoff sound V for the latter reading. If the first two readings vary by more than 5 mm Hg, additional measurements should be made (1). Where blood pressure recordings document marked lability, the use of 24-hour ambulatory BP recording devices may be considered to guide therapeutic decisions. Such recordings may be particularly useful in persons classified in borderline groups (109). The circadian pattern and actual levels of BP are quite consistent between 24-hour study periods (110), and assessment of the duration of pharmacologic agents is facilitated with whole-day BP monitoring (111).

After adequate documentation of BP in the clinic, the patient may be encouraged to do home blood-pressure monitoring, if an accurate machine is obtained and adequate training is undertaken (112–114).

Labeling Phenomenon

Appropriate concern has been expressed regarding possible adverse effects of the detection of hypertension in some individuals. Transient increases in absenteeism from work have been reported after detection (115), and the potential impact on employment, job security, and health insurance have caused some to question the wisdom of hypertension screening at the workplace. In reply, investigators from several large-scale studies have suggested that vigorous, positive personal support and follow-up will minimize these effects (116), and that the advantages of early detection and treatment will far outweigh other considerations (117).

MANAGEMENT

Public and Health Professional Education

Much of the success of the campaign in the USA in the early 1970s to detect and control blood pressure can be attributed to wide dissemination of information to both the public (118) and health care professionals (119). Systematic BP screening within the community, coupled with effective immediate referral to health professionals, has been associated with improved blood pressure control of community members (120).

Hygienic Treatment

DIET AND EXERCISE

Weight reduction is an important first principle in the treatment of hypertension (121); for each kg of body weight lost, a 1 mm Hg drop in SBP and DBP may be expected (122). In addition to facilitating weight loss, vigorous physical activity can independently reduce blood pressure (123–125).

Restriction of sodium, when coupled

with weight loss, acts independently to reduce blood pressure in some individuals (126). This effect is particularly marked during the first week of weight reduction treatment (127). In several studies, approximately half of the hypertensive subjects have responded to sodium restriction (128). In a report that suggested that the BP of obese adolescents is sensitive to dietary sodium intake; the authors concluded that this sensitivity may be due to the combined effects of hyperinsulinemia, hyperaldosteronism, and increased sympathetic nervous system activity characteristic of obesity (129). Since considerable sodium intake for many persons comes through prepared foods, avoidance of added salt at the table may be insufficient to meet recommended guidelines for a diet containing 4 to 6 g salt (1.5 to 2.5 g sodium) (1).

Clinical trials of low fat and vegetarian diets in several countries showed significant decreases in blood pressure, which were apparently unrelated to sodium intake. Reducing fat content and/or increasing the polyunsaturated:saturated (P:S) ratio have been effective in reducing SBP and DBP within several weeks. These factors, along with increased fiber and protein may also explain the observed success of vegetarian diets in lowering blood pressure (42).

Rissanen and colleagues randomized obese persons with stable hypertension into three groups for a year-long trial. Meetings of the groups focused on weight reduction only, sodium restriction only, or both. BP changed little during the trial in the sodium-restriction-only group, but was significantly reduced in the other two groups. The investigators reported improved BP control in 12% of the sodium-restriction group compared with 63% of persons in the two groups that included a weight-reduction component (130).

A five-year randomized, controlled trial of nutritional-hygienic intervention reduced the incidence of hypertension from 19.2 to 8.8%. Treated subjects consumed less than 1800 mg of dietary sodium and less than 26 g of alcohol daily. They were also given dietary advice to reduce their intake of dietary cholesterol, total and saturated fat (131).

In three different analyses of the NHANES I data, dietary calcium was inversely related to blood pressure. A randomized clinical trial of 1500 mg of elemental calcium daily in black and white men showed a significant reduction in seated and supine measurements of SBP and DBP in the calcium group (132).

PSYCHOLOGICAL

Recent trials of relaxation therapy and biofeedback indicate modest success in blood pressure reduction in selected groups (133, 134). The magnitude of BP reduction with relaxation therapy appears to depend upon the initial BP (135). Both techniques lower oxygen consumption, respiration rate, and heart rate, in addition to blood pressure during short-term practice. The two methods appear to be synergistic (136).

Pharmacologic Treatment

Several types of drugs are available for reduction of blood pressure. Figure 4.1 indicates recommendations from the 1988 report from the USA of the Joint National Committee on Detection, Evaluation, and Treatment of High Blood Pressure. This document lists dosage ranges, adverse drug effects, and drug interactions among the agents approved for use in the USA (1).

HYPERTENSIVE CRISIS

When severe hypertension is associated with encephalopathy, papilledema, dissecting aortic aneurysm, eclampsia, head trauma, left ventricular failure with

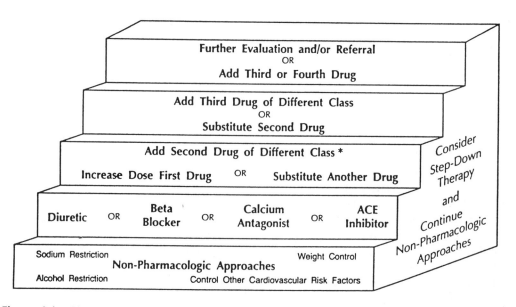

Figure 4.1. Pharmacologic, individualized, step-care therapy for hypertension. For some patients, nonpharmacologic therapy should be tried first. If the blood pressure goal is not achieved, add pharmacologic therapy. Other patients may require pharmacologic therapy initially. In these instances, nonpharmacologic therapy may be a helpful adjunct. ACE indicates angiotensin-converting enzyme; *, drugs such as diuretics, β-blockers, calcium antagonists, ACE inhibitors, α-blockers, centrally acting α_2-agonists, rauwolfia serpentina, and vasodilators.

pulmonary edema, or acute renal failure, immediate treatment of the elevated blood pressure is indicated. DeQuattro recommends intravenous sodium nitroprusside for patients with grade 4 retinopathy, hydralazine for women with toxemia of pregnancy, and nitroglycerin or labetalol if acute MI is accompanied by severe hypertension (137). In asymptomatic patients, recent studies have suggested that acute reduction of BP (138) has no benefit, and abrupt decreases in BP may adversely affect coronary artery blood flow and subendocardial perfusion, leading to myocardial ischemia and infarction (139, 140). Therefore, in the asymptomatic patient, an appropriate oral antihypertensive regimen should be started without loading; close surveillance will be necessary to lower BP within the subsequent week (141).

TREATMENT OF SEVERE HYPERTENSION

The Veterans Administration (VA) Cooperative Study Group reported, in 1967, a significant beneficial effect for treating persons with DBPs consistently between 115 and 129 mm Hg. The regular maintenance dose for men (randomized to the active regimen) was hydrochlorothiazide 100 mg, reserpine 0.2 mg, and hydralazine hydrochloride 150 mg. After 24 months of treatment, mean SBP and DBP were 43 and 30 mm Hg lower, respectively. Only 2 of 29 assessable morbid events occurred in the treatment group (142). Even with the availability of newer agents, many persons in this DBP category will not respond to only one drug. In such cases, the interval between changes in regimen should be decreased, and consideration should be given to higher doses of some drugs than in the treatment of milder hypertension (1).

TREATMENT OF MILD AND MODERATE HYPERTENSION

For the majority of patients with DBP between 90 and 114 mm Hg, one drug should suffice. Ideally, this drug should not only be effective in reducing BP but also it should not adversely affect other CAD risk indicators, nor should it interfere with one's quality of life. Other desirable features include a convenient dosage schedule, low cost, and compatibility with the pathophysiology of the patient's hypertension (143). In the paragraphs below, agents in the major categories of drugs will be discussed with these criteria in mind. In an extensive review published in 1989, Houston summarized the various features and usefulness of the major antihypertensive agents (95).

DIURETICS

For many years, most physicians chose diuretics as the first "step" (144). However, their biochemical consequences (hypokalemia and hyperglycemia) have lessened their appeal to clinicians. Further, in most studies, diuretics have not reversed left ventricular hypertrophy (LVH) (145). Most diuretics (indapamide being an exception (95)) also worsen the patient's lipid and lipoprotein profile, although the changes are most prominent during the early months of diuretic treatment (146). In most of the trials listed in Table 4.4, no significantly different changes occurred in blood total cholesterol levels after several years. Lower doses (12.5 to 25 mg of hydrochlorothiazide) in current use should further ameliorate concerns about diuretic-induced dyslipidemias.

These agents should be avoided in patients with gout and in those taking dig-

italis. They should not be the first drug of choice in persons with complex ventricular dysrhythmias, dyslipidemias, diabetes mellitus, or existing CAD. They do appear to be more effective in blacks (147) and persons over 50 (143).

β-ADRENERGIC BLOCKERS

β-blockers have also received wide usage for hypertension, and they continue to be useful in patients with concomitant angina or a history of MI. However, those without intrinsic sympathomimetic activity can increase serum triglycerides and LDL-cholesterol and may reduce HDL-cholesterol (95).

Some, but not all, studies have noted a decreased risk of first MI in persons taking β-blockers (148).

They should be avoided in persons with asthma, intermittent claudication, diabetes mellitus, congestive heart failure, and smokers. Their qualities may be effective in treating both conditions in hypertensives who also have migraine headaches, anxiety, or hyperthyroidism. They appear to be more effective in whites under the age of 50 (143). When β-blockers are prescribed in conjunction with an exercise training period, the β-1-selective agents (atenolol, metoprolol (149)) are preferred (150).

With their diverse characteristics, β-blockers display various capabilities for the regression of left ventricular hypertrophy (95, 103).

α- AND β-BLOCKER

Labetalol may have a neutral or slightly adverse effect on lipids and lipoproteins, serum uric acid, and glucose. Similarly, it appears to have no appreciable effect on exercise tolerance or on development or regression of left ventricular hypertrophy (95).

CONVERTING-ENZYME INHIBITORS

These agents (termed ACE inhibitors or CEIs) may be the drugs of choice in persons with diabetes mellitus, unilateral renal artery stenosis, or congestive heart failure secondary to systolic dysfunction. They should not be used in persons with bilateral renal artery stenosis or in patients taking nonsteroidal antiinflammatory agents (143). In the absence of congestive heart failure, all converting-enzyme inhibitors lower the total peripheral resistance, while causing little change in heart rate, cardiac output, or response to exercise, Valsalva, or cold-pressor tests. Regression of LVH has been documented with CEI treatment (151). The CEIs appear to have little effect on serum lipids, uric acid, or glucose levels (95).

CALCIUM-CHANNEL BLOCKERS

The calcium antagonists are preferable to diuretics in blacks and in elderly persons (152), and they are useful in persons with a vasospastic component to their angina pectoris. Unlike the diuretics and some β-blockers, they have no ill effects in patients with gout, diabetes, and asthma (143), nor do they adversely affect lipid and lipoprotein levels (95). Regression of LVH has been reported with some of these agents (103).

α-ADRENERGIC BLOCKERS

Prazosin and terazosin are useful in persons with gout, asthma, diabetes, or dyslipidemias, but should be avoided in patients with a history of dizziness or syncope (143). Prazosin has been demonstrated to regress LVH (153) and does not impair exercise tolerance. It may have a favorable effect on lipids, while terazosin is less effective in this regard (95).

α-ADRENERGIC AGONISTS

The agents clonidine, guanabenz, guanfacine, and methyldopa are useful antihypertensive agents that stimulate α-adrenergic receptors in the brain stem, resulting in reduced sympathetic outflow from the central nervous system (154). Transdermal clonidine has been associated with fewer side effects (155) and greater aerobic conditioning than other antihypertensive agents (156). Clonidine, guanabenz, and guanfacine have been associated with regression of LVH, have a favorable effect on lipids and lipoproteins, preserve the normal response to exercise, and have no significant effect on serum glucose or uric acid levels. Methyldopa may have an adverse effect on HDL-C and triglyceride levels, but otherwise it shares the beneficial effects on LVH regression, exercise, and levels of glucose and uric acid (95).

VASODILATORS

Agents such as hydralazine and minoxidil have been established components of hypertension treatment for many years (157), although they can be associated with headache, tachycardia, and fluid retention, and may actually increase left ventricular mass (1). However, they do not appear to adversely affect lipids, exercise tolerance, or serum levels of glucose and uric acid (95).

NITRATES

In patients with CAD, nitrates provide antianginal and antihypertensive effects, but little has been published on their use as primary agents in hypertension (158).

MAJOR DRUG TRIALS

Several large-scale trials have examined the effects on cardiovascular and all-cause mortality of treating hypertension with diuretics or β-blockers, plus adjunctive medication. These include the Veterans Administration trial (159) and Hypertension Detection and Followup Program trial (HDFP) (160) in the USA, the Australian Therapeutic Trial in Mild Hypertension (ATTMH) (161), the Oslo Study mild hypertension trial (162), the European Working Party on High Blood Pressure in the Elderly (EWPHE) (163), the UK Medical Research Council (MRC) trial of treatment of mild hypertension (164), the International Prospective Primary Prevention Study in Hypertension (IPPPSH) (165), the Heart Attack Primary Prevention in Hypertension trial (HAPPHY) (166), and the Metoprolol Atherosclerosis Prevention Hypertension Study (MAPHY) (167). Details of the study designs, inclusion and exclusion criteria, and principal results are summarized in Table 4.4.

Several authors have examined these

Table 4.4. Summary of Major Trials in Treatment of Mild Hypertension

Study Year (Ref)	Design[a] (n)	Criteria[b] Incl	Criteria[b] Excl	Mean F/U (yrs)	Drug Treatment[c] First	Drug Treatment[c] Supp	Group[d]	% Change DBP	Deaths/1000/yr CAD	Deaths/1000/yr CVD	Deaths/1000/yr All
VA 1970 (159)	RPC 380	DBP 90–114	CVA RET WMN	3.8	HCT+ RESor HYD		T C	−17.4 1.2	10.1 17.2	13.4 29.7	16.8 32.8
HDFP 1979 (160)	SCRC Open		DBP	4.9	CLT	5-step	S R	−5.0	4.9 5.6	7.3 9.1	13.0 15.8
ATTMH 1980 (161)	RPC 3427	DBP 95–109	SBP <200	4.0	CTZ	3-step	T C	−6.0	0.7 1.6	1.2 2.6	3.6 5.1
Oslo 1980 (162)	Open 785	SBP 150+	DBP >109 CAD WMN	5.5	HCT	MDP PRP	T C	−10.3	2.7 1.0	3.1 2.9	4.5 4.3
WWPHE 1985 (163)	RPC SB 840		CHF	4.7	HCT+ TMT		T C	−9.9	14.8 23.6	34.3 46.7	69.0 74.8
MRC 1985 (164)	RPC SB 17290	DBP 90–109	CHF	4.8	PRPor BEN	MDP GUA	B D	−11.7 −12.7	3.4 4.6	4.7 6.0	5.5 6.1
IPPPSH 1985 (165)	RPC 6357	DBP 100–125	CAD CHF	4.1	OXP	DIU MDP	B D	−17.6 −16.7	3.1 3.1	3.5 3.7	8.3 8.8
HAPPHY 1987 (166)	RC Open 6569	DBP 100–130	WMN	4.2	ATNor MET HCTor BEN		B D	−17.8 −16.8	4.3 4.1		7.7 8.3
MAPHY 1988 (167)	RC Open 3234	DB 100–130	WMN	4.2	MET HCTor BEN		B D	−17.6 −17.1	2.6 6.2		4.8 9.3
				5.4			B D		5.2 7.1		8.0 10.3

[a]Abbreviations: RPC = randomized placebo controlled; RC = Randomized control (open label); SCRC = Randomized to stepped care or referred care.
[b]Criteria abbreviations: CVA = cerebrovascular accident (stroke); RET = hypertensive retinopathy; WMN = women; CAD = coronary artery disease; CHF = congestive heart failure; CVD = cardiovascular disease.
[c]Drug abbreviations: HCT = hydrochlorothiazide; RES = reserpine; HYD = hydralazine; CLT = chlorthalidone; CTZ = chlorthiazide; TMT = triamterene; PRP = propranolol; BEN = bendrofluazide; OXP = oxprenolol; ATN = atenolol; MET = metoprolol; MDP = methyldopa; GUA = guanethedine; DIU = diuretic.
[d]Groups abbreviations: T = treatment; C = control.

trials, in some cases aggregating them to look for the overall benefit of pharmacologic treatment of mild hypertension. Using nine such trials, Cutler, MacMahon, and Furberg found a mean DBP decrease of 5.8 mm Hg in 43,000 subjects followed for an average of 5.6 years. All-cause mortality was reduced significantly (by 11%), but this was largely due to a 38% decrease in fatal strokes. CAD mortality was 8% lower in the treatment groups but, despite the large numbers of subjects, this result was not statistically significant (168).

The failure of most studies (HDFP and EWPHE being the exceptions) to demonstrate a statistically significant reduction in CAD mortality has led some to question the wisdom of routine treatment of mild hypertension and to examine further the factors that may have contributed to this uncertainty.

Among these factors is the possibility that a relatively long time period (compared to the lengths of most studies) is required for reduction of BP to have its effect on CAD (169). Further, CAD risk derives from many other factors besides hypertension, so subject selection and exclusion criteria will dramatically affect the expected number of CAD events (170). For example, the exclusion of individuals with evident CAD will reduce the number of outcome events (171). As noted in Table 4.4, the rates of CAD deaths (expressed per 1000 patient-years) vary widely among the studies. For example, the Australian and MRC studies had very low rates, while the European Working Party found high rates in their elderly subjects. The duration of the trials and the degree of blood pressure reduction are two other factors that must be considered in drawing generalizations, as noted in Table 4.4.

Another issue of great concern is the potentially adverse effect of some antihypertensive medications. Results of the Multiple Risk Factor Intervention Trial (MRFIT) have been explained in part by a lower than expected mortality in the intervention group (172, 173). However, more attention has been directed to subgroup analyses that show that subjects with baseline electrocardiographic abnormalities who were treated with diuretics had considerably higher mortality than expected. This has caused many clinicians to use agents other than diuretics as the first step in treatment, although others advise against discarding altogether this valuable category of drugs (174). Several of the large randomized trials have made direct comparisons of β-blockers and diuretics, including the MRC, HAPPHY, and IPPPSH studies. In each, investigators noted similar DBP, morbidity, and mortality reductions from treatment with the two drug categories. Investigators of the MAPHY study, a continuation of the metoprolol arm of the HAPPHY trial, suggested that metoprolol may be more effective than diuretics in reducing CAD and stroke deaths.

DRUG WITHDRAWAL

Persons whose mild hypertension has been satisfactorily controlled for at least one year may be candidates for a "step-down" of the drug regimen, particularly if they have improved their weight and their nutritional intake.

A lack of adherence to antihypertensive medications may result in abrupt blood pressure elevation. Centrally acting agents, guanethidine and reserpine, are most likely to exhibit this characteristic, alone or in combination with other agents. Weber and Drayer have postulated several mechanisms for this effect; these include increased levels of, and sensitivity to, circulating norepinephrine, increased renin-angiotensin system activity, and the breakthrough of cerebrovascular autoregulation (175).

QUALITY OF LIFE

The concept of "quality of life" received increased attention during the 1980s, and may be considered to include functional capacity, perceptions of one's general health status, and life satisfaction, as well as side effects from the treatment (176).

Physicians and patients often have

Table 4.5.   Average Wholesale Price to Pharmacies[a]

Medication Category	Unit Dose	Cost per Unit Dose (US $)	Typical Unit Doses per Day	Cost per Day
Diuretics				
Hydrochlorothiazide	25 mg		1–2	
Generic		0.01–0.03		0.01–0.06
Oretic		0.04		0.04–0.08
Hydrodiuril		0.10		0.10–0.21
Chlorthalidone	25 mg		1–2	
Generic		0.03		0.03–0.06
Baxter		0.10		0.10–0.20
Squibb		0.10		0.10–0.20
Furosemide	20 mg		1–2	
Generic		0.02–0.03		0.02–0.06
Lasix		0.11		0.11–0.23
Indapamide	2.5 mg	0.53	1	0.53
Potassium-sparing				
Triamterene	50 mg	0.27	4	1.07
β-Blockers	(See Table 16.2)			
α/β-Blocker				
Labetalol	100 mg	0.28	2	0.57
Converting-enzyme inhibitors				
Captopril	50 mg	0.67	1–2	0.67–1.34
Enalapril	10 mg	0.75	1–2	0.75–1.50
Lisinopril	10 mg		1–2	
Prinivil		0.63		0.63–1.26
Zestril		0.63		0.63–1.26
α-Blocker				
Prazosin	2 mg	0.47	1–3	0.47–1.40
Terazosin	2 mg	0.64	1–3	0.64–1.92
Central inhibitors				
Methyldopa	250 mg		2–3	
Generic		0.10		0.20–0.30
Aldomet		0.29		0.58–0.88
Clonidine	0.1 mg		1–3	
Generic		0.02		0.02–0.06
Squibb		0.16		0.16–0.48
Catapres		0.33		0.33–0.99
Guanabenz	8 mg	0.67	1–2	0.67–1.33
Guanfacine	1 mg	0.47	1	0.47
Vasodilators				
Hydralazine	50 mg		4	
Generic		0.024		0.10
Baxter		0.09		0.36
Apresoline		0.34		1.36

[a]Data from Annual Pharmacists' Reference. Orodell, NJ: Medical Economics, Inc., 1990.

different views of the side effects of antihypertensive medications. In one study, physicians reported almost no adverse effects on patients; in contrast, 40% of the patients reported feeling no better, and approximately 10% felt worse during therapy. All of the relatives queried reported that the patient's condition was worse during treatment (177).

Approximately 15 to 20% of patients receiving diuretics in the HDFP and MRC studies discontinued treatment, compared to 5% in the placebo groups. Similar rates were seen in the propranolol group of the MRC study. ACE inhibitors such as captopril appear to cause fewer side effects (178).

Sexual dysfunction or discomfort may also result from antihypertensive medication. In both men and women, decrease in libido may result from diuretics, guanethidine, methyldopa, β-blockers, and reserpine. Breast enlargment or tenderness can occur in both genders with clonidine, methyldopa, and spironolactone. Orgasmic and ejaculation difficulties have been reported with clonidine, guanethidine, methyldopa, and reserpine. Vaginal lubrication may be decreased in women taking diuretics, and menstrual irregularities may be seen with spironolactone. Impotence has been reported by patients taking almost all antihypertensive medications (45, 179).

COST OF TREATMENT

Stason reports results of a Gallup poll revealing that only 59% of all persons have health insurance that covers medications; for families with incomes under $15,000 in 1986, the percentage was only 44% (180). In a representative sample of households in the state of Georgia in 1981, investigators found that, compared with persons with mild or controlled high blood pressure, almost twice as many persons with uncontrolled moderate to severe hypertension reported economic barriers to filling and refilling antihypertensive prescriptions. This was particularly notable in black women (181).

Table 4.5 lists the average wholesale costs to pharmacies for agents in common use in the United States in 1990 (182).

INTEGRATED APPROACH TO TREATMENT

Results to date confirm the wisdom of combining individual and community treatment, educating both the public and health professionals, while encouraging action by governments, voluntary agencies, and industry to minimize the impact of hypertension on society (183).

REFERENCES

1. Joint National Committee. The 1988 report of the Joint National Committee on Detection, Evaluation, and Treatment of High Blood Pressure. Arch Intern Med 1988; 148:1023–1038.

2. Logan AG. Report of the Canadian Hypertension Society's consensus conference on the management of mild hypertension. Can Med Assoc J 1984;131:1053–1057.

3. Davies JW, Semenciw RM, Mao Y. Cardiovascular disease mortality trends and related risk factors in Canada. Can J Cardiol 1988;4(Suppl A):16A–20A.

4. Joint National Committee. Report of the Joint National Committee on Detection, Evaluation, and Treatment of High Blood Pressure. A cooperative study, JAMA 1977;237:255–261.

5. Joint National Committee. The 1980 report of the Joint National Committee on Detection, Evaluation, and Treatment of High Blood Pressure. Arch Intern Med 1980;140:1280–1285.

6. Applegate WB. Hypertension in elderly patients. Ann Intern Med 1989;110:901–905.

7. Drizd T, Dannenberg AL, Engel A. Blood pressure levels in persons 18–74 years of age in 1976–80, and trends in blood pressure from 1960 to 1980 in the United States. Hyattsville, MD: US Department of Health and Human Services, 1986. DHHS publication (PHS) 86-1684.

8. Siegel D, Kuller L, Lazarus NB, et al. Predictors of cardiovascular events and mortal-

ity in the Systolic Hypertension in the Elderly Program Pilot Project. Am J Epidemiol 1987;126:385–399.

9. Fiebach NH, Hebert PR, Stampfer MJ, et al. A prospective study of high blood pressure and cardiovascular disease in women. Am J Epidemiol 1989;130:646–654.

10. Bang KM, Greene EJ. Current epidemiologic status on aging in U.S. blacks: update on hypertension and diabetes. J Natl Med Assoc 1988;80:627–632.

11. Wenneker MB, Epstein AM. Racial inequalities in the use of procedures for patients with ischemic heart disease in Massachusetts. JAMA 1989;261:253–257.

12. Thomas J, Semenya KA, Neser WB, Thomas DJ, Green DR, Gillum RF. Risk factors and the incidence of hypertension in black physicians: the Meharry Cohort Study. Am Heart J 1985;110:637–645.

13. Cornoni-Huntley J, La Croix AZ, Havlik RJ. Race and sex differentials in the impact of hypertension in the United States. Arch Intern Med 1989;149:780–788.

14. Task Force on Black and Minority Health. Report of the Secretary's Task Force on Black and Minority Health, vol 4, pt 2. Washington, DC: Department of Health and Human Services, 1986.

15. Rowland M, Roberts J (eds). Blood pressure levels and hypertension in persons ages 6–74 years. United States 1976–80. National Center for Health Statistics Advance Data, 1982.

16. Hazuda HP, Stern MP, Gaskill SP, Haffner SM, Gardner LI. Ethnic differences in health knowledge and behaviors related to the prevention and treatment of coronary heart disease. The San Antonio Heart Study. Am J Epidemiol 1983;117:717–728.

17. Winklestein W, Kagan A, Kato H, Sacks S. Epidemiologic studies of coronary heart disease and stroke in Japanese men living in Japan, Hawaii, and California. Blood pressure distributions. Am J Epidemiol 1975;102:502–513.

18. Stavig GR, Igra A, Leonard AR. Hypertension among Asians and Pacific Islanders in California. Am J Epidemiol 1984;119:677–691.

19. Stavig GR, Igra A, Leonard AR, McCullough J, Oreglia A. Hypertension-related

mortality in California. Publ Health Reports 1986;101:39–49.

20. Rissanen AM, Nikkila EA. Aggregation of coronary risk factors in families of men with fatal and non-fatal coronary heart disease. Br Heart J 1979;42:373–380.

21. Wadsworth ME, Cripps HA, Midwinter RE, Colley JR. Blood pressure in a national birth cohort at the age of 36 related to social and familial factors, smoking, and body mass. Br Med J 1985;291:1534–1539.

22. Becker DM, Becker LC, Pearson TA, Fintel DJ, Levine DM, Kwiterovich PO. Risk factors in siblings of people with premature coronary heart disease. J Am Coll Cardiol 1988;12:1273–1280.

23. Heller RF, Robinson N, Peart WS. Value of blood pressure measurement in relatives of hypertensive patients. Lancet 1980; 1:1206–1208.

24. Thomas CB, Cohen BH. The familial occurrence of hypertension and coronary artery disease, with observations concerning obesity and diabetes. Ann Intern Med 1955;42:90–127.

25. Higgins M, Keller J, Moore F, Ostrander L, Metzner H, Stock L. Studies of blood pressure in Tecumseh, Michigan. Am J Epidemiol 1980;111:142–155.

26. Johnson CC, Nicklas TA, Arbeit ML, et al. Cardiovascular risk in parents of children with elevated blood pressure. Heart smart—family health promotion. J Clin Hypertens 1987;3:559–566.

27. Connor SL, Connor WE, Henry H, Sexton G, Keenan EJ. The effects of familial relationships, age, body weight, and diet on blood pressure and the 24 hour urinary excretion of sodium, potassium, and creatinine in men, women, and children of randomly selected families. Circulation 1984;70:76–85.

28. Hunt SC, Hasstedt SJ, Kuida H, Stults BM, Hopkins PN, Williams RR. Genetic heritability and common environmental components of resting and stressed blood pressures, lipids, and body mass index in Utah pedigrees and twins. Am J Epidemiol 1989;129:625–638.

29. Weber MA, Drayer JI. How extensive a workup for secondary hypertension? J Cardiovasc Med 1983;8:411–428.

30. Gifford RW Jr, Kirkendall W, O'Connor DT, Weidman W. Office evaluation of hypertension. Circulation 1989;79:721–731.

31. Chiang BN, Perlman LV, Epstein FH. Overweight and hypertension: a review. Circulation 1969;39:403–421.

32. Stamler R, Stamler J, Riedlinger WF, Algera G, Roberts RH. Weight and blood pressure. Findings in hypertension screening of 1 million Americans. JAMA 1978;240:1607–1610.

33. MacMahon SW, Blacket RB, Macdonald GJ, Hall W. Obesity, alcohol consumption and blood pressure in Australian men and women. The National Heart Foundation of Australia Risk Factor Prevalence Study. J Hypertens 1984;2:85–91.

34. Blair D, Habicht JP, Sims EA, Sylwester D, Abraham S. Evidence for an increased risk for hypertension with centrally located body fat and the effect of race and sex on this risk. Am J Epidemiol 1984;119:526–540.

35. Selby JV, Friedman GD, Quesenberry CP Jr. Precursors of essential hypertension. The role of body fat distribution pattern. Am J Epidemiol 1989;129:43–53.

36. Neser WB, Thomas J, Semenya K, Thomas DJ, Gillum RF. Obesity and hypertension in a longitudinal study of black physicians: the Meharry Cohort Study. J Chron Dis 1986;39:105–113.

37. Paffenbarger RS Jr, Wing AL, Hyde RT, Jung DL. Physical activity and incidence of hypertension in college alumni. Am J Epidemiol 1983;117:245–257.

38. Hickey N, Mulcahy R, Bourke GJ, Graham I, Wilson-Davis K. Study of coronary risk factors related to physical activity in 15,171 men. Br Med J 1975;3:507–509.

39. Sallis JF, Haskell WL, Wood PD, Fortmann SP, Vranizan KM. Vigorous physical activity and cardiovascular risk factors in young adults. J Chron Dis 1986;39:115–120.

40. Blair SN, Goodyear NN, Gibbons LW, et al. Physical fitness and incidence of hypertension in healthy normotensive men and women. JAMA 1984;252:487–490.

41. Criqui MH, Langer RD, Reed DM. Dietary alcohol, calcium, and potassium. Independent and combined effects on blood pressure. Circulation 1989;80:609–614.

42. Pietinen P, Huttunen JK. Dietary fat and blood pressure—a review. Eur Heart J 1987;8(suppl B):9–17.

43. Melby CL, Goldflies DG, Hyner GC, Lyle RM. Relation between vegetarian/nonvegetarian diets and blood pressure in black and white adults. Am J Public Health 1989;79:1283–1288.

44. Lian C. L'alcoolisme, cause d'hypertension arterielle. Bull Acad Med 1915;74:525–528.

45. Davidson DM. Cardiovascular effects of alcohol. West J Med 1989;151:430–439.

46. Saunders JB, Beevers DG, Paton A. Alcohol-induced hypertension. Lancet 1981;2:653–656.

47. Puddey IB, Beilin LJ, Vandongen R. Regular alcohol use raises blood pressure in treated hypertensive subjects: a randomized clinical trial. Lancet 1987;1:647–651.

48. Puddey IB, Beilin LJ, Vandongen R, Rouse IL, Rogers P. Evidence for a direct effect of alcohol consumption on blood pressure in normotensive men: a randomized clinical trial. Hypertension 1985;7:707–713.

49. Howes LG. Pressor effect of alcohol. Lancet 1985;2:835.

50. Klatsky AL, Friedman GD, Siegelaub AB, Gerard MJ. Alcohol consumption and blood pressure. Kaiser-Permanente Multiphasic Health Examination data. N Engl J Med 1977;296:1194–1200.

51. Criqui MH, Wallace RB, Mishkel M, Barrett-Connor E, Heiss G. Alcohol consumption and blood pressure. The Lipid Research Clinics Prevalence Study. Hypertension 1981;3:557–565.

52. Arkwright PD, Beilin LJ, Rouse I, Armstrong BK, Vandongen R. Effects of alcohol use and other aspects of lifestyle on blood pressure levels and prevalence of hypertension in a working population. Circulation 1982;66:60–66.

53. MacMahon SW, Norton RN. Alcohol and hypertension: implications for prevention and treatment. Ann Intern Med 1986;105:124–126.

54. Harburg E, Ozgoren F, Hawthorne VM, Schorck MA. Community norms of alcohol usage and blood pressure: Tecumseh, Michigan. Am J Public Health 1980;70:813–820.

55. Klatsky AL, Armstrong MA, Friedman GD. Relations of alcoholic beverage use to subsequent coronary artery disease hospitalization. Am J Cardiol 1986;58:710–714.

56. Criqui MH, Cowan LD, Heiss G, Haskell WL, Laskarzewski PM, Chambless LE. Frequency and clustering of nonlipid coronary

risk factors in dyslipoproteinemia. The Lipid Research Clinics Prevalence Study. Circulation 1986;73:140–150.

57. Trevisan M, Krogh V, Farinaro E, et al. Alcohol consumption, drinking pattern and blood pressure: analysis of data from the Italian National Research Council Study. Int J Epidemiol 1987;16:520–527.

58. Dyer AR, Stamler J, Paul O, et al. Alcohol, cardiovascular risk factors and mortality: the Chicago experience. Circulation 1981;64(suppl III):20–27.

59. Garrison RJ, Kannel WB, Stokes J III, Castelli WP. Incidence and precursors of hypertension in young adults: the Framingham Offspring Study. Prev Med 1985;16:235–251.

60. Kromhout D, Bosschieter EB, Coulander CD. Potassium, calcium, alcohol intake and blood pressure: the Zutphen Study. Am J Clin Nutr 1985;41:1299–1304.

61. Light KC. Psychosocial precursors of hypertension: experimental evidence. Circulation 1987;76(suppl I):I67–I76.

62. Dustan HP. Biobehavioral factors in hypertension. Circulation 1987;76(suppl I):I57–I59.

63. Franco LJ, Stern MP, Rosenthal M, Haffner SM, Hazuda HP, Comeaux PJ. Prevalence, detection, and control of hypertension in a biethnic community. The San Antonio Heart Study. Am J Epidemiol 1985;121:684–696.

64. Noppa H, Bengtson C. Obesity in relation to socioeconomic status. J Epidemiol Comm Health 1980;34:139–142.

65. Greenberg G. Psychosocial factors and hypertension. Br Med J 1988;296:591–592.

66. Marmot MG, McDowall ME. Mortality decline and widening social inequalities. Lancet 1986;2:274–276.

67. Syme SL. Psychosocial determinants of hypertension. In: Onesti E, Klimt C (eds): Hypertension determinants, complications and intervention. New York: Grune and Stratton, 1979:95–98.

68. James SA. Psychosocial precursors of hypertension: a review of the epidemiologic evidence. Circulation 1987;76 (suppl I):I60–I66.

69. Joseph JG, Prior IA, Salmond CE, Stanley D. Elevation of systolic and diastolic blood pressure associated with migration: the Tokelau Island migrant study. J Chron Dis 1983;36:507–516.

70. Elford J, Phillips AN, Thomson AG, Shaper AG. Migration and geographic variations in ischaemic heart disease in Great Britain. Lancet 1989;1:343–346.

71. Harburg E, Erfurt JC, Chape C, et al. Socioecological stressor areas and black-white blood pressure: Detroit. J Chron Dis 1973;26:595–611.

72. Broadhead WE, Kaplan BH, James SA, et al. The epidemiologic evidence for a relationship between social support and health. Am J Epidemiol 1983;117:521–537.

73. Strogatz DS, James SA. Social support and hypertension among blacks and whites in a rural, southern community. Am J Epidemiol 1986;124:949–956.

74. Anonymous. Controlling hypertension: community care and mutual aid through neighbourhood clubs. WHO Chronicle 1978;32:448–450.

75. Williams CA, Beresford SA, James SA, et al. The Edgecombe County High Blood Pressure Control Program. III. Social support, social stressors, and treatment dropout. Am J Public Health 1985;75:483–486.

76. Winnubst JA, Marcelissen FH, Kleber RJ. Effects of social support in the stressor-strain relationship: A Dutch sample. Soc Sci Med 1982;16:475–482.

77. Bandura A. Self-efficacy: toward a unifying theory of behavior change. Psychol Rev 1977;84:191–215.

78. Anonymous. Self-esteem. Lancet 1988;2:943–944.

79. Kaplan GA, Camacho T. Perceived health and mortality: a nine-year follow-up of the Human Population Laboratory cohort. Am J Epidemiol 1983;117:292–304.

80. King JB. Illness attributions and the health belief model. Health Educ Quart 1984;10:287–312.

81. Norman SA, Marconi KM, Schezel GW, Schechter CF, Stolley PD. Beliefs, social normative influences, and compliance with antihypertensive medication. Am J Prev Med 1985;1:10–17.

82. Chesney MA. Anger and hostility: future implications for behavioral medicine. In: Chesney MA, Rosenman RH (eds): Anger and hostility in cardiovascular and behavioral disorders. Washington: Hemisphere Publ Co, 1985:277–290.

83. Krantz DS, DeQuattro V, Blackburn HW, et al. Psychosocial factors in hypertension. Circulation 1987;76(suppl I):I84–I88.

84. Sallis JF, Johnson CC, Trevorrow TR, Kaplan RM, Hovell MF. The relationship between cynical hostility and blood pressure reactivity. J Psychosom Res 1987;31:111–116.

85. Babisch W, Ising H, Gallacher JE, Elwood PC. Traffic noise and cardiovascular risk. The Caerphilly Study, first phase. Outdoor noise levels and risk factors. Arch Environ Health 1988;43:407–414.

86. House JS, McMichael AJ, Wells JA, et al. Occupational stress and health among factory workers. J Health Soc Behav 1979;20:139–160.

87. Theorell T. Selected illnesses and somatic factors in relation to two psychosocial stress indices. A prospective study on middle-aged construction building workers. J Psychosom Res 1976;20:7–20.

88. Rosenman RH. The impact of anxiety on the cardiovascular system. Psychosomatics 1985;26(11(suppl)):6–17.

89. Theorell T, Hjemdahl P, Ericsson F, et al. Psychosocial and physiological factors in relation to blood pressure at rest—a study of Swedish men in their upper twenties. J Hypertens 1985;3:591–600.

90. Julius M, Harburg E, Cottington EM, Johnson EH. Anger-coping styles, blood pressure, and all-cause mortality; a follow-up in Tecumseh, Michigan (1971–1983). Am J Epidemiol 1986;124:220–233.

91. Culpepper L, Froom J. Incarceration and blood pressure. Soc Sci Med 1980;14A:571–574.

92. Dupree EA, Meyer MB. Role of risk factors in complications of diabetes mellitus. Am J Epidemiol 1980;112:100–112.

93. Ferrannini E, Buzzigoli G, Bonadonna R, et al. Insulin resistance in essential hypertension. N Engl J Med 1987;317:350–357.

94. Holm G, Johansson S, Vedin A, Wilhelmsson C, Smith U. The effect of β-blockade on glucose tolerance and insulin release in adult diabetes. Acta Med Scand 1980;208:187–191.

95. Houston MC. Treatment of hypertension in diabetes mellitus. Am Heart J 1989;118:819–829.

96. Freestone S, Ramsay LE. Effect of coffee and cigarette smoking on blood pressure of untreated and diuretic-treated hypertensive patients. Am J Med 1982;73:348–353.

97. Materson BJ, Reda D, Freis ED, Henderson WG. Cigarette smoking interferes with treatment of hypertension. Arch Intern Med 1988;148:2116–2119.

98. Douglas PS, Berko B, Lesh M, Reichek N. Alterations in diastolic function in response to progressive left ventricular hypertrophy. J Am Coll Cardiol 1989;13:461–467.

99. Devereux RB, Pickering TG, Harshfield GA, et al. Left ventricular hypertrophy in patients with hypertension: importance of blood pressure to regularly recurring stress. Circulation 1983;68:470–476.

100. Brush JE Jr, Cannon RO III, Schenke WH, et al. Angina due to coronary microvascular disease in hypertensive patients without left ventricular hypertrophy. N Engl J Med 1988;319:1302–1307.

101. Levy D, Garrison RJ, Savage DD, Kannel WB, Castelli WP. Left ventricular mass and incidence of coronary heart disease in an elderly cohort. The Framingham Heart Study. Ann Intern Med 1989;110:101–107.

102. Levy D, Labib SB, Anderson KM, Christiansen JC, Kannel WB, Castelli WP. Determinants of sensitivity and specificity of electrocardiographic criteria for left ventricular hypertrophy. Circulation 1990;81:815–820.

103. Hachamovitch R, Strom JA, Sonnenblick EH, Frishman WH. Left ventricular hypertrophy in hypertension and the effects of antihypertensive drug therapy. Curr Prob Cardiol 1988;13:375–422.

104. MacMahon SW, Wilcken DE, Macdonald GJ. The effect of weight reduction on left ventricular mass. A randomized controlled trial in young, overweight hypertensive patients. N Engl J Med 1986;314:334–339.

105. Pickering TG, James GD, Boddie C, Harshfield GA, Blank S, Laragh JH. How common is white coat hypertension? JAMA 1988;259:225–228.

106. White WB, Schulman P, McCabe EJ, Dey HM. Average daily blood pressure, not office blood pressure, determines cardiac function in patients with hypertension. JAMA 1989;261:873–877.

107. Petrie JC, O'Brien ET, Littler WA, de Swiet M. Recommendations on blood pressure measurement. Br Med J 1986;293:611–615.

108. Frolich ED, Grim C, Labarthe DR, Maxwell MH, Perloff D, Weidman WH. Recommendations for human blood pressure determination by sphygmomanometers. Circulation 1988;77:502A–514A.

109. Pickering TG, Harshfield GA, Kleinert HD, Blank S, Laragh JH. Blood pressure during normal daily activities, sleep, and exercise. JAMA 1982;247:992–996.

110. Weber MA, Drayer JI, Nakamura DK, Wyle FA. The circadian blood pressure pattern in ambulatory normal subjects. Am J Cardiol 1984;54:115–119.

111. Cheung DG, Gasster JL, Weber MA. Assessing duration of antihypertensive effects with whole-day blood pressure monitoring. Arch Intern Med 1989;149:2021–2025.

112. Padfield PL, Lindsay BA, McLaren JA, Pirie A, Rademaker M. Changing relation between home and clinic blood pressure measurements: do home measurements predict clinic hypertension? Lancet 1987;2:322–324.

113. Canadian Coalition for High Blood Pressure Prevention and Control. Recommendations on self-measurement of blood pressure. Can Med Assoc J 1988;138:1093–1096.

114. Evans CE, Haynes RB, Goldsmith CH, Hewson SA. Home blood pressure-measuring devices: a comparative study of accuracy. J Hypertension 1989;7:133–142.

115. Haynes RB, Sackett DL, Taylor DW, Gibson ES, Johnson AL. Increased absenteeism from work after detection and labeling of hypertensive patients. N Engl J Med 1979;299:741–744.

116. Polk BF, Harlan LC, Cooper SP, et al. Disability days associated with detection and treatment in a hypertension control program. Am J Epidemiol 1984;119:44–53.

117. Logan AG, Milne BJ, Achber C, Campbell WA, Haynes RB. A comparison of community and occupationally provided antihypertensive care. J Occup Med 1982;24:901–906.

118. Apostolides AY, Cutter G, Kraus JF, et al. Impact of hypertension information on high blood pressure control between 1973 and 1978. Hypertension 1980; 2:708–713.

119. Stross JK, Harlan WR. Dissemination of relevant information on hypertension. JAMA 1981;246:360–362.

120. Grimm RH Jr, Luepker RV, Taylor H, Blackburn H. Long-term effects of a blood pressure survey on patient treatment in a community. Circulation 1982;65:946–950.

121. Hovell MF. The experimental evidence for weight loss treatment of essential hypertension: a critical review. Am J Public Health 1982;72:359–368.

122. MacMahon S, Cutler J, Brittain E, Higgins M. Obesity and hypertension: epidemiological and clinical issues. Eur Heart J 1987;8(suppl B):57–70.

123. Boyer JL, Kasch FW. Exercise therapy in hypertensive men. JAMA 1970;211:1668–1671.

124. Kukkonen K, Rauramaa R, Voutilainen E, Lansimies E. Physical training of middle-aged men with borderline hypertension. Ann Clin Res. 1982;14(suppl 34):139–145.

125. Bjorntorp P. Effects of physical training on blood pressure in hypertension. Eur Heart J 1987;8(suppl B):71–76.

126. Gillum RF, Prineas RJ, Jeffrey RW, et al. Nonpharmacologic therapy of hypertension: the independent effects of weight reduction and sodium restriction in overweight borderline hypertensive patients. Am Heart J 1983;105:128–133.

127. Maxwell MH, Kushiro T, Dornfeld LP, Tucks ML, Waks AU. BP changes in obese hypertensive subjects during rapid weight loss. Comparison of restricted versus unchanged salt intake. Arch Intern Med 1984;144:1581–1584.

128. Schmieder RE, Messerli FH, Garavaglia GE, Nunez BD. Dietary salt intake. A determinant of cardiac involvement in essential hypertension. Circulation 1988;78:951–956.

129. Rocchini AP, Key J, Bondie D, et al. The effect of weight loss on the sensitivity of blood pressure to sodium in obese adolescents. N Engl J Med 1989;321:580–585.

130. Rissanen A, Pietinen P, Siljamaki-Ojansuu U, Piirainen H, Reissel P. Treatment of hypertension in obese patients: efficacy and feasibility of weight and salt reduction programs. Acta Med Scand 1985;218:149–156.

131. Stamler R, Stamler J, Gosch FC, et al. Primary prevention of hypertension

by nutritional-hygienic means. JAMA 1989;262:1801–1807.

132. Lyle RM, Melby CL, Hyner GC, Edmondson JW, Miller JZ, Weinberger MH. Blood pressure and metabolic effects of calcium supplementation in normotensive white and black men. JAMA 1987;257:1772–1776.

133. Health and Policy Committee, American College of Physicians. Biofeedback for hypertension. Ann Intern Med 1985;102:709–715.

134. Patel C, Marmot MG, Terry DJ, et al. Trials of relaxation in reducing coronary risk: four-year follow-up. Br Med J 1985;290:1103–1106.

135. Jacob RG, Kramer HC, Agras WS. Relaxation therapy in the treatment of hypertension. Arch Gen Psychiatry 1977;34:1417–1427.

136. Chesney MA, Agras WS, Benson H. Nonpharmacologic approaches to the treatment of hypertension. Circulation 1987;76(suppl I):I104–I109.

137. DeQuattro V. Treating hypertensive crises: which drug for which patient? J Crit Illness 1987;2:24–35.

138. Zeller KR, Kuhnert LV, Matthews C. Rapid reduction of severe asymptomatic hypertension. A prospective, controlled trial. Arch Intern Med 1989;149:2186–2189.

139. Stewart IM. Relation of reduction in pressure to first myocardial infarction in patients receiving treatment for severe hypertension. Lancet 1979;1:861–865.

140. Alderman MH, Ooi WL, Imadhavan S, Cohen H. Treatment-induced blood pressure reduction and the risk of myocardial infarction. JAMA 1989;262:920–924.

141. Fagan TC. Acute reduction of blood pressure in asymptomatic patients with severe hypertension. An idea whose time has come—and gone. Arch Intern Med 1989;149:2169–2170.

142. Veterans Administration Cooperative Study Group on Antihypertensive Agents. Effects of treatment on morbidity in hypertension. Results in patients with diastolic blood pressures averaging 115 through 129 mm Hg. JAMA 1967;202:116–122.

143. Black HR. Choosing initial treatment for hypertension. Hypertension. 1989;13(suppl I):I149–I153.

144. Havlik RJ, LaCroix AZ, Kleinman JC, Ingram DD, Harris T, Cornoni-Huntley J. Antihypertensive drug therapy and survival by treatment status in a national survey. Hypertension 1989;13(suppl I):I28–I32.

145. Kaplan NM. Maximally reducing cardiovascular risk in the treatment of hypertension. Ann Intern Med 1988;109:36–40.

146. Grimm RH Jr, Leon AS, Hunninghake DB, Lenz K, Hannan P, Blackburn H. Effects of thiazide diuretics on plasma lipids and lipoproteins in mildly hypertensive patients: a double-blind controlled trial. Ann Intern Med 1981;94:7–11.

147. Veterans Administration Cooperative Study Group on Antihypertensive Agents. Comparison of propranolol and hydrocholorothiazide for the initial treatment of hypertension. JAMA 1982;248:1996–2011.

148. Psaty BM, Koepsell TD, LoGerfo JP, Wagner EH, Inui TS. Beta-blockers and primary prevention of coronary heart disease in patients with high blood pressure. JAMA 1989;261:2087–2094.

149. Scott AK, Rigby JW, Webster J, Hawksworth GM, Petrie JC, Lovell HG. Atenolol and metoprolol once daily in hypertension. Brit Med J 1982;284:1514–1516.

150. Ades PA, Gunther PG, Meacham CP, Handy MA, LeWinter MM. Hypertension, exercise, and β-adrenergic blockade. Ann Intern Med 1988;109:629–634.

151. Williams GH. Converting-enzyme inhibitors in the treatment of hypertension. N Engl J Med 1988;319:1517–1525.

152. Dustan HP. Calcium channel blockers. Hypertension. 1989;13(suppl I):I137–I140.

153. Leenen FH, Smith D, Farkas RM, Reeves RA, Marquez-Julio A. Vasodilators and regression of left ventricular hypertrophy. Am J Med 1987;82:969–978.

154. Weber MA, Drayer JI. Central and peripheral blockade of the sympathetic nervous system. Am J Med 1984;77(suppl 4A):110–118.

155. Weber MA, Drayer JI, Brewer DD, Lipson JL. Transdermal continuous antihypertensive therapy. Lancet 1984;1:9–11.

156. Davies SF, Graif JL, Husebye DG, et al. Comparative effects of transdermal clonidine and oral atenolol on acute exercise perfor-

mance and response to aerobic conditioning in subjects with hypertension. Arch Intern Med 1989;149:1551–1556.

157. Chidsey CA, Gottleib TB. The pharmacologic basis of antihypertensive therapy: the role of vasodilator drugs. Prog Cardiovasc Dis 1974;17:99–113.

158. Fontanet H, Garcia JC, del Rio J, Martinez-Maldonado M. The use of isosorbide in the treatment of severe, uncontrolled hypertension. Arch Intern Med 1987;147:426–428.

159. Veterans Administration Cooperative Study Group on Antihypertensive Agents. Effects of treatment on morbidity in hypertension. II. Results of patients with diastolic blood pressure averaging 90 through 114 mm Hg. JAMA 1970;213:1143–1151.

160. Hypertension Detection and Follow-Up Program Cooperative Group. Five-year findings of the Hypertension Detection and Follow-up Program. I. Reduction in mortality of persons with high blood pressure, including mild hypertension. JAMA 1979;242:2562–2571.

161. Management Committee. The Australian therapeutic trial in mild hypertension. Lancet 1980;1:1261–1267.

162. Helgeland A. Treatment of mild hypertension: a five year controlled drug trial. Am J Med 1980;69:725–732.

163. Amery A, Birkenhager W, Brixko P, et al. Mortality and morbidity results from the European Working Party on High Blood Pressure in the Elderly trial. Lancet 1985;1:1349–1354.

164. Medical Research Council Working Party. MRC trial of treatment of mild hypertension: principal results. Br Med J 1985;291:97–104.

165. The IPPPSH Collaborative Group. Cardiovascular risk and risk factors in a randomized trial of treatment based on the β-blocker oxprenolol: the International Prospective Primary Prevention Study in Hypertension (IPPPSH). J Hypertens 1985;3:379–392.

166. Wilhelmsen L, Berglund G, Elmfeldt D, et al. Beta blockers versus diuretics in hypertensive men. Main results from the HAPPHY trial. J Hypertens 1987;5:561–572.

167. Wikstrand J, Warnold I, Olsson G, Tuomilehto J, Elmfeldt D, Berglund G. Primary prevention with metoprolol in patients with hypertension: mortality results from the MAPHY study. JAMA 1988;259:1976–1982.

168. Cutler JA, MacMahon SW, Furberg CD. Controlled clinical trials of drug treatment for hypertension. A review. Hypertension 1989;13(Suppl I):I36–I44.

169. MacMahon S, Cutler JA, Stamler J. Antihypertensive drug treatment. Hypertension 1989;13(suppl I):I45–I50.

170. Remington RD. Potential impact of exclusion criteria on results of hypertension trials. Hypertension 1989;13(suppl I):I66)–I68.

171. Browner WS, Hulley SB. Effect of risk status on treatment criteria. Implications of hypertension trials. Hypertension 1989;13(Suppl I):I51–I56.

172. Multiple Risk Factor Intervention Trial Research Group. Multiple Risk Factor Intervention Trial: risk factor changes and mortality results. JAMA 1982;248:1465–1477.

173. Multiple Risk Factor Intervention Trial Research Group. Coronary heart disease death, nonfatal acute myocardial infarction and other clinical outcomes in the Multiple Risk Factor Intervention Trial. Am J Cardiol 1986;58:1–13.

174. Moser M. Suppositions and speculations—their possible effects on treatment decisions in the management of hypertension. Am Heart J 1989;118:1362–1369.

175. Weber MA, Drayer JI. Withdrawal of antihypertensive therapy: physiological effects and therapeutic precautions. Practical Cardiol 1982;8(10):99–103, 107–109, 112–113.

176. Wenger NK, Mattson ME, Furberg CD, Elinson J. Assessment of quality of life in clinical trials of cardiovascular therapies. Am J Cardiol 1984;54:908–913.

177. Jachuck SJ, Brierley H, Jachuck S, et al. The effect of hypotensive drugs on the quality of life. J Royal Coll Gen Pract. 1982;32:103–105.

178. Croog SH, Levine S, Testa MA, et al. The effects of antihypertensive therapy on the quality of life. N Engl J Med 1986;314:1657–1664.

179. Papadopoulos C. Cardiovascular drugs and sexuality. Arch Intern Med 1980;140:1341–1345.

180. Stason WB. Cost and quality trade-offs in the treatment of hypertension. Hypertension 1989;13(suppl I):I145–I148.

181. Shulman NB, Martinez B, Brogan D, Carr AA, Miles CG. Financial cost as an obstacle to hypertension therapy. Am J Public Health 1986;76:1105–1108.

182. Annual Pharmacists' Reference. Oradell, NJ: Medical Economics Inc, 1990.

183. Blackburn H, Prineas R. Diet and hypertension: anthropology, epidemiology, and public health implications. Prog Biochem Pharmacol 1983;19:31–79.

5

smoking

In 1989, the surgeon general of the USA commemorated the 25th anniversary of his predecessor's first report on smoking and health. He noted that smoking is responsible for more than one in every six deaths in the USA, and it remains as the single most preventable cause of death. In 1985, more than 400,000 deaths in Canada and the USA were attributable to cigarette smoking. By 1986, lung cancer exceeded breast cancer as the leading cause of cancer death in women; the relative risk of lung cancer in women rose fourfold from the time of the first Report of the Surgeon General in 1964 (1).

However, two decades of public health information has made some impact. By 1987, the prevalence of smoking among adults in the USA had decreased from 40 to 29%, and during that interval, approximately 790,000 smoking-related deaths in the USA were avoided or postponed because of decisions to quit smoking or to not start. It has been estimated that another two million deaths will be avoided or postponed by the year 2000 (1).

The prevalence of smoking in 1990 varied widely within the United States, however, with California and some smaller states meeting goals of less than 25%. Other states, such as Kentucky and Nevada, remained among those with the highest prevalence (approximately 33%) (2). Internationally, the prevalence of smoking among women and men covers an even greater spectrum. For example, a majority of Glasgow residents of both genders smoke, as shown in Table 5.1 (3). In the following section, the epidemiology of smoking and cardiovascular disease will be further explored.

Epidemiology

The prevalence of daily smoking among adolescents in the USA is now higher in girls than in boys (4), despite improved programs to prevent smoking initiation by young persons of both genders. Although initiation of smoking has decreased at a more rapid rate in blacks than whites (5), adult black men still have the highest smoking rates, followed by Hispanic Americans and non-Hispanic whites (6). Mexican-American women have substantially lower smoking prevalence rates than other women (7). In Hispanics living in San Francisco, smoking was more common among less-acculturated men and among more-acculturated women (8).

In other industrialized countries, smoking prevalence varies widely. In 1966, more than 83% of Japanese men smoked; by 1980, this had decreased to 70%, while

83

Table 5.1. Smoking Prevalence (%) in 32 Selected Countries, 1981–1987

Country	Men	Women
Papua New Guinea	85	80
Swaziland	80	72
Nepal	79	58
Fiji (Melanesians)	76	44
Bangladesh	70	20
Venezuela	69	67
Japan	66	14
Poland	63	29
Tonga	62	38
Czechoslovakia	57	14
Yugoslavia	57	10
Greece	54	13
Nigeria	53	3
India	52	3
Denmark	49	38
France	49	26
USSR	48	11
Italy	46	18
Iraq	45	6
Federal Republic of Germany	44	29
Norway	42	32
Netherlands	41	33
Ireland	39	32
Australia	37	30
New Zealand	35	29
Belgium	35	21
Finland	35	17
Austria	33	22
Canada	31	28
USA	30	24
Sweden	26	30
Ivory Coast	24	1

approximately 15% of Japanese women were smokers. In Norway, where a goal of a smoke-free country by the year 2000 has been adopted, between 30 and 40% of adults smoked, but the prevalence of smoking among adolescents has decreased substantially (9).

In partially industrialized countries, the smoking prevalence continues to be very high. In some such nations, such as Brazil, Zimbabwe, and the Philippines, tobacco is a cash crop (10). To others, the USA aggressively markets tobacco prod-

ucts (11). In 1986, tobacco leaf export from Canada rose 23% (10).

In most countries, smokers are more likely to have lower levels of education and employment (12, 13). By the year 2000, it has been estimated that 30% of USA residents who have not attended college will be smokers, compared with less than 10% of college graduates (14). The highest rates of smoking for men are among blue collar workers, while professional and technical workers have the lowest rates (15).

However, educational and economic status, as well as knowledge of the health consequences of smoking, may be insufficient to encourage quitting and to prevent smoking uptake. Although a majority of physicians in the USA were smokers in 1945, only 12% of practicing pulmonary physicians smoked in 1983 (16). By that time, smoking among physicians in California was approximately 10% (17), and smoking ranged between 13 and 15% for female and male physicians in New Zealand. In contrast, prevalence rates among nurses were 31 to 39% in New Zealand (18) and approximately 25% in Canada, where smoking was most likely among critical care nurses, those who were widowed, divorced, or separated, and those with rotational schedules (19).

In Spain, however, a majority of cardiologists as well as most nurses were smokers in 1988 (20). That same year, the Spanish government introduced a smoking ban on all forms of public transport and in work areas containing pregnant women (21).

ACCURACY OF SMOKING LEVEL

Many smokers in the USA estimate their intake in packs or half-packs per day, leading to the digit preference of "tens" (10, 20, 30, 40 cigarettes per day) in self-report of smoking level. While cigarette packs in Canada have contained 25 cigarettes for some years, only recently has this practice been adopted in the USA (22).

The truthfulness of smokers' self-reports has been questioned (23), leading to the measurement of expired air carbon monoxide, saliva thiocyanate, or urinary cotinine during clinical investigations (24). Young adults tend to underreport current consumption when asked by telephone (25), while older, educated adults appear to have fairly accurate recall as far as 20 years in the past (26), particularly if their smoking level has not changed (27).

EXCESS CARDIOVASCULAR DISEASE IN SMOKERS

At least 10 major prospective studies in Canada, Europe, Japan, the United Kingdom, and the United States have found that all-cause mortality in smokers is approximately 1.7 times that of nonsmokers. Most studies show a strong dose-response relation of cigarettes smoked to deaths from CAD. In addition, smoking increases the risk of peripheral arterial occlusive disease, stroke, chronic obstructive pulmonary disease, and various forms of cancer (lung, larynx, oral, esophagus, bladder, pancreas, and others) (9, 28). Studies in Swedish and Finnish twins have confirmed the risks of developing these diseases as a consquence of smoking (29, 30).

In the Honolulu Heart Study of men of Japanese ancestry, those who continued to smoke during 12 years of follow-up had twice the risk of ischemic stroke as those who had never smoked. The risk of hemorrhagic stroke was fourfold in smokers (31). Investigators in the Framingham Study also confirmed the independent value of smoking in predicting strokes among their subjects (32). In the Coronary Artery Surgery Study (CASS), investigators prospectively followed 4165 smokers with angiographically documented CAD. Approximately one-third quit during the

follow-up period; these individuals had rates for MI-associated death and sudden cardiac death which were only half of those who continued to smoke (33).

Among individuals who survive an initial myocardial infarction (MI), those who quit smoking have a recurrence and mortality rate only half that of persons who persist, regardless of age or gender. Although the relative risk of smoking continuance is somewhat attenuated after the initial postinfarction years, (34, 35) Salonen has estimated that 28% of deaths in postinfarction patients are due to continuation of smoking (36). The risk of recurrent cardiac arrest is significantly higher in persons who continue smoking after successful cardiopulmonary resuscitation (37), and angina recurs after MI twice as often in continuing smokers (38). Approximately half of MI patients stop smoking at the time of their event, but half of these resume their habit later (39).

The association of smoking and CAD events is particularly striking in women. Between 1965 and 1985, the proportion of women in the USA who smoked 25 or more cigarettes per day nearly doubled (4). Nurses in the USA who smoked at that level had five times the risk of a coronary event as their nonsmoking contemporaries. Among heavy smokers, more than 80% of MIs were attributed to smoking. Even smoking 1 to 14 cigarettes per day was associated with a doubling of risk (40). In one study of cardiac rehabilitation program patients, only 14% of men were smoking six months after their cardiac event compared with 59% of women (41). Smoking by women is also associated with a significantly higher risk of sudden cardiac death (42–44).

The relative risk of all strokes for women smokers in that study was similar to that for coronary events, but women smoking 25 or more cigarettes per day had a relative risk of subarachnoid hemorrhage of 9.8 compared to never-smokers (45). In a study encompassing nearly one-quarter of the population of New Zealand, approximately 37% of strokes were attributed to smoking (46).

Smoking and Other CAD Risk Indicators

LIPIDS

LDL-cholesterol levels in young women are significantly higher in smokers, regardless of oral contraceptive use status (47). HDL-cholesterol is lower in smokers of both genders, decreases after smoking adoption (48) but it increases after smoking cessation (48, 49).

HYPERTENSION

In the USA Nurses Study, the prevalence of hypertension in smokers was compared with that in women who did not smoke. Women smoking 1–14 cigarettes per day were 1.4 times more likely to report themselves hypertensive, while heavier smokers were three times as likely as nonsmokers to have high blood pressure (40). Smoking may also interfere with the pharmacologic treatment of hypertension (50).

DIABETES MELLITUS

Among diabetics, smoking doubles the risk of CAD events; nearly two-thirds of cardiovascular disease deaths in diabetics may be attributed to smoking (51). Further, smoking accelerates peripheral atherosclerosis, increasing the risk of claudication, ulceration, and gangrene (52).

HORMONAL FACTORS

It has been suggested that the metabolism of estradiol is increased in women who smoke, and that estrogen production is decreased in postmenopausal smokers.

Several studies of postmenopausal women revealed no differences in enodogenous estrogen levels between smokers and nonsmokers. Khaw et al. found significantly higher levels of adrenal androgens in women who smoke, suggesting another mechanism for the adverse effect of smoking on CAD development in women (53).

HEMATOLOGIC PARAMETERS

Smoking can adversely affect platelet levels and other hematologic parameters in several ways. At the sites of endothelial damage, platelet adhesion in smokers is increased, along with the tendency for hyperaggregability. In turn, these factors can lead to further activation of the coagulation system, deposition of fibrin, and further occlusion of the arterial lumen (54). Plasma fibrinogen levels are often increased in smokers, along with reduced capacity for fibrinolysis (55).

WEIGHT

Smokers have an increasing CAD risk with increasing body weight; in the Evans County Study, smokers in the heaviest tertile had twice the CAD rate of smokers in the lightest tertile (56).

Cross-sectional associations between smoking habits, body mass index, and waist-to-hip ratio were examined in more than one thousand men in a longitudinal study on aging. Although weight and body mass index were lower in smoking men of a given age, waist-to-hip ratio was higher in smokers. The ratio in those who started smoking actually increased, despite their loss in weight (57). Investigators of a retirement community in southern California had similar findings, noting a dose-response relation between cigarettes smoked and waist-to-hip ratio (58).

Persistence of smoking despite successful therapeutic weight reduction negates the beneficial effects of weight loss on

HDL- and LDL-cholesterol levels, particularly in women (59).

ALCOHOL

Because the heaviest consumers of alcohol are often heavy smokers (60), recent trials have examined the independent contributions of the two addictions to CAD development. Each adds to CAD risk, as noted in a Swedish Multifactor Primary Prevention Study of middle-aged men. Risk was highest in those who smoked and drank heavily (relative risk = 4.2) (61).

Cardiovascular Effects

There are several possibilities for the effects of smoking on CAD. These include a direct atherogenic effect, disturbances of coagulation function, exacerbation of a tendency toward coronary artery spasm, chronic effects of nicotine, and acute effects of carbon monoxide ingestion (62).

DIRECT SMOKING

Smoking increases sympathetic discharge and leads to increases in the adrenomedullary hormone epinephrine and the sympathetic neurotransmitter norepinephrine (63). This neurohumoral response appears to result in the downregulation of β-adrenergic receptors in long-term smokers (64).

Benowitz and co-workers documented the vasoconstrictive effects of nicotine, and found that it could be antagonized with concurrent alcohol administration (65). Adrenergically mediated increases in coronary artery tone can also be prevented by calcium-channel blocking drugs and nitroglycerin (66). Recent advances in the sensitivity of ambulatory electrocardiographic monitoring for silent myocardial ischemia allowed Barry and her co-workers to document that smokers have significantly more myocardial ischemia during their daily activities than do nonsmoking CAD patients (67).

PASSIVE SMOKING

Exposure to smoke within confined spaces such as commercial airplane cabins can represent a significant health hazard (24, 68), leading the surgeon general of the USA to issue a report on the health consequence of such involuntary smoking (69).

Approximately 85% of involuntary smoking exposure is from sidestream smoke, that which emanates from the end of the cigarette between puffs. The concentration of carbon monoxide is 2.5 times higher in sidestream smoke than in mainstream smoke inhaled and exhaled by the smoker. Sidestream smoke particles are smaller and more likely to penetrate deeper in distal alveoli (70). The mechanisms of increased risk are probably similar to those who receive the smoke directly (71).

The use of urinary excretion of cotinine has facilitated assessment of the health consequences to infants and children of involuntary smoking (72, 73). Parental smoking impairs pulmonary function (74) and has been associated with increased lower respiratory illness (75), middle-ear effusions and related infection (24), as well as reduced height in children (76).

In adults, involuntary smoking can exacerbate angina pectoris (77), and increase the relative risk of CAD development (78). Among participants in the Multiple Risk Factor Intervention Trial, men whose wives smoked had twice the risk of fatal coronary event, nonfatal event, or both, compared with men with nonsmoking wives (79).

Passive intake of cigarette smoke by nonsmoking spouses increases the risk of lung cancer (80) and may exacerbate other lung conditions as well (24). The weight of the scientific evidence on passive smoking has led a majority of the United States to legislate smoking restrictions in public facilities such as mass transit, hospitals, and elevators (70).

SMOKELESS TOBACCO

Chewing tobacco and snuff use (placing tobacco between gum and cheek) has reemerged within the USA in recent years. Adoption of these habits by adolescent and young adult males (81), may be related to the more visible use by major-league baseball players and other well-known athletes (82). Bogalusa Heart Study investigators noted a rise in smokeless tobacco use which accompanied decreased cigarette smoking in their biracial study population of children and adolescents (83). The increased use has occurred despite the increased risk of oral and other cancers. Patterns of its use meet the criteria for tobacco dependence (84).

In one study of educated adult males, those who used smokeless tobacco were 2.5 times more likely to have a serum cholesterol level of 6.2 mmol/liter (240 mg/dl) or more (85). Smokeless tobacco use has also been associated with elevated blood pressure in men aged 18 to 25 (86), which may result, at least in part, from its very high sodium content (87). Like smoking, use of smokeless tobacco is associated with an increased resting heart rate (88).

Influences on Smoking Adoption and Maintenance

More than 90% of regular smokers begin their habit before they reach the age of 20; a majority of Canadian children have tried smoking or are current smokers by age 13 (89). These facts raise the possibility that young persons are ill-informed about the hazards of adopting cigarette smoking. One study found that those chil-dren at greatest risk for smoking were the misinformed; they also held different beliefs and attitudes than nonsmokers. They greatly overestimated the prevalence of adult and peer smoking, underestimated the negative attitudes of their peers toward smoking, and felt they were less likely than others to contract a smoking-related illness (90). A British study found that those who eventually smoked reported that they believed teachers and parents would not mind if they took up smoking, but parental smoking attitudes, strictness and beliefs about the effects of smoking on health did not predict subsequent smoking behavior (91).

In the past decade, considerable effort has been devoted to prevention of smoking adoption by children and adolescents (92). Components of successful programs have included greater emphasis on prevention within schools (93–95) including enhanced teacher training (96), participation by the community (97), mass media campaigns (98), and ongoing evaluative research (99). Altman and colleagues have designed a community and merchant education campaign that has reduced the sales of cigarettes to minors by 50% within six months (100). Given the higher rate of adoption by young girls, different aproaches may be necessary for female-specific patterns of smoking (101). Similarly, higher levels of smoking among students who drop out of school will require interventions outside the classroom (102).

ADVERTISING

In January 1971, cigarette advertising was banned on commerical television in the USA. Smoking by characters in television programs dropped over the next decade, including that by actors portraying physicians (103). Unfortunately, advertising restrictions do not extend to the print media. Such advertisements represent a considerable source of revenue to magazines, and their appearance has been correlated with a lack of editorial content on the health hazards of smoking (104, 105). Special targets of print advertising have been women, blacks, Hispanics, blue-collar workers, children, adolescents, military personnel, and prison inmates (106). Health warning labeling on advertisements has not been effective in changing the attitudes of smokers (107, 108).

The tobacco and advertising communities have denied that advertising leads to increased levels of tobacco consumption, but such claims did not dissuade the surgeon general of the USA from calling for an advertising ban (109). Further, the National Institutes of Health in the USA have published strategies for countering the media efforts of the tobacco manufacturers (1).

PUBLIC RESPONSE

Health activists in several countries have organized effective actions against their respective tobacco industries and governments, despite huge differences in financial resources (110). Among many creative antismoking efforts have been liability lawsuits against manufacturers (111), monetary incentives from employers for smoking cessation and abstinence (112), and removal of magazines containing cigarette advertisements from primary physicians' waiting rooms (113). Increasing taxes on cigarette purchases will help pay for smoking-related illnesses and may reduce smoking adoption and maintenance by adolescents and poor adults (114, 115). Lower insurance rates for nonsmokers may also encourage avoidance of smoking.

PHYSICIANS

While the influence of physicians in antismoking efforts is clearly acknowledged by the public, pessimism continues among physicians regarding the effective-

ness of such efforts. However, the importance of physician intervention in this regard cannot be overstated. Physicians in the United Kingdom and the United States have contact with at least 70% of all smokers each year, including a majority of those smokers who consider themselves to be in excellent health (116).

In recent years, the USA government has provided extensive literature on opportunities for smoking intervention for the "busy physician" (69) and a review and evaluation of smoking cessation methods in Canada and United States (117). In addition, studies have demonstrated that strategies for improving physicians' effectiveness in antismoking counseling have produced results that are both statistically and clinically significant (118, 119).

Ockene and colleagues use a three-hour training program that teaches physicians a patient-centered counseling approach. Their recommended techniques include elicitation from the patient of desire and motivation to change smoking behavior, past experiences in such changes, resources and barriers to change, ways of coping with obstacles, and establishment of a firm plan for change and careful follow-up. Open-ended questioning allows exploration of these issues more readily than the simple provision of factual information about the health hazards of smoking (120).

Prior unsuccessful attempts can be reframed as successes of limited duration and analyzed for expected obstacles and resources for the next attempt. Several techniques may aid the quitting smoker. These include maintenance of a diary in which times, places, and feelings are recorded when the urge to smoke appears. One can also make cigarettes inaccessible, such as buying one pack at a time and placing it in the refrigerator or on a high shelf, to minimize the ease of smoking the next cigarette. The patient is encouraged to choose a quitting date and then agree to (and sign) a structural plan for quitting. Copies of the agreement are given to the patient and placed in the patient's chart.

Techniques such as proper prescription of nicotine gum and the labeling of smokers' charts have facilitated smoking cessation by patients in a city-county teaching hospital (121). In general, frequent reinforcement by the physician and office staff members appears to be the single most important determinant in helping patients remain abstinent (122).

Advocacy by physicians for establishing smoke-free hospitals can also result in a significant reduction in exposure of children and adults to smoke (123), particularly when implemented on a system-wide basis, such as in the Indian Health Service (124).

EMPLOYMENT

Although most smokers establish their habit before they begin their working careers, the environment of the workplace can reinforce their smoking behavior. Smokers coalesce during breaks, meals, and meetings. Peer modeling and social pressure often interrupt quitting attempts (125). Blue-collar workers have the highest smoking prevalence and display the least interest in quitting (126). Persons receiving less peer support at the worksite have higher smoking rates, as do those with lower status, greater conflict, and longer working hours (127).

The introduction of women into male-dominated workplaces has had little or no effect on the womens' smoking adoption and maintenance. Unemployment among both genders is associated with higher smoking rates (128).

FAMILY

Significant smoking concordance exists among marriage partners, particularly among younger couples with the least education (129). Partner support is the primary predictor of smoking cessation maintenance among married women (130). Adults who are divorced or separated have the highest prevalance of smoking, while never-married adults are least likely to have ever adopted smoking (131).

In low-income families, smoking appears to provide a way of coping for mothers with preschool children. Since the smoking behavior of parents is a significant predictor of smoking adoption by children, this population represents an important target group for future efforts (132).

Smoking Reduction and Cessation

Ninety percent of smokers express a desire to quit, and one in six of these attempts to do so each year. A majority of persons who have quit smoking have done so on their own, but others have participated in education, behavior modification, hypnosis, or acupuncture or drug therapy programs with variable results (133).

Smokers who quit are qualitatively different from those who do not (134). The person who complies with medial advice, regardless of its content, is more likely to live longer. In the Coronary Drug Project, adherence to randomization to active drug or placebo was associated with improved survival compared to individuals who did not comply well to either regimen (135).

Prochaska and DiClemente have described several stages in quitting. These include preparation, quitting, early maintenance, late maintenance, and recycling (136).

CIGARETTE YIELD

Cigarette brands vary widely in tar, nicotine, and carbon monoxide content (137), and smokers commonly believe that changing to a brand lower in tar or nicotine will reduce their risks to health. While mortality from lung, oropharynx, esophagus, and bladder cancer is reduced with reduction in tar (138), no evidence is available suggesting a reduction in cardiovascular disease risk. Men smoking filter cigarettes have comparable CAD risk to those using nonfilter cigarettes (139), and those switching to cigars or pipes remain at the same risk (140). Smokers of lower nicotine cigarettes tend to smoke more cigarettes per day; other compensation is achieved by deeper inhalation and smoking more of each cigarette (141). In a case-control study of women experiencing their first MI, there was no lower risk among women smoking cigarettes with lower yields of carbon monoxide and nicotine (142).

CLINICAL TRIALS

Several large-scale trials have successfully reduced smoking among participants in the intervention groups, including the North Karelia Project in Finland (133), the Belgian Heart Disease Prevention Project (143), the Oslo Study Diet and Antismoking Trial (144), and the Whitehall Study of London civil servants (145). In the Multiple Risk Factor Intervention Trial, antismoking therapy consisted of 8 to 10 weeks of educational group sessions and individual treatment. After six years, 46% were abstinent at four years. Of those who remained abstinent at four months, 56% were abstinent at all visits through the 48-month follow-up period (146).

In large observational studies, such as the Framingham Study, persons who quit smoking have been noted to have CAD event rates only one-half of those who continue smoking (147). Investigators from the Coronary Artery Surgery Study (CASS) found that older persons benefited from smoking cessation as much as younger subjects (35).

USE OF NICOTINE GUM

Continued smoking is due, at least in part, to dependence on nicotine (148). The use of nicotine gum as a prescription drug to facilitate smoking cessation has been based on several hypotheses: that persons smoke to obtain the psychoactive properties of nicotine, that smokers experience nicotine withdrawal upon cessation, and that gradual withdrawal of nicotine would minimize symptoms. When chewed, the 2 mg pieces release nicotine at a uniform rate. The full effects are noted approximately 15 to 20 minutes after chewing begins, thus prophylactic use (before the urge for a cigarette) may be necessary. When subjects are confident of their ability to abstain from smoking, they should begin to taper gum use over a three- to four-week period (149). Nicotine gum use is most effective in combination with group counseling (150), and its cost-effectiveness is similar to that of pharmacologic treatment of hypertension or dyslipidemias (151). Its use, coupled with physical activity, can minimize weight gain after smoking cessation (152), which results from a decreased energy expenditure (153, 154).

REDUCTION IN RISK AFTER CESSATION

Many early reports indicated that one's CAD risk reverted to that of nonsmokers within two years after smoking cessation. These studies include the Western Collaborative Group Study (155), the Framingham Study (147), a study of British female physicians (156), an investigation of men under 55 years of age (157), and a study of women under age 65 in the United States (158). These findings suggest that the effect of smoking is less on atherogenesis and more on thrombosis or coronary artery spasm (159). Meade and colleagues noted that clotting factor levels in ex-smokers remained higher than those in never-smokers for up to five years after cessation (160).

However, not all investigations have noted a quick reduction in CAD risk. In the British Regional Heart Study, risk persisted for up to 20 years after quitting (161). In a retrospective study of Irish women and men admitted for a first episode of MI or unstable angina, investigators noted that ex-smokers tended to be slightly older and had a considerably higher prevalence of hypertension, which accounted for the small difference in calculated risk between current smokers and ex-smokers (162). In almost every study of post-MI patients subsequent mortality is cut in half among those who quit smoking and remain abstinent (163).

RELAPSE

Relapse prevention components include motivation, social support, coping skills, and pharmacotherapy. Motivation is particularly important during the early maintenance phase, and can be facilitated by social support from family members and co-workers. Coping skills include avoidance of high-risk situations and resistance to the cravings that may last for years and may result in a majority of relapse incidents. Nicotine gum facilitates maintenance when used as described above, while reports of the use of clonidine in smoking cessation have mixed results (164, 165).

SMOKING AND PREGNANCY

Among women 20 to 44 years of age in the United States, approximately 27% quit smoking upon learning they were pregnant; another 12% quit smoking later in pregnancy. Women smoking fewer than 20 cigarettes per day were five times more likely to quit than those smoking more. Women with 16 years or more of education were four times more likely to quit than women with less than 12 years of educa-

tion. Of those women who quit, half resumed smoking within three months after delivery, and another 20% relapsed within the following nine months, but there was no educational difference in smoking resumption rates (166).

REFERENCES

1. US Department of Health and Human Services. Reducing the health consequences of smoking: 25 years of progress. A report of the surgeon general. Washington: Public Health Service, 1989, DHHS Publication no. (CDC) 89-8411.

2. Remington PL, Novotny TE, Williamson DF, Anda RF. State-specific progress toward the 1990 objective for the nation for cigarette smoking prevalence. Am J Public Health 1989;79:1419-1421.

3. Masironi R, Rothwell K. Tendances et effets due tabagisme dans le monde. World Health Statistics Quarterly 1988;41:228-241.

4. Fielding JE. Smoking and women. Tragedy of the majority. N Engl J Med 1987;317:1343-1345.

5. Fiore MC, Novotny TE, Pierce JP, Hatziandreu EJ, Patel KM, Davis RM. Trends in cigarette smoking in the United States. The changing influence of gender and race. JAMA 1989;261:49-55.

6. Orleans CT, Schoenbach VJ, Salmon MA, et al. A survey of smoking and quitting patterns among black Americans. Am J Public Health 1989;79:176-181.

7. Rogers RG, Crank J. Ethnic differences in smoking patterns: findings from NHIS. Public Health Rep 1988;103:387-393.

8. Marin G, Perez-Stable EJ, Marin BV. Cigarette smoking among San Francisco Hispanics: the role of acculturation and gender. Am J Public Health 1989;79:196-199.

9. Fielding JE. Smoking: health effects and control. N Engl J Med 1985;313:491-498, 555-565.

10. Tobacco Reporter. World leaf trade: exports fall to 1.35 million tons. Tobacco Reporter. 1988;115(2):36-38,40.

11. American Public Health Association. Limiting the exportation of tobacco products. Am J Public Health 1988;78:195-196.

12. Hay DR, Foster FH. Intercensal trends in cigarette smoking in New Zealand. 2. Social and occupational factors. NZ Med J 1984;97:395–398.

13. Statistics Canada. Health and social support, 1985. Ottawa: Canadian Government Publishing Centre, 1987.

14. Pierce JP, Fiore MC, Novotny TE, Hatziandreu EJ, Davis RM. Trends in cigarette smoking in the United States. Projections to the year 2000. JAMA 1989;261:61–65.

15. McGinnis JM, Shopland D, Brown C. Tobacco and health: trends in smoking and smokeless tobacco consumption in the United States. Ann Rev Public Health 1987;8:441–467.

16. Sachs DP. Smoking habits of pulmonary physicians. N Engl J Med 1983;309:799.

17. Enstrome JE. Trends in mortality among California physicians after giving up smoking: 1950–79. Br Med J. 1983;286:1101–1105.

18. Hay DR. Intercensal trends in cigarette smoking by New Zealand doctors and nurses. NZ Med J 1984;97:253–255.

19. Dore K, Hoey J. Smoking practices, knowledge and attitudes regarding smoking of university hospital nurses. Can J Public Health 1988;79:170–174.

20. Sande L, Casariego J, Posada I, Llorian A. Asturias study: smoking habits in health professionals. Eur Heart J 1988;9(Suppl A):143.

21. Anonymous. Cigarette smoking around the world. Lancet. 1988;2:117–118.

22. Kozlowski LT. Pack size, reported cigarette smoking rates, and public health. Am J Public Health 1986;76:1337–1338.

23. Kozlowski LT, Herman CP, Frecker RC. What researchers make of what cigarette smokers say: filtering smokers' hot air. Lancet 1980;1:699–700.

24. Fielding JE, Phenow KJ. Health effects of involuntary smoking. N Engl J Med 1988;319:1452–1460.

25. Luepker RV, Pallonen UE, Murray DM, Pirie PL. Validity of telephone surveys in assessing cigarette smoking in young adults. Am J Public Health 1989;79:202–204.

26. Krall EA, Valadian I, Dwyer JT, Gardner J. Accuracy of recalled smoking data. Am J Public Health 1989;79:200–206.

27. Persson PG, Norell SE. Retrospective versus original information on cigarette smoking. Implications for epidemiologic studies. Am J Epidemiol 1989;130:705–712.

28. Gill JS, Shipley MJ, Tsementzis SA, et al. Cigarette smoking. A risk factor for hemorrhagic and nonhemorrhagic stroke. Arch Intern Med 1989;149:2053–2057.

29. Floderus B, Cederlof R, Friberg L. Smoking and mortality: a 21-year follow-up based on the Swedish Twin Registry. Int J Epidemiol 1988;17:332–340.

30. Haapanen A, Koskenvuo M, Kaprio J, Kesaniemi YA, Heikkila K. Carotid arteriosclerosis in identical twins discordant for cigarette smoking. Circulation 1989;80:10–16.

31. Abbott RD, Yin Y, Reed DM, Yano K. Risk of stroke in male cigarette smokers. N Engl J Med 1986;315:717–720.

32. Wolf PA, D'Agostino RB, Kannel WB, et al. Cigarette smoking as a risk factor for stroke: the Framingham Study. JAMA 1988;259:1025–1029.

33. Vlietstra RE, Kronmal RA, Oberman A, Frye RL, Killip T III. Effect of cigarette smoking on survival of patients with angiographically documented coronary artery disease. Report from the CASS registry. JAMA 1986;255:1023–1027.

34. Wilhelmsen L. Cessation of smoking after myocardial infarction: effects on mortality after ten years. Br Heart J 1988;49:416–422.

35. Hermanson B, Omenn GS, Kronmal RA, et al. Beneficial six-year outcome of smoking cessation in older men and women with coronary artery disease. Results from the CASS Registry. N Engl Med 1988;319:1365–1369.

36. Salonen JT. Stopping smoking and long-term mortality after acute myocardial infarction. Br. Heart J 1980;43:463–469.

37. Hallstrom AP, Cobb LA, Ray R. Smoking as a risk factor for recurrence of sudden cardiac arrest. N Engl J Med 1986;314:271–275.

38. Daly LE, Graham IM, Hickey N, Mulcahy R. Does stopping smoking delay onset of angina after infarction? Br Med J 1985;291:935–937.

39. Blumenthal JA, Levenson RM. Behavioral approaches to secondary preven-

tion of coronary heart disease. Circulation 1987;76(Suppl I):I130–I137.

40. Willett WC, Green A, Stampfer MJ, et al. Relative and absolute excess risks of coronary heart disease among women who smoke cigarettes. N Engl J Med 1987;317:1303–1309.

41. Higgins C, Schweiger MJ. Smoking termination patterns in a cardiac rehabilitation program. J Cardiac Rehabil 1983;3:55–59.

42. Spain DM, Siegel H, Bradess VA. Women smokers and sudden death. JAMA 1973;224:1005–1007.

43. Schatzkin A, Cupples LA, Heeren T, Morelock S, Kannel WB. Sudden death in the Framingham Heart Study. Am J Epidemiol 1984;120:888–899.

44. Suhonen O, Reunanen A, Knekt P, Aromaa A. Risk factors for sudden and nonsudden coronary death. Acta Med Scand 1988;223:19–25.

45. Coldtiz GA, Bonita R, Stampfer MJ, et al. Cigarette smoking and risk of stroke in middle-aged women. N Engl J Med 1988;318:937–941.

46. Bonita R, Scragg R, Stewart A, Jackson R, Beaglehole R. Cigarette smoking and risk of premature stroke in men and women. Br Med J 1986;293:6–8.

47. Willett W, Hennekens CH, Castelli W, et al. Effects of cigarette smoking on fasting triglyceride, total cholesterol, and HDL-cholesterol in women. Am Heart J 1983;105:417–421.

48. Fortmann SP, Haskell WL, Williams PT. Changes in plasma high density lipoprotein cholesterol after changes in cigarette use. Am J Epidemiol 1986;124:706–710.

49. Stubbe I, Eskilsson J, Nilsson-Ehle P. High-density lipoprotein concentrations after stopping smoking. Br Med J 1982;284:1511–1513.

50. Materson BJ, Reda D, Freis ED, Henderson WG. Cigarette smoking interferes with treatment of hypertension. Arch Intern Med 1988;148:2116–2119.

51. Suarez L, Barrett-Connor E. Interaction between cigarette smoking and diabetes mellitus in the prediction of death attributed to cardiovascular disease. Am J Epidemiol 1984;120:670–675.

52. Beach KW, Brunzell JD, Strandness DE Jr. Prevalence of severe arteriosclerosis obliterans in patients with diabetes mellitus. Relation to smoking and form of therapy. Arteriosclerosis 1982;2:275–280.

53. Khaw KT, Tazuke S, Barrett-Connor E. Cigarette smoking and levels of adrenal androgens in postmenopausal women. N Engl J Med 1988;318:1705–1709.

54. Belch JJ. The effects of acute smoking on platelet behavior, fibrinolysis, and hemorheology in habitual smokers. Thromb Haemost 1984;51:6–8.

55. Iso H, Folsom AR, Wu KK, et al. Hemostatic variables in Japanese and Caucasian men. Am J Epidemiol 1989;130:925–934.

56. Heyden S, Cassel JC, Bartel A, Tyroler HA, Hames CG, Cornoni JC. Body weight and cigarette smoking as risk factors. Arch Intern Med 1971;128:915–919.

57. Shimokata H, Muller DC, Andres R. Studies in the distribution of body fat. III. Effects of cigarette smoking. JAMA 1989;261:1169–1173.

58. Barrett-Connor E, Khaw KT. Cigarette smoking and increased central adiposity. Ann Intern Med 1989;111:783–787.

59. Van Gaal LF, DeLeeuw IH. Effects of smoking on lipid parameters during therapeutic weight loss. Atherosclerosis 1986;60:287–290.

60. Gordon T, Doyle JT. Alcohol consumption and its relationship to smoking, weight, blood pressure, and blood lipids. Arch Intern Med 1986;146:262–265.

61. Rosengren A, Wilhelmsen L, Wedel H. Separate and combined effects of smoking and alcohol abuse in middle-aged men. Acta Med Scand 1988;223:111–118.

62. Davidson DM. Carbon monoxide effects in persons with symptomatic coronary artery disease. Thesis, University of California, Irvine, 1987, 93 pp.

63. Cryer PE, Haymond MW, Santiago JV, Shah SD. Norepinephrine and epinephrine release and adrenergic mediation of smoking-associated hemodynamic and metabolic events. N Engl. J Med 1976;295:573–577.

64. Laustiola KE, Lassila R, Kaprio J, Koskenvuo M. Decreased β-adrenergic receptor density and catecholamine response in male cigarette smokers. Circulation 1988;78:1234–1240.

65. Benowitz NL, Jones RT, Jacob P III. Additive cardiovascular effects of nicotine and alcohol. Clin Pharmacol Ther 1986;40:420–424.

66. Winniford MD, Jansen DE, Reynolds GA, Apprill P, Black WH, Hillis LD. Cigarette smoking-induced coronary vasoconstriction in atherosclerotic coronary artery disease and prevention by calcium antagonists and nitroglycerin. Am J Cardiol 1987;59:203–207.

67. Barry J, Mead K, Nabel EG, et al. Effect of smoking on the activity of ischemic heart disease. JAMA 1989;261:398–402.

68. Mattson ME, Boyd G, Byar D, et al. Passive smoking on commercial airline flights. JAMA 1989;261:867–872.

69. US Department of Health and Human Services. The health consequences of involuntary smoking. A report of the surgeon general. Washington: Public Health Service, 1986. DHHS Publication no. (CDC) 87-8398.

70. Byrd JC, Shapiro RS, Schiedermayer DL. Passive smoking: a review of medical and legal issues. Am J Public Health 1989;79:209–215.

71. Davis JW, Shelton L, Watanabe IS, Arnold J. Passive smoking affects endothelium and platelets. Arch Intern Med 1989;149:386–389.

72. Greenberg RA, Haley NJ, Etzel RA, Loda FA. Measuring the exposure of infants to tobacco smoke. N Engl J Med 1984;310:1075–1078.

73. Jarvis MJ, McNeill AD, Russell MA, West RJ, Bryant A, Feyerabend C. Passive smoking in adolescents: one-year stability of exposure in the home. Lancet 1987;1:1324–1325.

74. Tager IB, Weiss ST, Munoz A, Rosner B, Speizer FE. Longitudinal study of the effects of maternal smoking on pulmonary smoking in children. N Engl J Med 1983;309:699–703.

75. Fergusson DM, Horwood LJ, Shannon FT, Taylor B. Parental smoking and lower respiratory illness in the first three years of life. J Epidemiol Comm Health 1981;35:180–184.

76. Rona RJ, Florey C, Clarke GC, Chinn S. Parental smoking at home and height of children. Br Med J 1981;283:1363.

77. Aronow WS. Effect of passive smoking on angina pectoris. N Engl J Med 1978;299:21–24.

78. Garland C, Barrett-Connor E, Suarez L, Criqui MH, Wingard DL. Effects of passive smoking on ischemic heart disease mortality of nonsmokers. A prospective study. Am J Epidemiol 1985;121:645–650.

79. Svendsen K, Kuller LH, Martin MJ, Ockene JK. Effects of passive smoking in the Multiple Risk Factor Intervention Trial. Am J Epidemiol 1987;126:783–795.

80. Hirayama T. Non-smoking wives of heavy smokers have a higher risk of lung cancer: a study from Japan. Br Med J 1981;282:183–185.

81. Koop CE. The campaign against smokeless tobacco. N Engl J Med 1986; 314:1042–1044.

82. Connolly GN, Orleans CT, Kogan M. Use of smokeless tobacco in major-league baseball. N Engl J Med 1988;318:1281–1285.

83. Hunter SM, Croft JB, Burke GL, Parker FC, Webber LS, Berenson GS. Longitudinal patterns of cigarette smoking and smokeless tobacco use in youth: the Bogalusa Heart Study. Am J Public Health 1986;76:193–195.

84. Connolly GN, Winn DM, Hecht SS, Henningfield JE, Walker B Jr, Hoffman D. The reemergence of smokeless tobacco. N Engl J Med 1986;314:1020–1027.

85. Tucker LA. Use of smokeless tobacco, cigarette smoking, and hypercholesterolemia. Am J Public Health 1989;79:1048–1050.

86. Schroeder KL, Chen MS Jr. Smokeless tobacco and blood pressure. N Engl J Med 1985;312:919.

87. Hampson NB. Smokeless is not saltless. N Engl J Med 1985;312:919–920.

88. Benowitz NL, Jacob P III, Yu L. Daily use of smokeless tobacco: systemic effects. Ann Intern Med 1989;111:112–116.

89. Brown KS, Cherry WH, Forbes WF. The 1978 national survey of smoking habits of Canadian school children. Can J Public Health 1986;77:139–146.

90. Leventhal H, Glynn K, Fleming R. Is the smoking decision an "informed choice"? Effect of smoking risk factors on smoking beliefs. JAMA 1987;257:3373–3376.

91. McNeill AD, Jarvis MJ, Stapleton JA, et al. Prospective study of factors predicting uptake of smoking in adolescents. J Epidemiol Comm Health 1988;43:72–78.

92. Silvestri B, Flay BR. Smoking education: comparison of practice and state-of-the-art. Prev Med 1989;18:257–266.

93. Vartiainen E, Fallonen U, McAlister AL, Puska P: Eight-year follow-up results of an adolescent smoking prevention program: the North Karelia Youth Project. Am J Public Health 1990;80:78–79.

94. Pentz MA, Brannon BR, Charlin VL, Barrett EJ, MacKinnon DP, Flay BR. The power of policy: the relationship of smoking policy to adolescent smoking. Am J Public Health 1989;79:1372–1376.

95. Flay BR, Koepke D, Thomson SJ, Santi S, Best JA, Brown KS. Six-year followup of the first Waterloo school smoking prevention trial. Am J Public Health 1989;79:1371–1376.

96. Tortu S, Botvin GJ. School-based smoking prevention: the teacher training process. Prev Med 1989;18:280–289.

97. Becker SL, Burke JA, Arbogast RA, Naughton MJ, Bachman I, Spohn E. Community programs to enhance in-school anti-tobacco efforts. Prev Med 1989;18:221–228.

98. Pentz MA, MacKinnon DP, Flay BR, Hansen WB, Johnson CA, Dwyer JH. Primary prevention of chronic diseases in adolescence: effects of the Midwestern Prevention Project on tobacco use. Am J Epidemiol 1989;130:713–724.

99. Pirie PL, Thomson SJ, Mann SL, et al. Tracking and attrition in longitudinal school-based smoking prevention research. Prev Med 1989;130:249–256.

100. Altman DG, Foster V, Rasenick-Douss L, Tye JB. Reducing the illegal sale of cigarettes to minors. JAMA 1989;261:80–83.

101. Gilchrist LD, Schinke SP, Nurius P. Reducing onset of habitual smoking among women. Prev Med 1989;18:235–248.

102. Pirie PL, Murray DM, Luepker RV. Smoking prevalence in a cohort of adolescents, including absentees, dropouts, and transfers. Am J Public Health 1988;78:176–178.

103. Breed W, DeFoe JR. Cigarette smoking on television, 1950–1982. N Engl J Med 1983;309:617.

104. Kitchens CS. Cigarette ads in the *Ladies' Home Journal.* N Engl J Med 1984;311:51–52.

105. Warner KE. Cigarette advertising and media coverage of smoking and health. N Engl J Med 1985;312:384–388.

106. Davis RM. Current trends in cigarette advertising and marketing. N Engl J Med 1987;316:725–732.

107. Fischer PM, Richards JW Jr, Berman EJ, Krugman DM. Recall and eye tracking study of adolescents viewing tobacco advertisements. JAMA 1989;261:84–89.

108. Davis RM, Kendrick JS. The surgeon general's warnings in outdoor cigarette advertising. JAMA 1989;261:90–94.

109. Koop CE. A parting shot at tobacco. JAMA 1989;262:2894–2895.

110. Jacobson B. Smoking and health: a new generation of campaigners. Br Med J 1983;287:483–484.

111. Charney ML. Tobacco-products liability lawsuits as an anti-smoking strategy. N Engl J Med 1986;314:587.

112. Warner KE, Hurt HA. Economic incentives for health. Ann Rev Public Health 1984;5:107–133.

113. Radovsky L, Barry PP. Tobacco advertisements in physicians' offices: a pilot study of physician attitudes. Am J Public Health 1988;78:174–175.

114. Manning WG, Keeler EB, Newhouse JP, Sloss EM, Wasserman J. The taxes of sin. Do smokers and drinkers pay their way? JAMA 1989;261:1604–1609.

115. Leigh JP. Cigarette taxes—regressive or progressive? West J Med 1989;150:467.

116. British Thoracic Society. Comparison of four methods of smoking withdrawal in patients with smoking-related diseases. Br Med J 1983;286:595–597.

117. US Department of Health and Human Services. Review and evaluation of smoking cessation methods: the United States and Canada, 1978–1985. Washington: Public Health Service, 1987. NIH Publication no. 87-2940.

118. Ockene JK. Physician-delivered interventions for smoking cessation: strategies for increasing effectiveness. Prev Med 1987;16:723–737.

119. Prochazka AV, Boyko EJ. How physicians can help their patients quit smoking. A practical guide. West J Med 1988;149:188–194.

120. Ockene JK, Quirk ME, Goldberg RJ, et al. A residents' training program for the development of smoking intervention skills. Arch Intern Med 1988;148:1039–1045.

121. Cohen SJ, Stookey GK, Katz BP, Drook CA, Smith DM. Encouraging primary care physicians to help smokers quit. A randomized controlled trial. Ann Intern Med 1989;110:648–652.

122. Kottke TE, Battista RN, DeFriese GH, Brekke ML. Attributes of successful smoking cessation interventions in medical practice. A meta-analysis of 39 controlled trials. JAMA 1988;259:2883–2889.

123. Becker DM, Conner HF, Warnach HR, et al. The impact of a total ban on smoking in the Johns Hopkins Childrens' Center. JAMA 1989;262:799–802.

124. Rhoades ER, Fairbanks LL. Smoke-free facilities in the Indian Health Service. N Engl J Med 1985;313:1548.

125. Schilling RF II, Gilchrist LD, Schinke SP. Smoking in the workplace: review of critical issues. Public Health Reports 1985;100:473–479.

126. Sorensen G, Pechacek T. Occupational and sex differences in smoking and smoking cessation. J Occup Med 1986;28:360–364.

127. Westman M, Eden D, Shirom A. Job stress, cigarette smoking and cessation: the conditioning effects of peer support. Soc Sci Med 1985;20:637–644.

128. Waldron I, Lye D. Employment, unemployment, occupation and smoking. Am J Prev Med 1989;5:142–149.

129. Venters MH, Jacobs DR Jr, Leupker RV, Maiman LA, Gillum RF. Spouse concordance of smoking patterns: the Minnesota Heart Survey. Am J Epidemiol 1984;120:608–616.

130. Coppotelli HC, Orleans CT. Partner support and other determinants of smoking cessation maintenance among women. J Consult Clin Psychol 1985;53:455–460.

131. Waldron I, Lye D. Family roles and smoking. Am J Prev Med 1989;5:136–141.

132. Graham H. Women's smoking and family health. Soc Sci Med 1987;25:47–56.

133. Health and Public Policy Committee of the American College of Physicians. Methods for stopping cigarette smoking. Ann Intern Med 1986;105:281–291.

134. Kabat GC, Wynder EL. Determinants of quitting smoking. Am J Public Health 1987;77:1301–1305.

135. Coronary Drug Project Research Group. Influence of adherence to treatment and response of cholesterol on mortality in the Coronary Drug Project. N Engl J Med 1980;303:1038–1041.

136. Prochaska JO, DiClements CC. Stages and processes of self-change of smoking: toward an integrative model of change. J Consult Clin Psychol 1983;51:390–395.

137. US Federal Trade Commission. Report of tar, nicotine, and carbon monoxide of the smoke of 200 varieties of cigarettes. Washington: Federal Trade Commission, 1981.

138. Lee PN, Garfinkel L. Mortality and type of cigarette smoked. J Epidemiol Comm Health 1981;35:16–22.

139. Castelli WP, Garrison RJ, Dawber TR, McNamara PM, Feinleib M, Kannel WB. The filter cigarette and coronary heart disease: the Framingham Study. Lancet 1981;2:109–113.

140. Pechacek TF, Folsom AR, de Gaudermaris R, et al. Smoke exposure in pipe and cigar smokers: serum thiocyanate measures. JAMA 1985;254:3330–3332.

141. Maron DJ, Fortmann SP. Nicotine yield and measures of cigarette smoke exposure in a large population: are lower-yield cigarettes safer? Am J Public Health 1987;77:546–549.

142. Palmer JR, Rosenberg L, Shapiro S. Low yield cigarettes and the risk of nonfatal myocardial infarction in women. N Engl J Med 1989;320:1569–1573.

143. Kornitzer M, Dramaix M, Kittel F, DeBacker G. The Belgian Heart Disease Prevention Project: changes in smoking habits after two years of intervention. Prev Med 1980;9:496–503.

144. Hjermann I, Holme I, Leren P. Oslo Study Diet and Antismoking Trial. Results after 102 months. Am J Med 1986;80(suppl 2A):7–11.

145. Rose G, Hamilton PJ, Colwell L, Shipley MJ. A randomised controlled trial of anti-smoking advice: 10-year results. J Epidemiol Comm Health 1982;36:102–108.

146. Hughes GH, Hymowitz N, Ockene JK, Simon N, Vogt TM. the Multiple Risk Factor Intervention Trial (MRFIT). V. Intervention on smoking. Prev Med 1981;10:476–500.

147. Gordon T, Kannel WB, McGee D, Dawber TR. Death and coronary attacks in men

after giving up cigarette smoking. Lancet 1974;2:1345–1348.

148. US Department of Health and Human Services. Smoking: nicotine addiction. A Report of the Surgeon General. Washington: Public Health Service, 1988. DHHS Publication no. (CDC)88–8406.

149. Hughes JR, Miller SA. Nicotine gum to help stop smoking. JAMA 1984;252:2855–2858.

150. Tonnesen P, Fryd V, Hansen M, et al. Effect of nicotine chewing gum in combination with group counseling on the cessation of smoking. N Engl J Med 1988;318:15–18.

151. Oster G, Huse DM, Delea TE, Colditz GA. Cost-effectiveness of nicotine gum as an adjunct to physician's advice against cigarette smoking. JAMA 1986;256:1315–1318.

152. Perkins KA, Epstein LH, Marks BL, Stiller RL, Jacob RG. The effect of nicotine on energy expenditure during light physical activity. N Engl J Med 1989;320:898–903.

153. Hoftstetter A, Schutz Y, Jequier E, Wahren J. Increased 24-hour energy expenditure in cigarette smokers. N Engl J Med 1986;314:79–82.

154. Rigotti NA. Cigarette smoking and body weight. N Engl J Med 1989;320:931–933.

155. Jenkins CD, Rosenman RH, Zyzanski SJ. Cigarette smoking: its relationship to coronary heart disease and related risk factors in the Western Collaborative Study. Circulation 1968;38:1140–1155.

156. Doll R, Gray R, Hafner B, Peto R. Mortality in relation to smoking: 22 years observation on female British doctors. Br Med J 1980;1:967–971.

157. Rosenberg L, Kaufman D, Helmrich S, Shapiro S. The risk of myocardial infarction after quitting smoking in men under 55 years of age. N Engl J Med 1985;313:1511–1514.

158. Rosenberg L, Palmer JR, Shapiro S. Decline in the risk of myocardial infarction among women who stop smoking. N Engl J Med 1990;322:213–217.

159. Hartz AJ, Barboriak PN, Anderson AJ, Hoffman RG, Barboriak JJ. Smoking, coronary artery occlusion and nonfatal myocardial infarction. JAMA 1981;246:851–853.

160. Meade TW, Imeson J, Stirling Y. Effects of changes in smoking and other characteristics on clotting factors and the risk of ischaemic heart disease. Lancet 1987;2:986–988.

161. Cook DG, Shaper AG, Pocock SJ, Kussick SJ. Giving up smoking and the risk of heart attacks: a report from the British Regional Heart Study. Lancet 1986;2:1376–1380.

162. Robinson K, Conroy RM, Mulcahy R. When does the risk of acute coronary heart disease in ex-smokers fall to that in non-smokers? Br Heart J 1989;62:16–19.

163. Mulcahy R. Influence of cigarette smoking on morbidity and mortality after myocardial infarction. Br. Heart J 1983;49:410–415.

164. Ornish SA, Zisook S, McAdams LA. Effects of transdermal clonidine treatment on withdrawal symptoms associated with smoking cessation. Arch Intern Med 1988;148:2027–2031.

165. Franks P, Harp J, Bell B. Randomized controlled trial of clonidine for smoking cessation in a primary care setting. JAMA 1989;262:3011–3013.

166. Fingerhut LA, Kleinman JC, Kendrick JS. Smoking before, during and after pregnancy. Am J Public Health 1990;80:541–544.

6

family history

Among the risk indicators for coronary artery disease (CAD), several have familial components (1–3), such as the dyslipidemias (4, 5), hypertension (6, 7), diabetes (8), and obesity (9). Shared environment also accounts for familial patterns in smoking, eating habits (10), and physical activity (11).

While these associations are discussed further in the specific chapters on those topics, this chapter focuses at the epidemiologic level on the relation of family history to CAD. In some cases, the length of parental life has been the outcome measure (regardless of cause of death). Even with this coarse indicator, offspring of persons who die young are significantly more likely to die themselves from cardiovascular and cerebrovascular disease (12, 13). In an early study, Hammond and colleagues arrayed parental and grandparental longevity into seven discrete categories (e.g., class 1: both parents still living and over 70 or they both survived to 80, at least one grandparent over 80; class 7: both parents died before age 70). Differences among groups were significant for mortality from CAD, hypertensive heart disease, and stroke (14). Such findings reemphasize the need to not only document the presence of CAD in the family history but also record the age of onset (15).

Research to date may be grouped in three main areas, depending on the age of the subjects. Within each age group, studies have looked both at persons with documented CAD and at those at high risk for its development. With these propositi, events and risk in parents, siblings, grandparents, children, and spouses have been investigated.

YOUNG ADULTS

Several studies have documented myocardial infarction (MI) in adults at an early age (commonly defined as men younger than 45, women under the age of 55), so these age limits will arbitrary define "young adults" in this chapter unless other noted.

CAD in Parents and Siblings

In a Canadian study of male MI survivors, subjects aged 50 and below were twice as likely to have a history of parental CAD (16). In a British study of 121 men and 96 women with CAD and 209 controls, the ages and causes of death for all first-degree relatives were determined. Women with documented CAD before age 65 were seven times more likely than control women to have a history of CAD death in a male relative younger than 55 or in a female relative below the age of 65. For male propositi under 55, their male and female relatives were 5 and 2.5 times more likely to have experienced CAD death, respectively (17). Dolder and Oliver reported results from a nine-country study of male MI survivors age 40 or less; 15% reported CAD deaths of their fathers. 7% reported maternal deaths, and 3% indicated sibling death due to CAD. This was particularly prevalent in Edinburgh, Scotland and Auckland, New Zealand, but much less so in Bombay and Singapore. Of their 240 subjects, 80% were smokers, 25% had a serum total cholesterol of 280 mg/dl or greater, and 15% were hypertensive (18).

In the prospective Western Collaborative Group study of type A behavior in men aged 39–59, those reporting a positive family history of CAD (no ages listed) more often developed angina pectoris during the ensuing 8.5 years. Men aged 39 to 49 with a positive family history were more likely to experience MI or sudden coronary death. The significance of this finding persisted after adjustment for other CAD risk indicators (19).

In the Tromsö, Norway, population survey of men aged 20 to 49, a family history of MI was obtained along with other CAD risk indicators. Of 1647 men, 25 had already experienced MI. Compared with healthy men, they were 3.9 times more likely to have a male relative with MI and 10.5 times more likely to have a female relative with that diagnosis (20).

In a series of studies of Finnish men with angina (21) and MI, Rissanen and colleagues found that the younger the MI patient, the more likely CAD also existed in his parents and siblings. When the index subject's MI had occured at age 45 or earlier, his brother was nine times more likely to also have CAD than was the brother of a control subject. Hypertension and dyslipidemias were most common among relatives of the youngest patients;

their prevalence diminished with increasing age of the study subject (22). Sisters of case subjects were twice as likely to have CAD. Cardiac deaths were most common in sibs of men with fatal MI; uncomplicated angina pectoris was more common in sibs of subjects who had angina without MI (23).

Studies in Air Force (24) and Navy (25) men in the USA who had experienced MI before the ages of 40 and 36, respectively, revealed that a majority of men had a positive family history of MI. However, ages at which relatives experienced MI were not given. Among British soldiers with MI before the age of 40, 22 of 45 had a history of a relative with MI before the age of 60. Smoking prevalence was 93%, and mean serum total cholesterol was 264 mg/dl (26).

In a study of 1671 men and 520 women undergoing coronary arteriography, fewer persons with minimal or no disease had a parental MI history (no age specified). Multiple linear regression confirmed that family history had independent predictive value for determining occlusive CAD (27).

Nora and colleagues noted that a family history of MI at an early age was strongly associated with MI in men younger than 55. Risk ratio when the relative was also younger than 55 was 10.4; 48% of subjects had such a history (28).

In a Mayo Clinic study of 435 women and men with coronary arteriography before the age of 50, a positive family history was defined as CAD in a first-degree relative age 50 or less. Multivariate analysis showed that the man or woman with significant CAD by angiography was best predicted by family history, smoking, and serum total cholesterol level. Occlusive disease was present in 90% of those with a positive family history, compared with a prevalence of 25% in persons with none of the three risk indicators (29).

In a study of a southern California residential community, women with a family history of CAD were more likely to smoke cigarettes than other women (30). During a nine-year surveillance, investigators found that 68% of the excess deaths in men with a family history of MI were attributable to the interaction of smoking and family history, suggesting that some of the risk associated with family history may be modifiable (31).

In the prospective Nurses' Health Study in the USA, women with a parental history of MI at age 60 or less had relative risks of fatal MI, nonfatal MI, and angina pectoris of 5.0, 2.8, and 3.4, respectively. When parental MI occurred after age 60, the relative risks dropped to 1.0, 2.6, and 1.9. These associations were only slightly altered by adjustment for other CAD risk indicators, including oral contraceptive and replacement estrogen use, suggesting an independent role for parental MI history in the genesis of CAD (32).

Investigators in the Framingham Heart Study examined 186 pairs of brothers in their cohort, noting the presence of CAD and its major risk indicators. CAD in the older brother is predictive of CAD in the younger, even after adjustment for lipids, blood pressure, and smoking (33). From the Kaiser Permanente Twin Registry, data from 434 adult female twin pairs were analyzed. Despite adjustment for shared environmental and behavioral effects, significant genetic associations were noted for HDL- and LDL-cholesterol, triglycerides, and relative weight (34). Johns Hopkins investigators studied 150 siblings of 86 persons with documented CAD before the age of 60. More than 40% were hypertensive, and more than 30% had a lipid abnormality, but less than half of these high-risk siblings were aware of their risk (35). Also distressing is the finding that most sibs had not changed their health habits four months after definite documentation of their family member's CAD (36).

Risk Factors in Children of Young CAD Patients

Copenhagen investigators studied 177 children and young adults whose fathers had died from CAD before age 45. Familial hypercholesterolemia was 10 times more likely in them than in a reference population. Significantly more children had total cholesterol levels above the 95th percentile (37). Spanish scientists had similar findings in children with a parental history of MI before age 56 (38).

In Iowa, CAD risk indicators were determined in 173 progeny of fathers with documented CAD before age 50. A majority of the children had elevated LDL-cholesterol or triglyceride levels, low HDL-cholesterol levels, or combinations of these abnormalities. Lipid and lipoprotein distribution in children closely resembled those of their fathers (39).

Apolipoproteins were measured in children participating in the Bogalusa Heart Study (Louisiana). Children whose fathers reported MI had significantly lower apoA-I levels and higher ratios of apoB:apoA-I. It was also noted in this biracial community that children whose fathers reported MI were more likely themselves to be older, cigarette smokers, and obese (40). Dutch investigators also noted a significant difference in apolipoprotein levels in children of persons with MI before age 50 and control children (41).

In Malmö, Sweden, 140 7-year-old children reported a first-degree relative with CAD before age 50 (men) or 55 (women); 79 of these children and their parents were studied. More than 14% of children had total and LDL-cholesterol levels above the 95th percentile (42). In the Tromsö, Norway, study, children of men at increased CAD risk were followed for six years. These children displayed significant lipid and lipoprotein differences from control children; their total and LDL-cholesterol values were higher, while HDL-cholesterol values were lower. Differences in blood pressure between the two groups were not noted (43).

OLDER ADULTS

In large measure, the familial relations discussed above hold true for men older than 55 and women over 65, although the correlation may be weaker.

In an Icelandic study, first-degree relatives of MI patients were at threefold CAD risk themselves. In first-degree relatives of male propositi, relative risk was five, and was similarly high in male relatives of female propositi (44). In a study of affluent whites in southern California, men with a first-degree relative with stroke were themselves at a relative risk of 3.3 for CAD, indicating susceptibility to generalized atherosclerosis (45).

In other studies, first-degree relatives of Swiss MI patients have displayed lower HDL-cholesterol levels (46). French investigators noted this as well as elevated levels of LDL-cholesterol and apolipoprotein B in subjects with parental history of MI (47). However, some geneticists have concluded that familial aggregation of CAD is not entirely explained by the familial clustering of currently known coronary risk factors (48).

CAD RISK IN PARENTS OF SCREENED CHILDREN

Several large-scale studies of risk-indicator screening in children have investigated parents and siblings of the study children, including those in Bogalusa (Louisiana) (49) and Muscatine (Iowa) (50). In a study of adolescent twins, those with a family history of CAD before the age of 55 had significantly lower HDL_2 levels,

as did those children with smoking mothers (51).

It also appears that approximately 10% of children of all racial and ethnic groups in the USA have blood total cholesterol levels exceeding 200 mg/dl (52), placing them above the desirable zone for adults. These findings have led to advocacy for school-based risk-indicator screening (53) and family-based health promotion programs (54). Such programs serve a "case-finding" function in reaching young adult parents who may not have a regular source of medical care, in addition to motivating these parents to change the health habits of the entire family (55).

REFERENCES

1. Thomas CB, Cohen BH. The familial occurrence of hypertension and coronary artery disease, with observations concerning obesity and diabetes. Ann Intern Med 1955;42:90–127.

2. Deutscher S, Epstein FH, Kjelsberg MO. Familial aggregation of factors associated with coronary heart disease. Circulation 1966;33:911–924.

3. Hunt SC, Hasstedt SJ, Kuida H, Stults BM, Hopkins PN, Williams RR. Genetic heritability and common environmental components of resting and stressed blood pressures, lipids, and body mass index in Utah pedigrees and twins. Am J Epidemiol 1989;129:625–638.

4. Sosenko JM, Breslow JL, Ellison RC, Miettinen OS. Familial aggregation of total cholesterol, high density lipoprotein cholesterol and total triglyceride levels in plasma. Am J Epidemiol 1980;112:656–660.

5. Motulsky AG. Genetic aspects of familial hypercholesterolemia and its diagnosis. Arteriosclerosis 1989;9(suppl I):13–17.

6. Connor SL, Connor WE, Henry H, Sexton G, Keenan EJ. The effects of familial relationships, age, body weight, and diet on blood pressure and the 24 hour urinary excretion of sodium, potassium, and creatinine in men, women, and children of randomly selected families. Circulation 1984;70:76–85.

7. Anonymous. Genetics, environment, and hypertension. Lancet 1983;1:681–682.

8. Norris JM, Dorman JS, LaPorte RE, et al. Clustering of premature mortality in 1,761 insulin-dependent diabetics and their family members. Am J Epidemiol 1989;129:723–731.

9. Bray GA. Obesity. Part I—Pathogenesis. West J Med 1988;149:429–441.

10. Kolonel LN, Lee J. Husband-wife correspondence in smoking, drinking, and dietary habits. Am J Clin Nutr 1981;34:99–103.

11. Perusse L, Leblanc C, Tremblay A, et al. Familial aggregation in physical fitness, coronary heart disease risk factors, and pulmonary function measurements. Prev Med 1987;16:607–615.

12. Vandenbroucke JP, Matroos AW, van der Heide-Wessel C, van der Heide RM. Parental survival, an independent predictor of longevity in middle-aged persons. Am J Epidemiol 1984;119:742–750.

13. Sorensen TI, Nielsen GG, Andersen PK, Teasdale TW. Genetic and environmental influences on premature death in adult adoptees. N Engl J Med 1988;318:727–732.

14. Hammond EC, Garfinkel L, Seidman H. Longevity of parents and grandparents in relation to coronary heart disease and associated variables. Circulation 1971;43:31–44.

15. Limacher M, Brinson Y, Norvell N, Martin AD, Conti CR. Housestaff practice of preventive cardiology: who's not doing what? J Am Coll Cardiol 1989;13(2):37A.

16. Shanoff HM, Little A, Murphy EA, et al. Studies of the male survivors of myocardial infarction due to "essential" atherosclerosis. Can Med Assoc J 1961;84:519–530.

17. Slack J, Evans KA. The increased risk of death from ischaemic heart disease in first degree relatives of 121 men and 96 women with ischaemic heart disease. J Med Genet 1966;3:239–257.

18. Dolder MA, Oliver MF. Myocardial infarction in young men. Study of risk factors in nine countries. Br. Heart J 1975;37:493–503.

19. Sholtz RI, Rosenman RH, Brand RJ. The relationship of reported parental history to the incidence of coronary heart disease in the Western Collaborative Group study. Am J Epidemiol 1975;102:350–356.

20. Forde OH, Thelle DS. The Tromsö Heart Study: risk factors for coronary heart disease related to the occurrence of myocardial in-

farction in first degree relatives. Am J Epidemiol 1977;105:192–199.

21. Rissanen AM, Nikkila EA. Coronary artery disease and its risk factors in families of young men with angina pectoris and controls. Br Heart J 1977;39:875–883.

22. Rissanen AM. Familial occurrence of coronary heart disease: effect of age at diagnosis. Am J Cardiol 1979;40:60–66.

23. Rissanen AM. Familial occurrence of coronary heart disease according to manifestation. Acta Med Scand 1985;218:355–363.

24. Savran SV, Bryson AL, Welch TG, Zaret BL, McGowan RL, Flamm MD Jr. Clinical correlates of coronary cineangiography in young males with myocardial infarction. Am Heart J 1976;91:551–555.

25. Warren SE, Thompson SI, Vieweg WVR. Historic and angiographic features of young adults surviving myocardial infarction. Chest 1979;75:667–670.

26. Lynch P, Ineson N, Jones KP, Scott AW, Crawford IC. Risk profile of soldiers aged under 40 with coronary heart disease. Br Med J 1985;290:1868–1869.

27. Anderson AJ, Loeffler RF, Barboriak JJ, Rimm AA. Occlusive coronary artery disease and parental history of myocardial infarction. Prev Med 1979;8:419–428.

28. Nora JJ, Lortscher RH, Spangler RD, Nora AH, Kimberling WJ. Genetic-epidemiologic study of early-onset ischemic heart disease. Circulation 1980;61:503–508.

29. Chesebro JH, Fuster V, Elveback LR, Frye RL. Strong family history and cigarette smoking as risk factors of coronary artery disease in young adults. Br Heart J 1982;47:78–83.

30. Barrett-Connor E, Khaw KT. Family history of heart attack as an independent predictor of death due to cardiovascular disease. Circulation 1984;69:1065–1069.

31. Khaw KT, Barrett-Connor E. Family history of heart attack: a modifiable risk factor? Circulation 1986;74:239–244.

32. Colditz GA, Stampfer MJ, Willett WC, Rosner B, Speizer FE, Hennekens CH. A prospective study of parental history of myocardial infarction and coronary heart disease in women. Am J Epidemiol 1986;123:48–58.

33. Snowden CB, McNamara PM, Garrison RJ, Feinleib M, Kannel WB, Epstein FH.

Predicting coronary heart disease in siblings—a multivariate assessment. Am J Epidemiol 1982;115:217–222.

34. Austin MA, King MC, Bawol RD, Hulley S, Friedman GD. Risk factors for coronary heart disease in adult female twins. Genetic heritability and shared environmental influences. Am J Epidemiol 1987;125:308–318.

35. Becker DM, Becker LC, Pearson TA, Fintel DJ, Levine DM, Kwiterovich PO. Risk factors in siblings of people with premature coronary heart disease. J Am Coll Cardiol 1988;12:1273–1280.

36. Becker DM, Levine DM. Risk perception, knowledge, and lifestyles in siblings of people with premature coronary disease. Am J Prev Med 1987;3:45–50.

37. Ibsen KK, Lous P, Andersen GE. Coronary heart risk factors in 177 children and young adults whose fathers died from ischemic heart disease before age 45. Acta Paediatr Scand 1982;71:609–613.

38. Plaza I, Madero R, Baeza J, et al. Fuenlabrada Study: familial aggregation of coronary heart disease and coronary risk factors. Eur Heart J 1988;9(Suppl A):89.

39. Lee J, Lauer RM, Clarke WR. Lipoproteins in the progeny of young men with coronary artery disease: children with increased risk. Pediatrics 1986;78:330–337.

40. Freedman DS, Srinivasan SR, Shear CL, Franklin FA, Webber LS, Berenson GS. The relation of apolipoproteins A-I and B in children to parental myocardial infarction. N. Engl J Med 1986;315:721–726.

41. De Backer G, Hulstaert F, De Munck K, Rosseneu M, Van Parijs L. Dramaix M. Serum lipids and apoproteins in students whose parents suffered prematurely from a myocardial infarction. Am Heart J 1986;112:478–484.

42. Sveger T, Fex G, Borgfors N. Hyperlipidemia in school children with family histories of premature coronary artery disease. Acta Paediatr Scand 1987;76:311–315.

43. Knutsen SF, Knutsen R. Are children of men with high risk for CHD also at higher risk? The Tromsö Study. Eur Heart J 1988;9(suppl A):206.

44. Thordarson O, Fridriksson S. Aggregation of deaths from ischaemic heart disease among first and second degree relatives of 108 males and 42 females with myocardial infarction. Acta Med Scand 1979;205:493–500.

45. Khaw KT, Barrett-Connor E. Family history of stroke as an independent predictor of ischemic heart disease in men and stroke in women. Am J Epidemiol 1986;123:59–66.

46. Pometta D, Suenram A, Sheybani E, Grab B, James R. HDL cholesterol levels in patients with myocardial infarction and their families. Atherosclerosis 1986;59:21–29.

47. Cambien F, Warnet JM, Jacqueson A, Ducimetiere P, Richard JL, Claude JR. Relation of parental history of early myocardial infarction to the level of apoprotein B in men. Circulation 1987;76:266–271.

48. ten Kate LP, Boman H, Daiger SP, Motulsky AG. Familial aggregation of coronary heart disease and its relation to known genetic risk factors. Am J Cardiol 1982;50:945–953.

49. Cresanta JL, Burke GL, Downey AM, Freedman DS, Berenson GS. Prevention of atherosclerosis in children. Pediatr Clin North Am 1986;33:835–858.

50. Bucher KD, Schrott HG, Clarke WR, Lauer RM. The Muscatine Cholesterol Family Study: familial aggregation of blood lipids and relationship of lipid levels to age, sex and hormone use. J Chron Dis 1982;35:375–384.

51. Bodurtha JN, Schieken R, Segrest J, Nance WE. High-density lipoprotein-cholesterol subfractions in adolescent twins. Pediatrics 1987;79:181–189.

52. Davidson DM, Iftner CA, Bradley BJ, Landry SM, Rose MY, Wong ND. Family history predictors of high blood cholesterol levels in 4th grade school children. J Am Coll Cardiol 1989;13:36A.

53. Davidson DM, Bradley BJ, Landry SM, Iftner CA, Bramblett SN. School-based blood cholesterol screening. J Pediatr Health Care 1989;3:3–8.

54. Johnson CC, Nicklas TA, Arbeit ML, et al. Cardiovascular risk in parents of children with elevated blood pressure. "Heart Smart"—family health promotion. J Clin Hypertens 1987;3:559–566.

55. Davidson DM, Doyle EJ Jr. Family-directed preventive cardiology. J Fam Prac 1984;18:57–64.

7

diabetes mellitus

In 1979, the National Diabetes Data Group published a classification of diabetes and other categories of glucose intolerance. Their framework has facilitated further epidemiologic and clinical research (1).

EPIDEMIOLOGY

The development of type I, insulin-dependent diabetes mellitus (IDDM) appears to have two peaks, the first near puberty and a second after the age of 40. Both are the result of immunologically mediated destruction of the pancreatic beta cells, and both usually require insulin therapy (2). Persons in whom the disease arises early more often carry histocompatibility antigens HLA-DR3, DR4, or both, and insulin autoantibodies have been found in as many as half of children and adolescents with newly diagnosed IDDM. In North America, the incidence of newly diagnosed IDDM is approximately 10 to 15 children per 100,000 per year (3). IDDM is more common in whites than in blacks in North America (4). When the disease is first diagnosed in adulthood, it is characterized by a longer symptomatic period before diagnosis and by better preservation of pancreatic beta-cell function (5).

Eisenbarth has proposed that IDDM can be divided into six stages: genetic susceptibility, triggering of beta-cell immunity by environmental factors, active immunity, progressive loss of glucose-stimulated insulin secretion, overt diabetes with some residual insulin secretion, and complete beta-cell destruction (6). Studies to date have not conclusively proven a cause-and-effect relationship for the prevention of microvascular complications by optimal insulin control of type I diabetes (7).

Ketosis-resistant, or type II diabetes, has been termed non–insulin dependent (NIDDM). It may be treated with insulin, with oral agents, or with dietary therapy alone. It arises more often in obese persons, and it is present in approximately 90% of all diabetics. Rates in Mexican-Americans exceed those of their Anglo neighbors, but the differential shrinks as socioeconomic status differences narrow (8). The Pima Indians of central Arizona and the Mohawk Indians of Quebec have rates of NIDDM among the highest in the world (9, 10). Diabetes can also be associated with other medical conditions; the term gestational diabetes is reserved for those in whom glucose intolerance develops or is discovered during pregnancy.

Individuals with plasma glucose levels higher than normal, but less than those seen in frank diabetics, are said to have impaired glucose tolerance (1). The prevalence of impaired glucose tolerance in the United States is approximately 11% (11). In one study of persons over age 50 in southern California, nearly twice as many men as women had elevated levels of fasting plasma glucose (12). Levels rise in women after menopause, but are lower in users of replacement estrogens (13). While screening for diabetes is widespread, some investigators have suggested that only screening for gestational diabetes will result in net therapeutic benefit (14).

DIABETES AND CAD

The response-to-injury hypothesis described in Chapter 2 provides the foundation for understanding the role of diabetes in atherosclerosis. In their review, Colwell and Lopes-Virella focused on altered endothelial and platelet function in diabetics. They note many reports of increased plasma levels of von Willebrand factor, decreased prostacyclin release, decreased fibrinolytic activity, and decreased lipoprotein lipase activity, which may account for endothelial damage and altered function in diabetes. Their work adds to the growing body of evidence for altered platelet function as well. They report marked hyperaggregability of platelets, most apparent when advanced disease is present. This feature, due at least in part to platelet-plasma interactions and increased thromboxane synthesis, has stimulated several trials of antiplatelet drugs in patients with diabetes mellitus (15).

Autonomic neuropathy alters many cardiovascular symptoms and signs. Among these are increased heart rate, which has been ascribed to involvement of the vagus nerve before cardiac sympathetic nerve involvement (16). Norepinephrine-mediated vasoconstriction and epinephrine-induced rises in plasma glucose and free fatty acids are also attributable to the

neuropathy, along with a decrease in blood pressure that is not easily explained (17).

Myocardial ischemia is often silent in diabetic patients, so ambulatory electrocardiographic monitoring is useful in such individuals (18). In patients having coronary angiography, diabetics may have more severe disease, particularly those who are insulin-dependent (19). However, persons having angiography do not represent a cross-section of the general population. In this case, because diabetics experience less angina, it might be expected that their coronary disease would be more advanced before it was detected than that in patients who are symptomatic.

Myocardial infarction may be "silent" in as many as half of diabetic patients, particularly those with autonomic neuropathy. An increased likelihood of sudden cardiac death may result from this lack of symptoms (20).

Given the reduced sensitivity of pain for detecting CAD in persons with diabetes, noninvasive testing becomes even more important. Diabetic patients with ST segment changes or myocardial perfusion (thallium-201) defects on exercise testing had very high rates of CAD events in one prospective study (21).

After 18 years of follow-up in the Framingham Study, women with diabetes were found to have double the risk of developing myocardial infarction (MI), angina, and sudden cardiac death. Relative risk in men was lower (approximately 1.5 for each outcome measure) than in women, but this risk was significantly greater than that of nondiabetic men (22). These gender differences persist after controlling for age, hypertension, smoking, cholesterol, and left ventricular hypertrophy (23). Intermittent claudication is four times more likely in diabetics (24). In a southern California study of persons 40 to 79 years of age, the age-adjusted relative risk of death in diabetics attributed to ischemic heart disease was 3.4 in women and 2.5 in men (25).

In the Whitehall study of 18,403 British male civil servants, CAD mortality was doubled in those having a blood glucose level above 95 mg/dl (95th percentile) (26), but the excess mortality in diabetics could not be attributed to differences in other CAD risk indicators (27).

Hyperinsulinemia may be responsible for accelerated atherosclerosis in NIDDM, so that oral agents such as glipizide or gliclazide, which induce less diurnal hyperinsulinemia, may be advantageous (28). In otherwise healthy nondiabetic persons who have hyperinsulinemia, higher levels of other CAD risk indicators are present (29). Although diabetes doubles the risk of developing thrombotic stroke, it appears to pose no additional risk for hemmorhagic stroke (30). Altered risks of thrombotic disease may be related to the alterations in platelet survival and hypersensitivity noted in diabetics (31).

Diabetes has been reported in 6% to 31% of patients undergoing coronary artery bypass surgery (CABS). Perioperative mortality in diabetics is somewhat higher, but effective angina relief is obtained. However, long-term survival after CABS in diabetics depends upon the initial severity of the disease. In one study, 15-year survival was 53% in nondiabetics, 43% for diabetics not receiving drugs, 33% for those taking oral agents, and 19% for insulin-treated patients (32).

Among women who experience myocardial infarction, diabetics are four times more likely to develop congestive heart failure (CHF) than nondiabetics. If CHF develops, the woman is at double risk for a recurrent MI (33).

CAD RISK INDICATORS IN DIABETICS

Diabetes mellitus is frequently associated with other indicators of CAD risk (34); in some cases, it causes the increase in risk. These indicators include lipids, lipoproteins, nutrition patterns, hypertension, smoking, obesity, and exercise.

Lipids and Lipoproteins

Lipid metabolism may be altered by diabetes in several ways. In untreated type I diabetes, HDL-C is lower than in nondiabetics; much of this difference is due to lower values of HDL_2. In cross-sectional studies, persons with IDDM and coronary artery disease (CAD) have significantly lower HDL-C and HDL_2 than individuals with IDDM alone; this effect is particularly true in women (35). Both values are enhanced with insulin treatment (36), probably as a result of elevated lipoprotein lipase levels, but the improvement is independent of the degree of metabolic control (37). LDL-C and triglyceride levels are higher in IDDM patients, particularly in women (38). Cases have been reported of myocardial infarction in young IDDM women, ages 18 and 19, who have coexisting dyslipidemias (39).

In a recent study, better blood glucose control, as reflected in the hemoglobin A_1 level, was correlated with improvement in lipid and lipoprotein levels in whites and black men with type I diabetes, but not in black women. In whites, a reduction of 1% in hemoglobin A_1 was associated with a decrease of 6 to 7 mg/dl in plasma total cholesterol and a reduction in LDL-C of 4 to 5 mg/dl (40). Glucose and lipid levels are lower in type I diabetic patients with some residual insulin secretion (41). However, it appears that strict glucose control and normalization of lipid levels do not favorably influence the development of diabetic retinopathy (42).

In type II diabetes, HDL-C is also lower in the untreated state, even after adjustment for other factors affecting HDL-C, such as obesity, smoking, alcohol, exercise, and postmenopausal estrogens (43). Again, these lower values occurred predominantly in those patients with established CAD (44). Because type II patients are often obese and have high triglyceride levels, restoration of normal HDL-C levels may not appear after treatment with insulin or oral agents, particularly in women (37). LDL-C levels are also higher in NIDDM patients of both genders (45). Medications can improve these dyslipidemic states, but some drugs may unfavorably alter glucose levels, while others may have side effects of particular relevance in diabetics (46).

Despite these factors, a minority of diabetics with dyslipidemias are aware of their lipid disorders, and even fewer are currently being treated specifically for that condition (47). As with dyslipidemias in nondiabetics, diet optimization is the cornerstone of treatment. In earlier years, prescription of a low-carbohydrate, high-fat, and higher cholesterol diet for diabetics resulted in higher blood cholesterol levels than are currently seen (48). At present, a diet with 20 to 30% of calories from fat, 55 to 65% from carbohydrates, and 15% from protein and with high fiber content is considered appropriate for treating both insulin-dependent diabetes and dyslipidemias (49, 50). The necessity of a very low fat diet for NIDDM patients has been questioned; it has been suggested that replacing saturated fats with monounsaturated and polyunsaturated fats would be optimal (51, 52).

Anderson and Geil have documented the benefits of an optimal caloric intake, a high percentage of complex carbohydrates, and limited saturated fat and cholesterol intake. They review their own studies along with those of others in emphasizing the importance of fiber in the diabetic's diet. Guar, pectin, and oat bran have favorably influenced postprandial glycemic and insulin responses as well as improving lipid profiles. They recommend doubling current fiber intake in North American adults (from 20 g to 40 g daily), focusing on both soluble and insoluble forms of fiber-rich foods rather than supplements (53).

In healthy women, fasting plasma insulin has been correlated with elevated triglycerides and reduced HDL (54). In type II diabetes, elevated levels of insulin stimulate hepatic synthesis of triglycerides. In addition, insulin regulates lipoprotein lipase activity, so IDDM may be accompanied by reduced conversion of VLDL to LDL. Hyperglycemia and consequent glycosylation can alter the LDL molecule, interfering with receptor binding and slowing LDL catabolism in diabetics (55).

Improved glycemic control with sulfonylureas has generally resulted in decreases in LDL-C and triglycerides, with either no change or slight improvement in HDL-C levels. However, some reports indicated that HDL-C levels were lower in patients receiving sulfonylurea treatment than in those taking insulin (given comparable levels of glycemic control). Changes from one agent to another, or addition of one medication to another, may alter HDL-C levels (56).

Hypertension

Diabetics of both types and of both genders have higher blood pressures than controls; more diabetics are under treatment for hypertension, but control of their hypertension is often more difficult than in nondiabetics (57).

Among the several categories of antihypertensive drugs, β-adrenergic blockers are most likely to disturb diabetic control, particularly those which block both β_1 and β_2 receptors (58). Diuretics also worsen diabetic control, and both categories of drugs worsen lipid and lipoprotein values. In contrast, α-adrenergic blockers, central α-agonists, and ACE inhibitors apparently have no adverse effects on blood glucose and lipid control, so they represent choices for the hypertensive diabetic (59).

Clinical and subclinical neuropathies associated with diabetes may be exacerbated by some antihypertensive medications. Investigators have suggested that such patients may be more sensitive to the sexual dysfunction sometimes noted with centrally acting medications, and they have documented alleviation of impotence in a majority of hypertensive diabetic men switched from these medications to prazosin (55).

Smoking

The risk for cardiovascular mortality in smoking diabetic patients is double that of nonsmoking diabetics. It has been estimated that 65% of cardiovascular disease deaths in diabetics could be attributed to smoking (60). In addition, smoking further accelerates the process of atherosclerosis in peripheral arteries, leading to claudication, ulceration, and gangrene (61).

Obesity

In the prospective Framingham Heart Study, the development of glucose intolerance was directly related to relative body weight (62). Others have demonstrated that upper body fat in women is correlated with the development of diabetes. However, in a study of black and white male US Army veterans, obesity did not explain an increased prevalence of fasting hyperglycemia and diagnosed diabetes in black men (63).

Dietary management as described above is appropriate, and it also appears that low-energy ("very low calorie") diets can be used safely in NIDDM patients, reducing blood pressure, glucose, cholesterol, and triglycerides (64).

Physical Activity

In obese NIDDM patients, regular exercise can significantly decrease peripheral insulin resistance, leading to lower fasting plasma glucose levels and hemoglobin A_{1c} levels, in addition to beneficial effects on lipids, blood pressure, and body weight. To date, however, better diabetic control has not been noted in type I patients who exercise regularly. However, IDDM patients may wish to exercise for the other salutogenic benefits.

For both type I and type II diabetics, exercise can be undertaken with a few key precautions. The presence of proliferative retinopathy is a contraindication to strenuous exercise. Autonomic neuropathy may limit one's exercise capacity, and care must be taken to avoid foot injuries in such patients. Finally, proteinuria may be increased with vigorous exercise. Warm-up and cool-down should be included in the exercise period, which should be 30 to 40 minutes, at least three times weekly. Beneficial effects on the heart, lipids, and weight will be noted when exercise heart rates in the range of 60 to 75% of maximum are maintained.

In the well-controlled insulin-treated diabetic, the following guidelines are helpful. The optimal time to exercise is one to three hours after a meal; extra carbohydrates can be consumed before, during, and after exercise to avoid hypoglycemia. Persons taking a single daily dose of intermediate-acting insulin can decrease the dose by ⅓ on exercise days. If short-acting insulin is used on nonexercise days, it can be omitted before exercise, but may need to be given later in the day. Patients using infusion therapy should reduce the basal rate by one-third until the exercise period is complete (65).

Electrocardiographic Abnormalities

In a study of 2223 women and men aged 50–69 years, those with NIDDM were nearly twice as likely to have resting electrocardiographic abnormalities as those with euglycemia (66).

DIABETIC CARDIOMYOPATHY

Both clinical and pathological studies indicate that diabetes may be associated with a cardiomyopathic state. Investigators have employed a variety of noninvasive techniques to document systolic impairment, diastolic dysfunction, or both, in type I diabetics. In almost all studies, impairment of myocardial function did not correlate with the duration of diabetes or microvascular complications (67).

Possible etiologic mechanisms for decreased ventricular compliance include myocardial fibrosis and interstitial accumulation of collagen. These processes appear to exist independent of coronary atherosclerosis in diabetics (68). Other pathogenetic possibilities include diabetic autonomic neuropathy, growth hormone–induced angiopathy, and interactions of diabetes and hypertension that produce myocardial alterations. A clearer understanding of these factors will require further investigation (67).

REFERENCES

1. National Diabetes Data Group. Classification and diagnosis of diabetes mellitus and other categories of glucose intolerance. Diabetes 1979;28:1039–1057.

2. Krolewski AS, Warram JH, Rand LI, Kahn CR. Epidemiologic approach to the etiology of type I diabetes mellitus and its complications. N Engl J Med 1987;317:1390–1398.

3. Cahill GF Jr. McDevitt HO. Insulindependent diabetes mellitus: the initial lesion. N Engl J Med 1981;304:1454–1465.

4. Winter WE, Maclaren NK, Riley WJ, Clark DW, Kappy MS, Spillar RP. Maturityonset diabetes of youth in black Americans. N Engl J Med 1987;316:285–291.

5. Karjalainen J, Salmela P, Ilonen J, Surcel HM, Knip M. A comparison of childhood and adult type I diabetes mellitus. N Engl J Med 1989;320:881–886.

6. Eisenbarth GS. Type I diabetes mellitus. A chronic autoimmune disease. N Engl J Med 1986;314:1360–1368.

7. Zinman B. The physiologic replacement of insulin. An elusive goal. N Engl J Med 1989;321:363–370.

8. Stern MP, Rosenthal M, Haffner SM, Hazuda HP, Franco LJ. Sex difference in the effects of sociocultural status on diabetes and cardiovascular risk factors in Mexican Americans. The San Antonio Heart Study. Am J Epidemiol 1984;120:834–851.

9. Saad MF, Knowler WC, Pettitt DJ, Nelson RG, Mott DM, Bennett PH. The natural history of impaired glucose tolerance in the Pima Indians. N Engl J Med 1988;319:1500–1506.

10. Macaulay AC, Montour LT, Adelson N. Prevalence of diabetic and atherosclerotic complications among Mohawk Indians of Kahnawake, PQ. Can Med Assoc J 1988;139:221–224.

11. Harris MI, Hadden WC, Knowler WC, Bennett PH. Prevalence of diabetes and impaired glucose tolerance and plasma glucose levels in U.S. population aged 20–74 yr. Diabetes 1987;36:523–534.

12. Barrett-Connor E. The prevalence of diabetes mellitus in an adult community as determined by history of fasting hyperglycemia. Am J Epidemiol 1980;111:705–712.

13. Barrett-Connor E. Factors associated with the distribution of fasting plasma glucose in an adult community. Am J Epidemiol 1980;112:518–523.

14. Singer DE, Samet JH, Coley CM, Nathan DM. Screening for diabetes mellitus. Ann Intern Med 1988;109:639–649.

15. Colwell JA, Lopes-Virella MF. A review of the development of large-vessel disease in diabetes mellitus. Am J Med 1988;85(suppl A):113–118.

16. Ewing DJ, Campbell IW, Clarke BF. Heart rate changes in diabetes mellitus. Lancet 1981;1:183–186.

17. Hilsted J, Richter E, Madsbad S, et al. Metabolic and cardiovascular responses to epinephrine in diabetic autonomic neuropathy. N Engl J Med 1987;317:421–426.

18. Nesto RW, Phillips RT. Asymptomatic myocardial ischemia in diabetic patients. Am J Med 1986;80:40–47.

19. Lemp GF, VanderZwaag R, Hughes JP, et al. Association between the severity of di-

abetes mellitus and coronary arterial athero-sclerosis. Am J Cardiol 1987;60:1015–1019.

20. Niakan E, Harati Y, Rolak LA, Comstock JP, Rokey R. Silent myocardial infarction and diabetic cardiovascular autonomic neuropathy. Arch Intern Med 1986;146:2229–2230.

21. Rubler S, Gerber D, Reitano J, Chokshi V, Fisher VJ. Predictive value of clinical and exercise variables for detection of coronary artery disease in men with diabetes mellitus. Am J Cardiol 1987;59:1310–1313.

22. Kannel WB. Contributions of the Framingham Study to the conquest of coronary artery disease. Am J Cardiol 1988;62:1109–1112.

23. Kannel WB, McGee DL. Diabetes and cardiovascular disease: the Framingham Study. JAMA 1979;241:2035–2038.

24. Garcia MJ, McNamara P, Gordon T, Kannel WB. Morbidity and mortality in diabetics in the Framingham population. Sixteen year follow-up study. Diabetes 1974;23:105–111.

25. Barrett-Connor E, Wingard DL. Sex differential in ischemic heart disease mortality in diabetics: a prospective population-based study. Am J Epidemiol 1983;118:489–496.

26. Fuller JH, Shipley MJ, Rose G, Jarrett RJ, Keen H. Coronary heart disease and impaired glucose tolerance. The Whitehall Study. Lancet 1980;1:1373–1376.

27. Jarrett RJ, Shipley MJ. Mortality and associated risk factors in diabetics. Acta Endocrinol Suppl 1985;272:21–26.

28. Stolar MW. Atherosclerosis in diabetes: the role of hyperinsulinemia. Metabolism 1988;37:1–9.

29. Zavaroni I, Bonora E, Pagliara M, et al. Risk factors for coronary artery disease in healthy persons with hyperinsulinemia and normal glucose tolerance. N Engl J Med 1989;320:702–706.

30. Abbot RD, Donahue RP, MacMahon SW, Reed DM, Yano K. Diabetes and the risk of stroke. The Honolulu Heart Program. JAMA 1987;257:949–952.

31. Mustard JF, Packham MA. Platelets and diabetes mellitus. N Engl J Med 1984;311:665–667.

32. Lawrie GM, Morris GC Jr Glaeser DH. Influence of diabetes mellitus on the results of coronary artery bypass surgery. Follow-up of 212 diabetic patients ten to 15 years after surgery. JAMA 1986;256:2967–2971.

33. Abbot RD, Donahue RP, Kannel WB, Wilson PW. The impact of diabetes on survival following myocardial infarction in men vs women. The Framingham Study. JAMA 1988;260:3456–3460.

34. Wingard DL, Barrett-Connor E. Family history of diabetes and cardiovascular disease risk factors and mortality among euglycemic, borderline hyperglycemic, and diabetic adults. Am J Epidemiol 1987;125:948–958.

35. Laakso M, Pyorala K, Sarlund H, Voutilainen E. Lipid and lipoprotein abnormalities associated with coronary heart disease in patients with insulin-dependent diabetes mellitus. Arteriosclerosis 1986;6:679–684.

36. Falko JM, O'Dorisio TM, Cataland S. Improvement of high-density lipoprotein cholesterol levels. Ambulatory type I diabetics treated with the subcutaneous insulin pump. JAMA 1982;247:37–39.

37. Bergman M, Gidez LI, Eder HA. High-density lipoprotein subclasses in diabetes. Am J Med 1986;81:488–492.

38. Walden CE, Knopp RH, Wahl PW, Beach KW, Strandness E. Sex differences in the effect of diabetes mellitus on lipoprotein triglyceride and cholesterol concentrations. N Engl J Med 1984;311:953–959.

39. Declue TJ, Malone JI, Root AW. Coronary artery disease in diabetic adolescents. Clin Pediatr 1988;27:587–590.

40. Semenkovich CF, Ostlund RE, Schechtman KB. Plasma lipids in patients with type I diabetes mellitus. Influence of race, gender, and plasma glucose control: lipids do not correlate with glucose control in black women. Arch Intern Med 1989;149:51–56.

41. Sjoberg S, Gunnarson R, Rossner S, Ostman J. Serum lipid and lipoprotein levels in long-term insulin-dependent diabetes mellitus. Relation to residual insulin secretion, microvascular lesions and environmental factors. Acta Med Scand 1987;222:445–451.

42. Agardh CD, Agardh E, Bauer B, Nilsson-Ehle P. Plasma lipids and plasma lipoproteins in diabetics with and without proliferative retinopathy. Acta Med Scan 1988;223:165–169.

43. Barrett-Connor E, Witzwum JL, Holdbrook M. A community study of high den-

sity lipoproteins in adult noninsulin-dependent diabetics. Am J Epidemiol 1983;117:186–192.

44. Laakso M, Voutilainen E, Pyorala K, Sarlund H. Association of low HDL and HDL₂ cholesterol with coronary heart disease in non-insulin-dependent diabetics. Arteriosclerosis 1985;5:653–658.

45. Fuh MM, Shieh SM. Association of low plasma high density lipoprotein (HDL)-cholesterol concentration with documented coronary artery disease in males with non-insulin dependent mellitus. Horm Metab Res 1987;19:267–270.

46. Garg A, Grundy SM. Lovastatin for lowering cholesterol levels in non-insulin-dependent diabetes mellitus. N Engl J Med 1988;318:81–86.

47. Stern MP, Patterson JK, Haffner SM, Hazuda HP, Mitchell BD. Lack of awareness and treatment of hyperlipidemia in type II diabetes in a community survey. JAMA 1989;262:360–364.

48. Wood FC Jr, Bierman EL. Is diet the cornerstone in management of diabetes? N Engl J Med 1986;315:1224–1227.

49. Simpson HC, Simpson RW, Lousley S, et al. A high carbohydrate leguminous fiber diet improves all aspects of diabetic control. Lancet 1981;1:1–5.

50. American Diabetes Association. Nutritional recommendations and principles for individuals with diabetes mellitus: 1986. Diabetes Care 1987;10:126–132.

51. Garg A, Bonanome A, Grundy SM, Zhang ZJ, Unger RH. Comparison of a high-carbohydrate diet with a high-monounsaturated diet in patients with non-insulin-dependent diabetes mellitus. N Engl J Med 1988;319:829–834.

52. Reaven GM. Dietary therapy for non-insulin-dependent diabetes mellitus. N Engl J Med 1988;319:862–864.

53. Anderson JW, Geil PB. New perspectives in nutrition management of diabetes mellitus. Am J Med 1988;85(suppl 5A):159–165.

54. Wing RR, Bunker CH, Kuller LH, Matthews KA. Insulin, body mass index, and cardiovascular risk factors in premenopausal women. Arteriosclerosis 1989;9:479–484.

55. Tzagournis M. Interaction of diabetes with hypertension and lipids—patients at high risk. Am J Med 1989;86(suppl 1B):50–54.

56. Gerich JE. Oral hypoglycemic agents. N Engl J Med 1989;321:1231–1245.

57. Dupree EA, Meyer MB. Role of risk factors in complications of diabetes mellitus. Am J Epidemiol 1980;112:100–112.

58. Holm G, Johansson S, Vedin A, Wilhelmsson C, Smith U. The effect of β-blockade on glucose tolerance and insulin release in adult diabetes. Acta Med Scand 1980;208:187–191.

59. Houston MC. Treatment of hypertension in diabetes mellitus. Am Heart J 1989;118:819–829.

60. Suarez L, Barrett-Connor E. Interaction between cigarette smoking and diabetes mellitus in the prediction of death attributed to cardiovascular disease. Am J Epidemiol 1984;120:670–675.

61. Beach KW, Brunzell JD, Strandness DE Jr. Prevalence of severe arteriosclerosis obliterans in patients with diabetes mellitus. Relation to smoking and form of therapy. Arteriosclerosis 1982;2:275–280.

62. Wilson PF, McGee DL, Kannel WB. Obesity, very low density lipoproteins, and glucose intolerance over fourteen years. The Framingham Study. Am J Epidemiol 1981;114:697–704.

63. O'Brien TR, Flanders WD, Decoufle P, Boyle CA, Destefano F, Teutsch S. Are racial differences in the prevalence of diabetes in adults explained by differences in obesity? JAMA 1989;262:1485–1488.

64. Amatruda JM, Richeson JF, Welle SL, Brodows RG, Lockwood DH. The safety and efficacy of a controlled low-energy ("very-low-calorie") diet in the treatment of non-insulin-dependent diabetes and obesity. Arch Intern Med 1988;148:873–877.

65. Devlin JT, Horton ES. Symposium on type II diabetics: diet and exercise: important therapeutic tools. Drug Therapy 1984;14:109–115.

66. Scheidt-Nave C, Barrett-Connor E, Wingard DL. Resting electrocardiographic abnormalities suggestive of asymptomatic ischemic heart disease associated with non-insulin-

dependent diabetes mellitus in a defined population. Circulation 1990;81:899–906.

67. Zarich SW, Nesto RW. Diabetic cardiomyopathy. Am Heart J 1989;118:1000–1012.

68. Ruddy TD, Shumak SL, Liu PP, et al. The relationship of cardiac diastolic dysfunction to concurrent hormonal and metabolic status in type I diabetes mellitus. J Clin Endocrinol Metab 1988;66:113–118.

8

physical activity

In recent years, numerous studies have examined the relation of habitual physical activity at work and leisure to the development of coronary artery disease (CAD). Because the conclusions of these studies have not been uniform, several articles and commentaries have been written to clarify the issue. After thorough reviews of the populations and methods used, most authors have concluded that physically active adults are at lower risk for CAD events than their sedentary counterparts (1–4).

Powell and colleagues found 43 studies that met their criteria for epidemiologic rigor. Four were case-control studies, three compared previous physical activity of persons from a specified population who had died from CAD, and 36 followed specific groups of individuals to determine the incidence of CAD events. They found an inverse association between physical activity and CAD in the various studies, consistent with biological plausibility, current knowledge, and a dose-response relation of the two measures. They concluded that the evidence was sufficient to support a causal link between physical activity and CAD. They further suggested that the magnitude of risk from physical inactivity is similar in magnitude to that from hypertension, dyslipidemias, and cigarette smoking. Given the large proportion of persons who

are physically inactive, they proposed that the proportion of CAD cases attributable, at least in part, to a sedentary life is large (5).

However, there have been no randomized clinical trials of physical activity and its effect on CAD development. Given the high costs of such investigations, and the methodological issues discussed below, it is unlikely that such a trial will be undertaken.

METHODOLOGY

Accurate quantitation of habitual physical activity has been a major limitation in most studies. Earlier studies tended to examine either occupational physical activity or leisure-time pursuits; more recent investigations have attempted to integrate the two. Studies of occupation-related physical activity have often used job titles or descriptions as a rough indicator of work demands. Categorization has been accomplished by questionnaire, corporate records, or death certificates. Quantitation of leisure physical activity often involves inquiring about time spent per week at various sports activities. Since such a crude measure serves to weaken the significance of any potential associations between caloric expenditure during physical activity and CAD, devices have been designed that can record body movement, giving a surrogate measure of physical activity. In general, however, use of these instruments is limited to smaller-scale research studies, leading investigators to continue work to develop self-report questionnaire items with increased reliability (6).

Several studies have measured physical fitness, suggesting it as a surrogate for habitual physical activity. Although they are more quantitative, measurements of fitness (such as treadmill testing or bicycle ergometry) are usually prohibitively expensive for large-scale population studies.

In addition to the possibility of its direct causal effect on CAD, physical activity may indirectly influence CAD events through its improvement of levels of the standard CAD risk indicators, such as blood pressure, lipids, and obesity. However, those studies that made statistical adjustments for such factors were just as likely to find an association between physical activity and CAD as those who made no such adjustments (5). A brief summary of the major studies to date follows.

EVIDENCE

Physical Activity

Morris and colleagues studied London busmen, noting more frequent CAD events amongst drivers than the more active conductors, who frequently climbed to the second story of the buses (7). Subsequent adjustments for age, initial level of fitness (as indicated in the waist size of uniforms issued upon employment), and other potentially confounding factors did not eliminate the significant associations between presumed (since they were not directly measured) physical activity levels of the two types of workers and CAD (8, 9). Later, Morris et al. questioned British,

male, civil service administrative workers about leisure-time physical activity during a sample weekend. Among these men whose occupations required little physical exertion, those who reported vigorous physical activity on the weekend had only half the fatal and nonfatal myocardial infarctions (MI) during the ensuing eight years as those who remained inactive on the weekend (10).

Paffenbarger and co-workers studied San Francisco longshoremen longitudinally. The energy expenditure on different jobs was quantified directly, and an adjustment was made annually for job transfers. Job energy requirements were inversely related to new CAD events; the relative risk associated with less active jobs varied (with age) between 1.5 and 3.0. Sudden cardiac death was even more strongly associated with relative physical inactivity than death occurring later after MI (11).

In another study, Paffenbarger et al. surveyed male alumni of Harvard University and the University of Pennsylvania whose college entrance (1916–1950) physical examination records had been reviewed. Leisure-time activities, including walking, sports play, and stair climbing, were assessed by self-report, then combined into a physical activity index expressed as kilocalories expended per week. College sports participation was not predictive, but men with current leisure-time activities requiring 2000 or more kilocalories per week did have a reduction of 25 to 30% in CAD risk and all-cause mortality compared to more sedentary alumni (12, 13).

In a given study population, the power of habitual activity to predict CAD events will depend upon a wide range of physical activity levels as well as the competing effects of other risk indicators. This is illustrated in the Framingham and Puerto Rico studies, which used the same physical activity questionnaire. In Framingham, most participants were sedentary and many had high levels of other CAD risk indicators. Little effect of physical activity on CAD events was observed in women; in men, the increased CAD risk noted with physical inactivity was much less important than other risk indicators (14). In contrast, there was a wide range of physical activity among the Puerto Rican participants, and it ranked immediately after hypertension as the most predictive CAD risk indicator (15). Other CAD risk indicators such as smoking were less prevalent in Puerto Rico than in mainland USA (16).

In a New Zealand case-control study, physical inactivity contributed as much of the attributable CAD risk as did hypertension and smoking. However, the decreased relative risk in subjects was largely found in those who had actively exercised for five years or more (17).

Studies in Finland have been particularly useful because of high CAD rates and wide variations in activity levels at leisure and during work. In one investigation of two rural male populations (east and southwestern Finland), work activity did not predict CAD incidence. Lumberjacks had the highest occupational energy expenditure, but did not have lower CAD rates. Examination of other CAD risk indicators revealed that their mean blood pressure and blood cholesterol levels were not different from men with more sedentary work, but they did have a higher percentage of cigarette smokers (18). In contrast, in a six-year follow-up study of women and men in two provinces of Eastern Finland (Kuopio and North Karelia), low physical activity at work was associated with an increased risk of MI, even after adjustment for other CAD risk indicators. Low levels of leisure-time activity also correlated significantly with MI; the association was weakened, but still signif-

icant, after adjustment for smoking, cholesterol, blood pressure, education, and social network participation (19).

In a third study conducted in four areas of Finland, leisure-time physical activity was inversely correlated with cardiovascular risk. Investigators employed an index that was the product of the number of exercise sessions per week and an indicator of session intensity (20).

A case-referent study of Dutch individuals suggests a protective effect from leisure-time physical activity (walking, cycling, or gardening), but only when performed more than eight months per year. CAD events that proved fatal within four months of onset were significantly higher in persons who were physically active less than four months per year (21). In a 12-year follow-up of women in Göteborg, Sweden, low physical activity at work was significantly related to overall mortality, and leisure-time inactivity was associated with increased stroke rates (22).

In the Multiple Risk Factor Intervention Trial (MRFIT) of middle-aged men in the upper 10 to 15% of CAD risk, participants in the lowest tertile of leisure-time physical activity (quantitated in mean minutes per day) had significantly more fatal and nonfatal CAD events, even after adjustment for possible confounding factors (23).

In men aged 45 to 69 years participating in the Honolulu Heart Program, those in the most active tertile had significantly lower rates of definite CAD during 12 years of follow-up (24).

In the Lipid Research Clinics (LRC) study, heart rate after completion of the second stage of the exercise test and the duration of exercise on baseline treadmill testing were used as measures of physical fitness. Lower levels of fitness were associated with higher CAD risk, independent of levels of other CAD risk indicators (25).

In addition to reducing the risk for

MI, regular vigorous exercise also decreases the overall risk of sudden cardiac death (26), although it may transiently raise that risk during the actual exercise periods (27).

Physical Fitness

A study of the Los Angeles Fire and Police Departments used cycle ergometry at baseline as an indicator of physical fitness; 2779 men were followed for approximately five years for development of a first MI. Those in the lower half of maximal oxygen uptake on ergometry had a relative risk of 2.2 for MI. Within this more sedentary half of the study population, those men with at least two other CAD risk indicators (smoking, hypertension, dyslipidemias) had a relative risk of 6.6 (28).

Some studies have measured both physical activity habits and physical fitness performance. In the Göteborg, Sweden study, for example, Wilhelmsen et al. noted increased CAD risk with leisure-time inactivity, but not with low physical activity at work (29).

EFFECTS ON CAD RISK INDICATORS

The positive benefits of physical activity on indicators of CAD event risk include improvement of lipid and lipoprotein profiles, enhanced blood-pressure control, and facilitation of weight reduction and maintenance. These topics will be discussed in detail below. While suggestive, evidence is not yet compelling for a positive effect of physical activity on smoking abstention maintenance and diabetes control. In addition, regular vigorous physical activity prevents post-menopausal bone loss (30) and may improve self-esteem and other indicators of psychological health (4).

Lipids and Lipoproteins

High-density lipoprotein (HDL) levels are directly related to physical activity. Endurance athletes typically have higher HDL levels than sedentary individuals, even after a year's training in the latter group, probably as a result of lower HDL-catabolism rates (31). In previously sedentary men, Stanford investigators found increased HDL levels after a year's training program, with changes proportional to the amount of exercise habitually performed (32). In this study, improved cardiovascular function determined by echocardiography also correlated with exercise duration per week (33).

In contrast, exercise effects on LDL-cholesterol have generally been small in the absence of weight change or dietary modification (34). In the Framingham Offspring Study, mean LDL-cholesterol levels were almost identical in persons categorized by quartiles of total yearly kilocalorie expenditure, while HDL levels were significantly inversely related (35).

Kramsch et al. fed monkeys an atherogenic diet, then allocated their animals to exercise conditioning and control groups for more than three years. Another group of monkeys ate a control diet and did not exercise. The exercise group had substantially reduced overall atherosclerotic involvement, lesion size, and collagen accumulation (36).

Hypertension

As part of an Irish Heart Foundation program, more than 15,000 men from industry and the general population were screened for CAD risk indicators. Different degrees of physical activity at work were not associated with blood pressure levels, but leisure-time physical activity was inversely related to systolic and diastolic blood pressure (37). Self-reported vigorous physical activity was inversely related to diastolic blood pressure in young adults from northern California communities (38). However, in the Framingham Offspring Study, there was no relation between yearly kilocalorie expenditure and either systolic or diastolic blood pressure. The investigators suggest that antihypertensive medication may have confounded the activity–blood pressure relationship in their study (35).

In healthy women who were self-referred for evaluation, the estimated maximal oxygen uptake on treadmill-test performance was inversely correlated with both systolic and diastolic blood pressures (39).

In longitudinal studies of individuals with baseline blood-pressure determination, low levels of self-reported physical activity and treadmill-test performance predict higher rates of hypertension development (40, 41). In studies of persons with borderline hypertension, physical training has been associated with significantly lower blood pressures (42–45).

Weight Reduction and Maintenance

Theoretically, an increased energy expenditure with constant caloric intake should result in weight loss. However, a moderate aerobic exercise program may add only 5 to 10% to one's weekly caloric expenditure, and weight loss from increased activity alone may seem slow to many patients. Some have suggested that the basal metabolic rate remains elevated after an acute bout of exercise, but data are conflicting (4). It is clear that increased physical activity coupled to dietary modification (lower saturated fats and calories) will result in weight reduction and maintenance.

In the Framingham Offspring Study (which included spouses of offspring of the original Framingham cohort as well), women and men in the least active quartile of yearly caloric expenditure had significantly higher mean values for body mass index (weight/height^2) (35). Of course, this observation may reflect the reluctance of obese persons to engage in vigorous activity.

EXERCISE PRESCRIPTION

The physician prescribes exercise for a wide variety of individuals, from the healthy, young, endurance athlete to the octogenarian recovering from MI. However, the principles of the exercise prescription remain the same. Frequency, duration, and intensity are the key parameters. In general, a frequency of 3 to 5 times weekly will provide adequate cardiovascular conditioning, while minimizing the risk of orthopaedic injury and maximizing adherence. Ideally, the prescription of exercise intensity is based on testing by treadmill or cycle ergometry. For those who cannot do leg exercise, stationary bicycles can be rotated 90° to provide an arm ergometry apparatus.

On the North American continent, treadmill testing is more common than cycle ergometry. Several protocols have been developed that adjust treadmill speed and inclination to provide varying workloads, which are usually calibrated in metabolic equivalents (METs). One MET activity (resting in sitting or supine position) involves an oxygen consumption of 3.5 mg/kg body weight/min. Depending on the patient's limitations and preferences, one or more of the protocols listed in Table 8.1 may be employed.

In the absence of indications of ischemia (electrocardiographic ST depression, angina, dysrhythmias, exertional hypotension), a training heart-rate range can be calculated which is 70 to 85% of the peak heart rate achieved on the treadmill test.

Table 8.1.   Treadmill Exericse Protocols[a] (Speed in Miles per Hour/Grade in %)

METs[b]	Balke	Bruce	Davidson-A	Davidson-B	Ellestad	Naughton
1.6		1.2/0	1.0/0	1.0/0		1.0/0
2.0			2.0/0	2.0/0		2.0/0
3.0	3.0/0	1.7/5	2.0/3.5	2.0/3.5		2.0/3.5
4.0	3.0/2.5		2.0/7	2.0/7		2.0/7
5.0	3.0/5.0	1.7/10	2.0/10	2.5/7	1.7/10	2.0/10.5
6.0	3.0/7.5		2.5/10	2.5/10		2.0/14
7.0	3.0/10	2.5/12	2.5/12.5	3.0/10	3.0/10	2.0/17.5
8.0	3.0/12.5		2.8/12.5	3.4/10		
9.0	3.0/15		3.0/15	3.8/10		
9.5		3.4/14			4.1/10	
10.0	3.0/17.5		3.0/17.5	4.1/10		
11.0	3.0/20		3.0/20	4.3/10		
12.0	3.0/22.5		3.0/22.5	4.5/10		

[a]Data from: DeBusk R. The value of exercise stress testing. JAMA 1975; 232:956–958. Davidson DM, Maloney CA. Recovery after cardiac events. Phys Ther 1985; 65:1820–1827.
[b]METs = Metabolic equivalents, where one MET equals an oxygen consumption of 3.5 ml/kg body weight/minute.

An alternative calculation recommended by Karvonen involves adding 60 to 70% of the heart rate (HR) increase during exercise to the resting heart rate. In equation form:

$$\text{Target Heart-Rate Range} = \text{Resting HR} + (60 \text{ to } 70\%)(\text{Peak HR} - \text{Resting HR})$$

Because the perception of effort varies among individuals with cardiac impairment, age (46), and other factors, an appropriate next step is to consider the individual's reports of exertion during each stage of the test, using the original Borg scale shown in Table 8.2 (47). To optimize adherence, the training heart-rate range should coincide with a perceived exertion rating of 11 to 13 ("fairly light" to "somewhat hard"). If one exercises at easier levels, cardiovascular conditioning is suboptimal; at much harder levels, exercise duration is frequently decreased as compensation.

Most patients find it convenient to monitor their heart rate while exercising for 10-second intervals, so the exercise prescription can also be expressed in those terms.

To demonstrate the value of habitual exercise, some programs have focused on preparing their participants for marathon races. For a brief period, some advocates asserted that no person who finished a

Table 8.2.   Borg Scale for Perceived Exertion[a]

Numerical Rating	Description
6	
7	Very, very light
8	
9	Very light
10	
11	Fairly light
12	
13	Somewhat hard
14	
15	Fairly hard
16	
17	Very hard
18	
19	Very, very hard
20	

[a]From Borg G. Perceived exertion as an indicator of somatic stress. Scand J Rehabil Med 1970; 2:92–98.

marathon ever died from CAD. As with all things in medicine, this was soon followed by a series of reports of autopsy-proved coronary atherosclerosis in marathoners. Other investigators have documented impaired left ventricular performance after an uninterrupted, competitive 24-hour run (48).

Even more modest levels of running may be accompanied by hazard. In addition to musculoskeletal injuries, frostbite, and heat stroke, joggers have been attacked by motor vehicles and buzzards (49).

In elderly individuals, walking often elevates heart rates into the training heart-rate range. As conditioning proceeds, the speed and length of walking can be increased to maintain a stimulus for cardiovascular adaptation.

Adoption of vigorous exercise habits has many determinants, including the genetic and environmental influences of one's parents, age, perceived barriers to exercise, support from friends, and exercise self-efficacy (the confidence that one can exercise at given levels in specific situations) (50, 51). After adoption, the critical factor becomes maintaining motivation and adherence to the healthier habits.

ADHERENCE

Oldridge has described factors associated with lack of adherence to exercise in cardiac patients. These include lack of interest, motivation, and spousal support; time and location inconvenience; and angina or other medical problems. The exercise dropout is likely to be an overweight blue-collar worker who continues to smoke cigarettes. Oldridge recommends program staff and structure adaptation to the individual's needs, making referrals as necessary to other health professionals, such as those specializing in nutrition, smoking cessation, and stress management coun-

seling (52). King and colleagues found that brief baseline instruction in self-monitoring, coupled with frequent telephone contact by program staff, allowed healthy individuals to successfully adopt and maintain a moderate-intensity, home-based exercise training program (53).

Several investigators have noted a decrease in preexisting depression with the adoption of a vigorous exercise program (54). In the USA, investigators in the first National Health and Nutrition Examination Study (NHANES) used the Center for Epidemiologic Studies Depression (CES-D) Scale, a sensitive measure of mild depressive symptoms. A lack of recreational physical activity at baseline was correlated with depressive symptoms in both men and women. Prospectively, women with a significant activity level at baseline had significantly fewer depressive symptoms eight years later (55). Differences in depression levels have been attributed to improved self-efficacy, social support and involvement, and increased neurotransmission of catecholamines and endogenous opiates in persons who exercise regularly (56).

Finally, it appears that habitual physical activity may be beneficial for the economy of the United States. Investigators from the Centers for Disease Control and the RAND Corporation have demonstrated net economic savings under certain scenarios for exercising adults (57, 58).

REFERENCES

1. Froelicher V, Battler A, McKirnan MD. Physical activity and coronary heart disease. Cardiology 1980;65:153–190.

2. LaPorte RE, Adams LL, Savage DD, Brenes G, Dearwater S, Cook T. The spectrum of physical activity, cardiovascular disease and health: An epidemiologic perspective. Am J Epidemiol 1984;120:507–517.

3. Curfman GD, Thomas GS, Paffenbarger RS Jr. Physical activity and primary pre-

vention of cardiovascular disease. Cardiol Clin 1985;3:203–222.

4. Phelps JR. Physical activity and health maintenance—exactly what is known? West J Med 1987;146:200–206.

5. Powell KE, Thompson PD, Caspersen CJ, Kendrick JS. Physical activity and the incidence of coronary heart disease. Ann Rev Public Health 1987;8:253–287.

6. Sallis JF, Haskell WL, Wood PD, et al. Physical activity assessment methodology in the Five-City Project. Am J Epidemiol 1985;121:91–106.

7. Morris JN, Heady JA, Raffle PA, Roberts CG, Parks JW. Coronary heart disease and physical activity of work. Lancet 1953;2:1053–1057,1111–1120.

8. Heady JA, Morris JN, Kagan A, Raffle PA. Coronary heart disease in London busmen: a progress report with special reference to physique. Br J Soc Prev Med 1961;15:143–153.

9. Morris JN, Kagan A, Pattison DC, Gardner MJ, Raffle PA. Incidence and prediction of ischaemic heart disease in London busmen. Lancet 1966;2:553–559.

10. Morris JN, Everitt MG, Pollard R, Chave SP. Vigorous exercise in leisure-time; protection against coronary heart disease. Lancet 1980;2:1207–1210.

11. Paffenbarger RS Jr, Hale WE. Work activity and coronary heart mortality. N Engl J Med 1975;292:545–550.

12. Paffenbarger RS Jr, Wing AL, Hyde RT. Physical activity as an index of heart attack risk in college alumni. Am J Epidemiol 1978;108:161–175.

13. Paffenbarger RS Jr, Hyde RT, Wing AL, Hsieh CC. Physical activity, all-cause mortality, and longevity of college alumni. N Engl J Med 1986;314:605–613.

14. Kannel WB, Sorlie P. Some health benefits of physical activity. The Framingham Study. Arch Intern Med 1979;139:857–861.

15. Garcia-Palmieri MR, Costas R Jr, Cruz-Vidal M, Sorlie PD, Havlik RJ. Increased physical activity. A protective factor against heart attacks in Puerto Rico. Prev Med 1982;50:749–755.

16. Sorlie PD, Garcia-Palmieri MR, Costas R, Cruz-Vidal M, Havlik R. Cigarette smoking and coronary heart disease in Puerto Rico. Prev Med 1982;11:304–316.

17. Scragg R, Stewart A, Jackson R, Beaglehole R. Alcohol and exercise in myocardial infarction and sudden coronary death in men and women. Am J Epidemiol 1987;126:77–85.

18. Punsar S, Karvonen MJ. Physical activity and coronary heart disease in populations from east and west Finland. Adv Cardiol 1976;18:196–207.

19. Salonen JT, Slater JS, Tuomilehto J, Rauramaa R. Leisure time and occupational physical activity: risk of death from ischemic heart disease. Am J Epidemiol 1988;127:87–94.

20. Tuomilehto J, Marti B, Salonen JT, Virtala E, Lahti T, Puska P. Leisure-time physical activity is inversely related to risk factors for coronary heart disease in middle-aged Finnish men. Eur Heart J 1987;8:1047–1055.

21. Magnus K, Matroos A, Strackee J. Walking, cycling or gardening with or without seasonal interruption, in relation to acute coronary events. Am J Epidemiol 1979;110:724–733.

22. Lapidus L, Bengtsson C. Socioeconomic factors and physical activity in relation to cardiovascular disease and death. A 12-year follow-up of participants in a population study of women in Gothenburg, Sweden. Br Heart J 1986;55:295–301.

23. Leon AS, Connett J, Jacobs DR Jr, Rauramaa R. Leisure-time physical activity levels and risk of coronary heart disease and death. The Multiple Risk Factor Intervention Trial. JAMA 1987;258:2388–2395.

24. Donahue RP, Abbott RD, Reed DM, Yano K. Physical activity and coronary heart disease in middle-aged and elderly men: the Honolulu Heart Program. Am J Public Health 1988;78:683–685.

25. Ekelund LG, Haskell WL, Johnson JL, Whaley FS, Criqui MH, Sheps DS. Physical fitness as a predictor of cardiovascular mortality in asymptomatic North American men. The Lipid Research Clinics Mortality Follow-up Study. N Engl J Med 1988;319:1379–1384.

26. Siscovick DS, Weiss NS, Fletcher RH, Schoenbach VJ, Wagner EH. Habitual vigorous exercise and primary cardiac arrest; effect of other risk factors on the relationship. J Chron Dis 1984;37:625–631.

27. Siscovick DS, Weiss NS, Fletcher RH, Lasky T. The incidence of primary cardiac arrest during vigorous exercise. N Engl J Med 1984;311:874–877.

28. Peters RK, Cady LD, Bischoff DP, Bernstein L, Pike MC. Physical fitness and subsequent myocardial infarction in healthy workers. JAMA 1983;249:3052–3056.

29. Wilhelmsen L, Tibblin G, Aurell M, Bjure J, Ekstrom-Jodal B, Grimby G. Physical activity, physical fitness and risk of myocardial infarction. Adv Cardiol 1976;18:217–230.

30. Smith R. Exercise and osteoporosis. Br Med J 1985;1:1163–1164.

31. Thompson PD, Cullinane EM, Sady SP, et al. Modest changes in high-density lipoprotein concentration and metabolism with prolonged exercise training. Circulation 1988;78:25–34.

32. Wood PD, Haskell WL, Blair SN, et al. Increased exercise level and plasma lipoprotein concentrations: A one-year randomized controlled study in sedentary middle-aged men. Metabolism 1983;32:31–39.

33. Davidson DM, Popp RL, Haskell WL, Wood PD, Blair S, Ho P. Echocardiographic changes during a one-year exercise program in previously sedentary normal middle-aged men. In: Rijsterborgh H(ed): Echocardiology. The Hague, Netherlands: Martinus Nijhoff Publishers, 1981:167–170.

34. Haskell WL. Exercise-induced changes in plasma lipids and lipoproteins. Prev Med 1984;13:23–36.

35. Dannenberg AL, Keller JB, Wilson PW, Castelli WP. Leisure time physical activity in the Framingham Offspring Study. Description, seasonal variation, and risk factor correlates. Am J Cardiol 1989;129:76–88.

36. Kramsch DM, Aspen AJ, Abramowitz BM, Kreimendahl T, Hood WB Jr. Reduction of coronary atherosclerosis by moderate conditioning exercise in monkeys on an atherogenic diet. N Engl J Med 1981;305:1483–1489.

37. Hickey N, Mulcahy R, Bourke GJ, Graham I, Wilson-Davis K. Study of coronary risk factors related to physical activity in 15,171 men. Br Med J 1975;3:507–509.

38. Sallis JF, Haskell WL, Wood PD, Fortmann SP, Vranizan KM. Vigorous physical activity and cardiovascular risk factors in young adults. J Chron Dis 1986;39:115–120.

39. Gibbons LW, Blair SN, Cooper KH, et al. Association between coronary heart disease risk factors and physical fitness in healthy adult women. Circulation 1983;67:977–983.

40. Paffenbarger RS Jr, Hyde RT. Exercise in the prevention of coronary heart disease. Prev Med 1984;13:3–22.

41. Blair SN, Goodyear NN, Gibbons LW, et al. Physical fitness and incidence of hypertension in healthy normotensive men and women. JAMA 1984;252:487–490.

42. Kukkonen K, Rauramaa R, Voutilainen E, Lansimies E. Physical training of middle-aged men with borderline hypertension. Ann Clin Res 1982;14(suppl 34):139–145.

43. Duncan JJ, Farr JE, Upton SJ, Hagan RD, Oglesby ME, Blair SN. The effects of aerobic exercise on plasma catecholamines and blood pressure in patients with mild essential hypertension. JAMA 1985;254:2609–2613.

44. DeBusk R. The value of exercise stress testing. JAMA 1975;232:956–958.

45. Davidson DM, Maloney CA. Recovery after cardiac events. Phys Ther 1985;65:1820–1827.

46. Shephard RJ. Habitual physical activity levels and perception of exertion in the elderly. J Cardiopulmonary Rehabil 1989;9:17–23.

47. Borg G. Perceived exertion as an indicator of somatic stress. Scand J Rehabil Med 1970;2:92–98.

48. Niemela KO, Palatsi IJ, Ikaheimo MJ, Takkunen JT, Vuori JJ. Evidence of impaired left ventricular performance after an uninterrupted competitive 24-hour run. Circulation 1984;70:350–356.

49. Itin P, Haenel A, Stalder H. From the heavens, revenge on joggers. N Engl J Med 1984;311:1703.

50. Perusse L, Tremblay A, Leblanc C, Bouchard C. Genetic and environmental influences on level of habitual physical activity and exercise participation. Am J Epidemiol 1989;129:1012–1022.

51. Sallis JF, Hovell MF, Hofstetter CR, et al. A multivariate study of determinants of vigorous exercise in a community sample. Prev Med 1989;18:20–34.

52. Oldridge NB. Compliance and dropout in cardiac exercise rehabilitation. J Cardiac Rehabil 1984;4:166–169, 173–177.

53. King AC, Taylor CB, Haskell WL, DeBusk RF. Strategies for increasing early adherence to and long-term maintenance of home-based exercise training in healthy middle-aged men and women. Am J Cardiol 1988;61:628–632.

54. Taylor CB, Sallis JF, Needle R. The relation of physical activity and exercise to mental health. Publ Health Reports 1985; 100:195–202.

55. Farmer ME, Locke BZ, Moscicki EK, Dannenberg AL, Larson DB, Radloff LS. Physical activity and depressive symptoms: the NHANES I Epidemiologic Follow-up Study. Am J Epidemiol 1988;128:1340–1351.

56. Hughes JR. Psychological effects of habitual aerobic exercise: A critical review. Prev Med 1984;13:66–78.

57. Hatziandreu EI, Koplan JP, Weinstein MC, Caspersen CJ, Warner KE. A cost-effectiveness analysis of exercise as a health promotion activity. Am J Public Health 1988;78:1417–1421.

58. Keeler EB, Manning WG, Newhouse JP, Sloss EM, Wasserman J. The external costs of a sedentary lifestyle. Am J Public Health 1989;79:975–981.

9

obesity

Until the past decade, most investigators of CAD development had concluded that obesity, while having a positive association with CAD events, was not an independent indicator of risk. Recognition of the negative influence on other CAD risk indicators was noted, however, leading to the general recommendation to achieve and maintain an ideal weight for one's height. In recent years, epidemiologists have refined measurements of obesity and their discriminative power in predicting CAD.

DEFINITIONS AND MEASURES

Obesity, a high proportion of body fat frequently resulting in an impairment of health, should be distinguished from overweight, a high value of body weight over some standard based on height (1, 2). Two persons of the same gender, height, and weight may have substantial differences in their percentages of fat and lean body tissue. Techniques for accurately determining body-fat percentage, such as isotopic dilution measurements or underwater weighing, are generally used only in research settings (3). Anthropometric measurements, including height, weight, waist and hip circumference, skinfold thicknesses, and skeletal measurements, are more appropriate for epidemiologic and office use. For adults, the estimation of relative weight and calculation of body mass index are most commonly used.

For more than 75 years, height and weight tables have been used in North America. The Metropolitan Life Insurance Company developed tables of ideal weights, noting evidence that adult overweight was associated with shortened life spans. In 1959, the company published desired weight tables, based on results from the Build and Blood Pressure Study reported that year (4, 5). Desirable weights were determined by choosing from 4.5 million policyholders whose relative weights were associated with the lowest all-cause mortality rates. Without specifying criteria for frame size, the tables were constructed by allocating those within the desired weight range into quartiles, with the lowest being designated "small frame" and the upper quartile as "large frame" (6).

In 1983, the same company published new tables, recommending that frame-size determination be based on the bicondylar breadth of the humerus, with reference values coming from the first National Health and Nutrition Examination Survey (NHANES I) done during 1971 to 1974. These tables, based on the 1979 Build and Blood Pressure studies, drew considerable comment from clinicians and public health officials because "desirable weights" had increased (1).

The methodology of the desirable or ideal weight concept has been questioned (7). Manson and colleagues found that they could not do a formal metaanalysis on the 25 major prospective studies on optimal weight, because each study had failed to control for at least one of the following: smoking, hypertension, hyperglycemia, or weight loss due to subclinical disease (8). Further, Gordon and Doyle point out that data from these studies were usually collected at least a decade before their publication, and they suggest that the health implications of a given weight for height may vary with one's position along the lifespan (9).

Of the possible permutations of height and weight relations, weight divided by the square of height (usually using kg and m) has been most widely accepted. Termed the body-mass index (BMI) by Keys and colleagues, this measure has the best correlation with body fat (body weight minus lean body mass) (10). While direct measurement is preferred, several studies have indicated that self-reported height and weight are reasonably accurate (11), although there is a tendency for heavy persons to underreport their weight and shorter individuals to overreport their height (12). A second NHANES was done from 1976 to 1980, also based on a representative sample of USA residents. From data collected, investigators found that BMI levels exceeding 27.8 for men and 27.3 for women describe the upper 15% of the population. The NIH Consensus Development Panel recommended weight reduction for persons above those levels, and at lower levels of BMI when hypertension or diabetes is present (2). As Jarrett points out (13), the panel did not specify whether the 1959 or 1983 tables were to be used, but in either case, "upper limit" values are substantially higher than those recommended by the Fogarty Center conference on obesity in 1973 or those recommended by the Royal College of Physicians (14). Given these ambiguities and the lack of familiarity of many patients in the USA with metric measurements of their height and weight, clinicians may find it difficult to communicate goals for weight reduction.

However, individual subjects can measure waist and hip girths with acceptable accuracy and reliability (15). Recent studies indicate that the proportions of these two measurements are indicative of CAD risk, so that a goal of reduction in "inches" may facilitate practitioner-patient dialogue.

PREVALENCE OF OBESITY

During the prepubertal years, body fat in both girls and boys is approximately 15 to 18%. After puberty, the body-fat percentage in girls increases substantially. Between the ages of 20 and 50, fat content often doubles, although total body weight increases only 10 to 15%, suggesting some reduction in lean body mass with aging. Body-fat percentage varies with current physical activity level, parity, smoking, cultural norms, socioeconomic conditions, and residence (1, 6, 16, 17) and the knowledge and attitudes that accompany these conditions (18), so it is difficult to determine exact prevalence levels without specifying the population subset of interest. Using the NHANES II criteria, a 1987 survey in the United States revealed an overweight prevalence of approximately 21%, ranging from 15% in New Mexico to 26% in Wisconsin (19).

OBESITY AND CAD

Adoption and genetic studies confirm that height shows multifactoral inheritance patterns, but data are conflicting regarding the relative contributions of heredity and environment to fatness in adult humans (20, 21).

Clearly, there are several potential causes of obesity, including defective thermogenesis (22), adipose tissue size and number (23), energy intake (24), and energy expenditure (25). Bogardus et al. demonstrated a familial tendency for resting metabolic rate within Native Americans in southwestern USA, but they found that persons from families with lower rates were no more likely to be obese (26).

Cardiac function changes have been associated with moderate to severe obesity, even in young persons. Left ventricular function impairment is correlated with the level of obesity (27). Left ventricular mass also increases; since hypertension so often coexists with obesity, the two effects are probably independent and additive (28, 29).

CAD Prevalence and Incidence

RELATIVE BODY WEIGHT

In morbid obesity (200% or more of ideal weight), all-cause mortality is 6 to 12 times greater in men under the age of 45 than in men of average weight. Most deaths in these obese men are cardiovascular (30).

In persons with lesser degrees of obesity, Keys et al. noted a higher prevalence of obesity in men of North America and southern Europe than in those in northern Europe, but they found no independent contribution of relative weight or obesity to future CAD after adjustment for other risk indicators (31). In Glostrup, Denmark, women and men with a relative weight of 120% had twice the risk of CAD events (32). In Honolulu, male residents of Japanese heritage who were in the upper quintile of BMI had significantly higher CAD rates (33). Adult residents of American Samoa have a high prevalence of obesity, but after controlling for diastolic blood pressure, obesity is no longer independently predictive of CAD deaths (34).

Hubert and colleagues found that baseline relative weight of Framingham Study participants was independently correlated with CAD events over 26 years in both men and women. They also noted that weight gain after early adulthood conveyed an increased CAD risk that was not attributable to either initial weight or the levels of CAD risk indicators associated with a weight gain (35). In the adult population studies of eastern Finland, BMI did not contribute significantly to the risk of either MI or CAD death in women, but men with BMI of 28.5 or more had a significantly higher incidence of MI. This effect was independent of smoking, but not of hypertension and dyslipidemia (36).

In the Nurses' Health Study, women in the heaviest decile (BMI>29) had fatal and nonfatal MI three times more frequently than women in the leanest quartile (37).

BODY WEIGHT CHANGE

Change in body weight has also been documented to reflect CAD risk. In comparing the 25-year mortality of middle-aged men by weight gain during that interval, investigators noted that subjects who had reported large gains (with or without large losses) were at double the risk for CAD death, even after adjustment for other CAD risk indicators (38). In the Göteborg, Sweden study of middle-aged women, the incidence of angina pectoris was significantly correlated with weight gain over a six-year period (39). In the Nurses' Health Study, women who had gained 20 kg or more had a relative risk of 2.5 for fatal and nonfatal MI (37).

BODY FAT DISTRIBUTION

The prevalence of CAD in men and women, blacks and whites, was higher in persons with greater abdominal:lower body fat ratios. Mean values of the upper:lower body fat distribution increased with age in all groups, was higher in men than in women, and was higher in black women than in white women (40). In a study of 41.837 Iowa women aged 55 to 69, the prevalence of a history of MI was 2.2 times higher in persons in the highest tertile of waist to hip circumference ratio versus those in the lowest tertile. This ratio was better correlated than BMI with MI prevalence (41).

Incidence studies have noted that the rate of new CAD events is likewise related to waist to hip circumference ratio. With 13-year follow-up of 975 randomly selected men with obesity in Göteborg, those in the upper quintile had CAD rates double those in the lowest quintile (42). In a 12-year follow-up of 1462 Göteborg women, similar findings were obtained; the incidence of MI continued to correlate highly with upper body fat predominance after multivariate adjustment for other CAD risk indicators (43). Central obesity also conferred an increased CAD risk on women in the Framingham Study (44).

In a 12-year study of 7692 male participants in the Honolulu Heart Study, the risk of incident CAD events was directly related to central obesity as measured with skinfold thicknesses. This effect persisted even after adjustment for age, cholesterol, triglycerides, glucose, hypertension, and smoking. However, the association of BMI with CAD events was not independent of these other CAD risks (45).

OBESITY AND CAD RISK INDICATORS

Lipids and Lipoproteins

Elevations of triglycerides and reductions in HDL-cholesterol have been associated with relative body weight (46, 47) and measures of central obesity (48–50). With a significant weight loss, HDL-cholesterol can increase, while triglycerides decrease (51, 52). Brownell and Stunkard found such changes to be more marked in men than in women (53), while Follick and colleagues found significant long-term changes in women, although they observed no changes during the 10-week treatment program for weight loss (54). Schwartz noted that elevations in HDL-cholesterol with weight loss were not accompanied by similar rises in HDL_2 or apoA-1, in contrast to the effects of physical activity (55), while Wood et al. did find significant increases in HDL_2 (52).

Hypertension

Data from several epidemiologic studies and clinical trials have confirmed the clinical observation of a direct relation between obesity and hypertension. Work continues, however, on several issues. These include the proportion of hypertension attributable to obesity, demographic differences in the obesity-hypertension association, the role of body fat distribution, and the effects of blood pressure treatment in obese persons (56).

The cross-sectional association between obesity and blood pressure is quite consistent, regardless of the specific obesity measures used. Chiang et al. reviewed more than 20 population studies, noting linear increases in both systolic and diastolic blood pressure with increasing body weight or relative weight. This was true despite the possibility of overestimating blood pressure by sphygmomanometry in persons with large arm circumferences (57). Using self-report as underweight, normal weight, or overweight, investigators of the Community Hypertension Evaluation Clinic program surveyed more than one million USA residents. Persons classifying themselves as overweight had prevalence rates of hypertension 1.5 to 3.0 times higher than other screenees (58).

Relative weight and BMI were both correlated with blood pressure in the Tecumseh, Framingham, and NHANES-I studies (59–61). More than 400 black physicians were enrolled in a prospective study while they were students at Meharry Medical College between 1958 and 1965. Their subsequent development of hypertension correlated both with initial body weight and with weight change over a 22.5-year follow-up period (62). In their study of Harvard University alumni, Paffenbarger et al. noted that those participants with 120% or more of desirable weight at baseline were 78% more likely to develop hypertension than leaner men. Those who had gained 25 pounds or more since entering college were 60% more likely to become hypertensive (63). In their 10-year study of Swedish women, Noppa and co-workers documented a positive correlation between the incidence of hypertension and both BMI and central fat preponderance (64).

Stallones and colleagues found body weight had a stronger statistical association with blood pressure than did body fat or fat patterns in USA adolescents (65), but studies in older women and men confirm the risk of higher waist:hip girth ratios. In NHANES-I, hypertension and hypertensive heart disease were more prevalent in men and women aged 18 to 79 with higher ratios (40). In a survey of more than 30,000 women who belonged to a national weight-reduction organization, the ratio was significantly associated with hypertension in women age 40 or older (66). Further studies in this population revealed that diabetes mellitus also correlated with fat distribution, with increased risk not only from abdominal preponderance, but from increased fat from various regions of the upper body (67). Progression from normotension to hypertension in members of the Kaiser Permanente Medical Care Program was more likely in those with centrally deposited body fat, independent of the overall level of obesity (68).

In the Hypertension Detection and Follow-up Program (HDFP), it was estimated that a majority of hypertensives in the USA are more than 20% overweight (69). In the Risk Factor Prevalence Study sponsored by the National Heart Foundation of Australia, obesity was defined as BMI of 26 or more in men, 25 or more in women. Investigators estimated that, in women and men aged 25 to 64, approximately one-third of the prevalence of hypertension was attributable to obesity. In men aged 25 to 44, that prevalence figure was doubled (70).

Results from some studies have suggested that obese hypertensives may have a lower rate of CAD development, but a prospective study of Japanese-American men showed that CAD risk associated with hypertension was similar across quintiles of BMI (71). Further study of this question may be limited by the availability of lean hypertensives.

Treatment of hypertension in obese persons should begin with weight reduction through diet and exercise (72); a 1 mm Hg drop in systolic and diastolic blood pressure may be seen with each kg body weight lost (56). Sodium restriction appears to have an independent effect from weight reduction in hypertension treatment (73). Its effects are particularly noticeable during the first week of weight reduction effort (74). With weight loss, plasma renin activity decreases, irrespective of sodium intake (75). Cardiac output decreases are directly related to a contracted total blood volume and decreased cardiopulmonary blood volume. Resting circulating levels of plasma norepinephrine also fall after a significant weight loss (76).

Among the HDFP, some voluntarily lost weight over the first two years. Compared to those who gained weight, those who lost weight had a 30% greater reduction in systolic blood pressure and a 77% greater drop in diastolic blood pressure (77). Even among normotensive men, weight loss can significantly decrease both clinic and ambulatory blood pressure readings (78).

Smoking

Smoking by the obese individual has confounded analyses of weight and cardiovascular mortality (79). Investigators in the Evans County (Georgia, USA) studies noted that smokers have an increasing CAD risk with increasing degrees of overweight (80). Persistence of smoking during successful therapeutic weight reduction minimizes the beneficial effects of weight loss on HDL- and LDL-cholesterol levels, especially in women (81).

TREATMENT OF OBESITY

Given the health hazards detailed above, the need becomes clear for treating what Brownell has described as a "serious, prevalent, and refractory disorder." He asserts that if "cure" from obesity is defined as reduction to, and maintenance at, ideal weight for five years, a person is more likely to recover from most forms of cancer than from obesity (82). Programs for weight loss have been mounted in the schools and at work sites as well as being offered through clinics and community organizations. Based on behavioral modification principles, many programs have helped their participants achieve weight reductions of 1 to 2 pounds per week, but individual responses are rather unpredictable. At the core of most programs is dietary adjustment, supplemented by advocacy for increased physical activity.

Diet

Despite interindividual variation, Bray and Gray assert that "no adult patient who has been studied in a metabolic chamber has needed fewer than 1200 kcal per day for maintaining weight" (1). Many studies show a predictable rate of weight loss when caloric intake is reduced below expenditure. Conventional diets can be defined as those with intake below energy expenditure but greater than 800 kcal intake per day. Very low calorie diets are those containing between 200 and 800 kcal per day, while starvation diets have intakes below 200 kcal daily.

An important component of dietary prescription is the distribution of calories. In one study of middle-aged men, systolic and diastolic blood pressures correlated inversely with monounsaturated fat intake (83). Although saturated fat restriction is important in CAD prevention, substitution of carbohydrates may lead to sodium retention and transient gains in body weight. Carbohydrate intake can also influence triiodothyronine and may alter metabolic rates (1). Brownell describes the animal experiments of Sciafani and Springer, who fed a "supermarket" diet of chocolate chip cookies, salami, cheese, bananas, marshmallows, milk chocolate, peanut butter, sweetened condensed milk, and a fat ration to rats, who gained three times as much weight as the control animals within two months (82). The resemblance of this diet to that consumed by many young people should not escape the reader.

To ensure an adequate intake of vitamins and minerals, it is important for a person following a restricted-calorie diet to avoid foods that have little or no nutritive value, such as alcohol and foods high in sucrose, choosing instead those that are "nutrient-dense." Meal frequency also appears to be important for weight loss and minimization of lipid-induced CAD risk. In one study, when the same number of calories were fed as 17 snacks per day rather than three meals daily, LDL-cholesterol and apo-B concentrations fell 10 to 15% (84).

Very low calorie diets have been effectively combined with behaviour therapy to produce a rate of weight loss that is satisfying for the patient, with some decline in long-term effectiveness but a minimum of complications (85). These diets should be carefully distinguished from one liquid-protein diet that contained collagen as its sole source of protein and resulted in at least 17 fatalities, often secondary to ventricular tachycardia and cardiac arrest (86). Later formulations that contain casein, egg albumin, or soy as high-quality proteins, along with adequate quantities of potassium, magnesium, vitamins, and minerals, have been used with no recurrences of the fatal dysrhythmias (87, 88).

Important behavioral modification principles in dietary adjustment include self-monitoring, stimulus control, and self-reward. Patients should record the location, frequency, and emotional setting during eating, as well as attempting to identify events that prompted the meal or snack. Physical constraints to food access or rapidity of eating can be designed and implemented for the individual patient. Finally, a system of self-rewards will reinforce positive steps towards healthier eating behaviors.

An increased rate of gallstone formation has been described in women and men during weight loss (89, 90).

Exercise

Concomitant exercise may facilitate adherence to dietary modification (91), although vigorous activity that increases lean body mass may obscure real losses of body fat, if only total body weight is monitored. However, monitoring "inches" at waist and hip regions should eliminate that concern.

In moderately obese persons, a decrease in fat-cell size is noted along with a reduction of body fat content during physical training. In contrast, persons with a large number of relatively small fat cells, termed hyperplastic obesity, respond less favorably to physical activity programs (1).

Drug and Invasive Treatments

Bray and Gray have recently reviewed the evidence for the use of drugs and invasive procedures in the treatment of obesity. Appetite-suppressing drugs include those that act on catecholamine or serotonin neurotransmitters, phenylpropanolamine, phenytoin, and opioid antagonists. Thermogenic drugs include thyroid hormone, ephedrine, and β-adrenergic agonists. Invasive techniques include placement of the gastric bubble, jaw wiring, vagotomy, liposuction, and a variety of other gastrointestinal surgical procedures. They conclude that behavior modification is a key element of long-term maintenance of weight loss, even with the excellent surgical results (1).

REFERENCES

1. Bray GA, Gray DS. Obesity. West J Med 1988;149:429–441,555–571.

2. National Institutes of Health Consensus Development Panel. Health implications of obesity: National Institutes of Health Consensus Development Conference statement. Ann Intern Med 1985;103:1073–1077.

3. Noppa H, Andersson M, Bengtsson C, Bruce A, Isaksson B. Longitudinal studies of anthropometric data and body composition. The population study of women in Goteborg, Sweden. Am J Clin Nutr 1980;33:155–162.

4. Metropolitan Life Insurance Company. New weight standards for men and women. Stat Bull 1959;40:1–4.

5. Build and Blood Pressure Study, vol 1 and 2. Chicago: Society of Actuaries, 1959.

6. Van Itallie TB. When the frame is part of the picture. Am J Publ Health 1985;75:1054–1055.

7. Knapp TR. A methodological critique of the "ideal weight" concept. JAMA 1983;250:506–510.

8. Manson JE, Stampfer MJ, Hennekens CH, Willett WC. Body weight and longevity. A reassessment. JAMA 1987;257:353–358.

9. Gordon T, Doyle JT. Weight and mortality in men: the Albany Study. Int J Epidemiol 1988;17:77–81.

10. Keys A, Fidanza F, Karvonen MJ, Kimura N, Taylor HL. Indices of relative weight and obesity. J Chron Dis 1972;25:329–343.

11. Stewart AL. The reliability and validity of self-reported weight and height. J Chron Dis 1982;35:295–309.

12. Schlichting P, Hoiland-Carlsen PF, Quaade F. Comparison of self-reported height and weight with controlled height and weight in women and men. Int J Obesity 1981;5:67–76.

13. Jarrett RJ. Is there an ideal body weight? Br Med J 1986;293:493–495.

14. Royal College of Physicians. Obesity: a report. J R Coll Physicians, Lond 1983;17:3–58.

15. Kushi LH, Kaye SA, Folsom AR, Soler JT, Prineas RJ. Accuracy and reliability of self-measurement of body girths. Am J Epidemiol 1988;128:740–748.

16. Noppa H, Bengtsson C. Obesity in relation to socioeconomic status. A population study of women in Goteborg, Sweden. J Epidemiol Comm Health 1980;34:139–142.

17. Heliovaara M, Aromaa A. Parity and obesity. J Epidemiol Comm Health 1981;35:197–199.

18. Stern MP, Pugh JA, Gaskill SP, Hazuda HP. Knowledge, attitudes and behavior related to obesity and dieting in Mexican Americans and Anglos: the San Antonio Heart Study. Am J Epidemiol 1982;115:917–928.

19. Anonymous. Prevalence of overweight—Behavioral Risk Factor Surveillance System 1987. MMWR 1989;38:421–423.

20. Karlin S, Williams PT, Jensen S, Farquhar JW. Genetic analysis of the Stanford LRC family study data. Am J Epidemiol 1981;113:307–324.

21. Stunkard AJ, Sorensen TI, Hanis C, et al. An adoption study of human obesity. N Engl J Med 1986;314:193–198.

22. Himms-Hagen J. Thermogenesis in brown adipose tissue as an energy buffer. Implications for obesity. N Engl J Med 1984;311:1549–1558.

23. Noppa H, Bengtsson C, Isaksson B, Smith U. Adipose tissue cellularity—metabolic aspects. Acta Med Scand 1979;206:501–506.

24. Garrow JS, Blaza SE, Warwick PM, Ashwell MA. Predisposition to obesity. Lancet 1980;1:1103–1104.

25. Ravussin E, et al. Reduced rate of energy expenditure as a risk factor for body-weight gain. N Engl J Med 1988;318:467–472.

26. Bogardus C, Lillioja S, Ravussin E, et al. Familial dependence of the resting metabolic rate. N Engl J Med 1986;315:96–100.

27. deDivitis O, Fazio S, Petitto M, Maddalena G, Contaldo F, Mancini M. Obesity and cardiac function. Circulation 1981;64:477–482.

28. MacMahon SW, Wilcken DE, Macdonald GJ. The effect of weight reduction on left ventricular mass: a randomized controlled trial in young, overweight hypertensive patients. N Engl J Med 1986;314:334–339.

29. Hammond IW, Devereaux RB, Alderman MH, Laragh JH. Relation of blood pressure and body build to left ventricular mass in normotensive and hypertensive employed adults. J Am Coll Cardiol 1988;12:996–1004.

30. Drenick EJ, Bale GS, Seltzer F, Johnson DG. Excessive mortality and causes of death in morbidly obese men. JAMA 1980;243:443–445.

31. Keys A, Aravanis C, Blackburn H, et al. Coronary heart disease: overweight and obesity as risk factors. Ann Intern Med 1972;77:15–27.

32. Schroll M. A longitudinal epidemiologic survey of relative weight at age 25, 50 and 60 in the Glostrup population of men and women born in 1914. Dan Med Bull 1981;28:106–116.

33. Rhoads GG, Kagan A. The relation of coronary disease, stroke and mortality to weight in youth and in middle age. Lancet 1983;1:492–495.

34. Crews DE. Multivariate prediction of total and cardiovascular mortality in an obese Polynesian population. Am J Publ Health 1989;79:982–986.

35. Hubert HB, Feinleib M, McNamara PM, Castelli WP. Obesity as an independent risk factor for cardiovascular disease: A 26-year followup of participants in the Framingham Heart Study. Circulation 1983;67:968–977.

36. Tuomilehto J, Salonen JT, Marti B, et al. Body weight and risk of myocardial infarction and death in the adult population of eastern Finland. Br Med J 1987;295:623–627.

37. Manson JE, Colditz GA, Stampfer MJ, et al. A prospective study of obesity and risk of coronary heart disease in women. N Engl J Med 1990;322:882–889.

38. Hamm P, Shekelle RB, Stamler J. Large fluctuations in body weight during young adulthood and 25-year risk of coronary death in men. Am J Epidemiol 1989;129:312–318.

39. Noppa H. Body weight change in relation to incidence of ischemic heart disease and change in risk factors for ischemic heart disease. Am J Epidemiol 1980;111:693–704.

40. Gillum RF. The association of body fat distribution with hypertension, hypertensive heart disease, coronary heart disease, diabetes and cardiovascular risk factors in men and women aged 18-79 years. J Chron Dis 1987;40:421–428.

41. Folsom AR, Prineas RJ, Kaye SA, Soler JT. Body fat distribution and self-reported prevalence of hypertension, heart attack and other heart disease in older women. Int J Epidemiol 1989;18:361–367.

42. Krotkiewski M, Bjorntorp P, Sjostrom L, Smith V. Impact of obesity on metabolism in men and women. Importance of regional adipose tissue distribution. J Clin Invest 1983;72:1150–1162.

43. Lapidus L, Bengtsson K, Larsson B, et al. Distribution of adipose tissue and risk of cardiovascular disease and death—a 12-year followup of participants in the population study. Br Med J 1984;289:1257–1261.

44. Kannel WB. Metabolic risk factors for coronary heart disease in women; perspective from the Framingham Study. Am Heart J 1987;114:413–419.

45. Donahue RP, Abbott RD, Bloom E, Reed DM, Yano K. Central obesity and coronary heart disease in men. Lancet 1987;1:821–824.

46. Berchtold P, Berger M, Jorgens V, et al. Cardiovascular risk factors and HDL-cholesterol levels in obesity. Int J Obesity 1981;5:1–10.

47. Berns MA, deVries JH, Katan MB. Increase in body fatness as a major determinant of changes in serum total cholesterol and high density lipoprotein cholesterol in young men over a 10-year period. Am J Epidemiol 1989;130:1109–1122.

48. Albrink MJ, Krauss RM, Lindgrem FT, von der Groeben J, Pan S, Wood PD. Intercorrelations among plasma high density lipoprotein, obesity and triglycerides in a normal population. Lipids 1980;15:668–676.

49. Terry RB, Wood PD, Haskell WL, Stefanick ML, Krauss RM. Regional adiposity patterns in relation to lipids, lipoprotein cholesterol, and lipoprotein subfraction mass in men. J Clin Endocrinol Metab 1989;68:191–199.

50. Ostlund RE Jr, Staten M, Kohrt WM, Schultz J, Malley M. The ratio of waist-to-hip circumference, plasma insulin level, and glucose intolerance as independent predictors of the HDL_2 cholesterol level in older adults. N Engl J Med 1990;322:229–234.

51. Streja DA, Boyko E, Rabkin SW. Changes in plasma high-density lipoprotein cholesterol concentration after weight reduction in grossly obese subjects. Br Med J 1980;281:770–772.

52. Wood PD, Stefanick ML, Dreon DM, et al. Changes in plasma lipids and lipoproteins in overweight men during weight loss through dieting as compared with exercise. N Engl J Med 1988;319:1173–1179.

53. Brownell KD, Stunkard AJ. Differential changes in plasma high-density lipoprotein cholesterol levels in obese men and women during weight reduction. Arch Intern Med 1981;141:1142–1146.

54. Follick MJ, Abrams DB, Smith TW, Henderson LO, Herbert PN. Contrasting short- and long-term effects of weight loss on lipoprotein levels. Arch Intern Med 1984;144:1571–1574.

55. Schwartz RS. The independent effects of dietary weight loss and aerobic training on high density lipoproteins and apoliproteins A-I concentrations in obese men. Metabolism 1987;36:165–171.

56. MacMahon S, Cutler J, Brittain E, Higgins M. Obesity and hypertension: epidemiological and clinical issues. Eur Heart J 1987;8(suppl B):57–70.

57. Chiang BN, Perlman LV, Epstein FH. Overweight and hypertension: a review. Circulation 1969;39:403–421.

58. Stamler R, Stamler J, Riedlinger WF, Algera G, Roberts RH. Weight and blood pressure. Findings in hypertension screening of one million Americans. JAMA. 1978;240:1607–1610.

59. Higgins M, Keller J, Moore F, Ostrander L, Metzner H, Stock L. Studies of blood pressure in Tecumseh, MI. Am J Epidemiol 1980;111:142–155.

60. Havlik RJ, Hubert HB, Fabsitz RR, Feinleib M. Weight and hypertension: Nutrition and blood pressure control. Ann Intern Med 1983;98:855–859.

61. Harlan WR, Hull AL, Schmouder RL, Landis JR, Thompson FE, Larkin FA. Blood pressure and nutrition in adults: the National Health and Nutrition Examination Survey. Am J Epidemiol 1984;120:17–28.

62. Neser WB, Thomas J, Semenya K, Thomas DJ, Gillum RF. Obesity and hypertension in a longitudinal study of black physicians: the Meharry Cohort Study. J Chron Dis 1986;39:105–113.

63. Paffenbarger RS Jr, Wing AL, Hyde RT, Jung DL. Physical activity and incidence of hypertension in college alumni. Am J Epidemiol 1983;117:245–257.

64. Noppa H, Bengtsson C, Wedel H, Wilhelmsen L. Obesity in relation to morbidity and mortality from cardiovascular disease. Am J Epidemiol 1980;111:682–692.

65. Stallones L, Mueller WH, Christensen BL. Blood pressure, fatness and fat patterning among USA adolescents from two ethnic groups. Hypertension 1982;4:483–486.

66. Hartz AJ, Rupley DC, Rimm AA. The association of girth measurements with disease in 32,856 women. Am J Epidemiol 1984;119:71–80.

67. Freedman DS, Rimm AA. The relation of body fat distribution, as assessed by six girth measurements, to diabetes mellitus in women. Am J Public Health 1989;79:715–720.

68. Selby JV, Friedman GD, Quesenberry CP Jr. Precursors of essential hypertension. The role of body fat distribution pattern. Am J Epidemiol 1989;129:43–53.

69. Hypertension Detection and Followup Program Cooperative Group. Race, education and prevalence of hypertension. Am J Epidemiol 1977;106:351–361.

70. MacMahon SW, Blacket RB, Macdonald GJ, Hall W. Obesity, alcohol consumption and blood pressure in Australian men and women. The National Heart Foundation of Australia Risk Factor Prevalence Study. J Hypertens 1984;2:85–91.

71. Bloom E, Reed D, Yano K, MacLean C. Does obesity protect hypertensives against cardiovascular disease? JAMA 1986;256:2972–2975.

72. Bjorntorp P. Hypertension in obesity. Acta Med Scand 1982;211:241–242.

73. Gillum RF, Prineas RJ, Jeffrey RW, et al. Nonpharmacologic therapy of hypertension: the independent effects of weight reduction and sodium restriction in overweight borderline hypertensive patients. Am Heart J 1983;105:128–133.

74. Maxwell MH, Kushiro T, Dornfeld LP, Tuck ML, Waks AU. BP changes in obese hypertensive subjects during rapid weight loss. Comparison of restricted versus unchanged salt intake. Arch Intern Med 1984;144:1581–1584.

75. Tuck ML, Sowers J, Dornfeld L, Kledzik G, Maxwell M. The effect of weight reduction on blood pressure, plasma renin activity, and plasma aldosterone levels in obese patients. N Engl J Med 1981;304:930–933.

76. Reisin E, Frolich ED, Messerli FH, et al. Cardiovascular changes after weight reduction in obesity hypertension. Ann Intern Med 1983;98:315–319.

77. Heyden S, Borhani NO, Tyroler HA, et al. The relationship of weight change to changes in blood pressure, serum uric acid, cholesterol and glucose in the treatment of hypertension. J Chron Dis 1985;38:281–288.

78. Fortmann SP, Haskell WL, Wood PD, and the Stanford Weight Control Project Team.

Effects of weight loss on clinic and ambulatory blood pressure in normotensive men. Am J Cardiol 1988;62:89–93.

79. Garrison RJ, Feinleib M, Castelli WP, et al. Cigarette smoking as a cofounder of the relationship between relative weight and long-term mortality: the Framingham Heart Study. JAMA 1983;249:2199–2203.

80. Heyden S, Cassel JC, Bartel A, Tyroler HA, Hames CG, Cornoni JC. Body weight and cigarette smoking as risk factors. Arch Intern Med 1971;128:915–919.

81. Van Gaal LF, DeLeeuw IH. Effects of smoking on lipid parameters during therapeutic weight loss. Atherosclerosis 1986;60:287–290.

82. Brownell KD. Obesity: understanding and treating a serious, prevalent, and refractory disorder. J Consult Clin Psychol 1982;50:820–840.

83. Williams PT, Fortmann SP, Terry RB, et al. Associations of dietary fat, regional adiposity, and blood pressure in men. JAMA 1987;257:3251–3256.

84. Jenkins DJ, Wolever TM, Vuskan V, et al. Nibbling versus gorging: metabolic advantages of increased meal frequency. N Engl J Med 1989;321:929–934.

85. Wadden TA, Stunkard AJ, Liebschutz J. Three-year follow-up of the treatment of obesity by very low calorie diet, behavior therapy, and their combination. J Consult Clin Psychol 1988;56:925–928.

86. Sours HE, Frattali VP, Brand CD, et al. Sudden death associated with very low calorie weight reduction regimens. Am J Clin Nutr 1981;34:453–461.

87. Amatruda JM, Biddle TL, Patton ML, et al. Vigorous supplementation of a hypocaloric diet prevents cardiac arrhythmias and mineral depletion. Am J Med 1983;74:1016–1022.

88. Wadden TA, Van Italie TB, Blackburn GL. Responsible and irresponsible use of very-low-calorie diets in the treatment of obesity. JAMA 1990;263:83–85.

89. Maclure KM, Hayes KC, Colditz GA, Stampfer MJ, Speizer FE, Willett WC. Weight, diet and the risk of symptomatic gallstones in middle-aged women. N Engl J Med 1989;321:563–569.

90. Liddle RA, Goldstein RB, Saxton J. Gallstone formation during weight reduction dieting. Arch Intern Med 1989;149:1750–1753.

91. King AC, Frey-Hewitt B, Dreon DM, Wood PD. Diet vs exercise in weight maintenance. Arch Intern Med 1989;149:2741–2746.

10

sociobehavioral and environmental factors

In analyzing the rise in coronary artery disease (CAD) during the first two-thirds of this century and its decline in incidence in the past 20 years, epidemiologists have estimated that at least half of the variance in CAD rates remains unexplained after accounting for the physiological risks discussed in earlier chapters (1). In recent years, attention has been directed toward socioeconomic and behavioral factors (2–5). These include chronic (6), recurrent, and major acute stimuli (7) such as community economic conditions, daily hassles and conflicts, loss of a spouse (8, 9), or an earthquake (10). Each person encounters these stimuli equipped with a certain personality and capability for self-appraisal, as well as a repertoire of resources to cope with these stimuli. Responses to these stressful stimuli may include fear, anxiety, depression, anger, or hostility, which may, in turn, affect the incidence of cardiovascular events such as myocardial infarction, congestive heart failure, and sudden cardiac death (11, 12).

For several centuries, clinicians have written of these factors (13). In his classic book published in 1628, William Harvey describes the case of a man "who, having received an injury from one more powerful than himself, and upon whom he could not have his revenge, was so overcome with hatred and spite and passion, which he yet communicated to no one, that at last he fell into a strange distemper, suffering from extreme oppression and pain of the heart and breast." He concluded that "every affection of the mind that is attended with either pain or pleasure, hope or fear, is the cause of an agitation whose influence extends to the heart" (14).

It is reported that the English surgeon John Hunter, who was susceptible to chest discomfort during emotional upset, and who commented, "My life is at the mercy of any fool who shall put me in a passion," died during a heated discussion at a hospital board meeting (15). In 1910, Osler noted in his classic lecture that the typical person with angina pectoris is "not the delicate neurotic but the robust, the vigorous in mind and body, the keen ambitious man, the indicator of whose engine is always full speed ahead" (16).

In this chapter, the epidemiology and pathophysiology of these factors are discussed in detail.

135

SOCIOECONOMIC STATUS AND CONDITIONS

Earlier in this century, CAD was largely a disease of the more affluent, better-educated segments of industrialized societies. In succeeding decades, CAD became more equally distributed until now, in industrialized countries, persons in upper socioeconomic classes are at lower risk (17, 18). Several indices of education, income, and social class have been derived for epidemiologic studies (19).

Jenkins and associates examined death certificates in Massachusetts and compared them with social and demographic data. They found that excess hypertensive disease mortality was found in geographic areas where most men had low occupational status, where the median years of schooling for adults was very low, and in impoverished families. Of these factors, measures of low educational level and occupational status had the highest association with hypertension and CAD deaths (20).

Kitagawa and Hauser compared whites with various levels of education, finding that those with less than eight years had higher CAD risks than those with one or more years of college education (relative risk was 1.25 for middle-aged men, 2.40 for similarly aged women) (21). A similar study in Chicago showed that persons from census tracts in the lower quintile of socioeconomic status in that city had age-adjusted CAD mortality ratios of 1.22 for men and 2.40 for women when compared to the upper quintile of tracts classified by social and income levels (22).

Why should persons in lower social and educational classes die more often from CAD? Remembering that at least half of all CAD deaths occur before persons arrive at a hospital, the ability to seek medical attention promptly becomes a possible explanatory factor. Croog and Levine showed that persons in the upper socioeconomic strata are more likely to report pain and correctly identify its source (23). Financial access to care may also play an important part in reluctance to seek medical attention when symptoms of CAD arise.

Marmot and colleagues found that male civil servants in London (UK) who were in the lowest employment grades had a relative risk of 3.6 compared to those in the highest grade. The significant differences persisted despite adjustment for other CAD risk indicators. Similarly, they found that age-adjusted mortality among married women under the age of 65 was higher in the lowest social class than in the highest (24, 25). A later British study showed that manual workers had a 7 to 38% increased risk of CAD mortality, depending on their smoking status (26).

Similar findings arose in Finland when all death certificates for a 6-year period were examined. CAD incidence was lowest in farmers and the higher professional classes and highest in the lower professional classes and unskilled workers (27). In Oslo, those in the lowest quintiles of education and income had much higher CAD rates than those in the uppermost quintiles (28, 29).

The Framingham investigators found that the women in their study most susceptible to CAD were those who were married to blue-collar workers, had children at home, and worked outside the home in a clerical job for an employer they did not like (30).

How early might the susceptibility to CAD be manifest? Burr and Sweetnam interviewed men with myocardial infarction (MI) during their stay in Welsh hospitals. They noted that in each of three social class groupings, MI patients came from larger families than controls and that a higher percentage of their fathers had been unemployed (31).

COMMUNITY AND CULTURAL FACTORS

Although improvements in socioeconomic status may make a wider variety of foods affordable, many people continue to prefer traditional, customary diets. In some cases, such as immigrants from Asian, Central American, or Mediterranean countries, choices of rice, beans, and olive oil are far healthier than the "all-American" diet of fried hamburgers and deep-fried potatoes.

A classic study of these effects was the Ni-Hon-San study, which matched Japanese men with Japanese-American men (living in Hawaii and California) whose ancestors came from the same prefectures in Japan. California men ranked highest in body weight, percentage of calories from saturated fat, blood pressure, serum cholesterol, and CAD mortality; residents of Japan had the lowest values in each category (32, 33). Among those residing in California, CAD risk was much lower in men who had remained within a Japanese-based culture rather than being assimilated into the mainstream of California life (34).

Economic changes within a culture can also affect CAD rates. Brenner has described an association between national and regional economic changes, such as recessions, and increased mortality rates in nine industrialized countries (35).

WORK ENVIRONMENT

In addition to the individual's social class, education, and gender, several other aspects of a particular job and jobsite can influence the probability of developing CAD (36, 37). These latter factors include the physical activity required by the job (Chapter 8) (38–49), the physical environment (noise, temperature, exposure to chemicals), the psychological aspects of one's occupation, migration, unemployment, and retirement (50). These factors may affect CAD directly, as well as influencing standard physiological risk indicators such as cholesterol, blood pressure, and smoking. Most studies have been done in men, but attention to the relation of women, work, and health has been increasing (51).

Physical Environment

Noise (52) and high temperatures (53, 54) are known to alter hemodynamics to a degree that may upset a tenuous balance between the myocardial oxygen supply and demand in a worker with CAD. The effects of occupational exposure to nitrates have been well studied, following notation of weekend symptoms in workers that were relieved upon reexposure to nitrates on Monday mornings (55). Antimony trisulfide, sulfurous oxides, and carbon disulfide (in viscose rayon) have also been related to heart disease (56). Jappinen found an excess of deaths from CAD among Finnish workers at sulfite, sulfate, and paper mills compared with persons working at sawmills (57).

Psychological Factors

Perceived job stress may take several forms, such as undesirable job pace, shift work, role ambiguity or conflict, lack of autonomy, and poor social support from seniors, colleagues, and subordinates (58).

Both blue- and white-collar workers report that they must often work in haste. This time pressure translates into increased heart rates and catecholamine levels, such as those noted in surgeons while operating (59), and workers doing piecework or being paced by machine (9). High work demand, coupled with low control or decision latitude, resulted in the highest rates of CAD events in a Swedish study (60).

The stresses of motorcar driving were documented by Taggart and Carruthers and their colleagues (15, 61). β-Adrenergic blockade can attenuate blood pressure rises during stressful driving (62). Bus drivers have been extensively studied in several countries (63), with unusually high rates of hypertension and other forms of cardiovascular disease (64). Commuting by individuals on congested urban roads has also been correlated with electrocardiographic changes (65) and elevations in blood pressure (66).

Russek and Russek compared job stress and CAD prevalence in groups of physicians, dentists, attorneys, and other professionals. They found that dermatologists, patent lawyers, and periodontists had the lowest CAD prevalence rates, while anesthesiologists, general practice attorneys, and security traders had the highest rates (67). Perceived stress levels are also reported to be high by a vast majority of teachers (68) and clergymen (69), although mortality rates in these two professions is often lower than that of the general population (68, 70–72).

Monotony and shift work were associated with significant excess CAD risk in a case-control study of Stockholm men below age 65 (73). In a prospective study of papermill workers in Sweden, those with an 11- to 15-year history of shift work had a relative risk of 2.2 for CAD development, compared with day workers. For persons with a 16- to 20-year history, the relative risk was 2.8. These associations were independent of age and smoking history (74). Orth-Gomer found that clockwise rotation of shifts favorably influenced serum glucose and triglyceride levels, systolic blood pressure, and urinary excretion of catecholamines, compared with counterclockwise shift-change patterns (75).

Workers who are unclear about their job role or who encounter conflicting job demands are more susceptible to stress and related illnesses, although personality differences might mitigate the effects of such ambiguity or conflict. Karasek and colleagues have compared perceived work demands with the amount of decision latitude offered to workers. Where autonomy is high, job demands may be high without the perception of job stress. When job demands are high and latitude is low, CAD rates were found to be highest (60, 73, 76, 77). However, not all studies have agreed. In a study of 8006 men of Japanese ancestry in Hawaii, no associations between the aforementioned factors and CAD rates were noted (78).

In four Dutch communities, self-employed persons had CAD incidence rates much higher than others; for men, the relative risk was two, while in women, CAD rates were seven times higher than in housewives. Men who "feel driven to all their work with great intensity and against the clock" had MI seven times more often than others and were more than twice as likely to have fatal MI (79).

Repetti has noted that men with heavy daily workloads tend toward withdrawal from family members during times of acute job stress, leading to potential conflict at home (80).

Job Change and Migration

It has become common for workers in the USA to change jobs frequently. The Evans County Study showed that, while mobility of persons in the upper two social classes did not increase their CAD rates, such changes in the lower two classes did raise CAD risk (81). An earlier study in North Dakota revealed a doubling of CAD prevalence in men with several job changes and frequent geographic moves, compared with peers who remained in one place. The relative risk of CAD was highest (threefold) among men who were reared on farms but later took white-collar jobs in the city

(82). Similar findings were obtained by investigators in a California study (83).

In Chapter 1, an adverse effect on CAD risk was described for persons migrating from rural to urban environments in lesser-developed countries, as well as for immigration to the United Kingdom from Bangladesh and other Asian countries. Differences in diet, smoking, and hypertension were often dramatic.

Unemployment

The psychologic response to unemployment has been described as having three phases. First comes shock and denial, followed by feelings of optimism and a well-deserved holiday. These are followed by increasing distress, as the person becomes more acutely aware of the magnitude of the problem. Finally, if persons become dispirited, the "unemployed identity" may be assumed. Feelings of inferiority and submissiveness arise, along with feelings of inadequacy about providing financially for the family (84).

Kasl and colleagues found that blood pressure, serum cholesterol, and uric acid all increased in conjunction with depression, irritability, and decreased self-esteem after a person lost a job. These abnormalities persisted until reemployment was achieved (85). In Scotland, unemployment and classification in the two lowest social classes were independent predictors of CAD incidence in men (86). The World Health Organization has made recommendations for policies to minimize these effects (87).

Retirement

Cascelles and colleagues interviewed wives of men who died in two counties in Florida. They matched men by occupational history, prevalence of CAD risk factors, and retirement status. They found that the risk of CAD death was 80% greater in retirees compared with men of the same age who were still working. The authors suggest that for many men, anxiety and depression increase after retirement, self-esteem is lost, and there are diminished opportunities to deal with stress through other activities (88).

Occupation and CAD Risk Indicators

Pieper and colleagues noted associations of lipid and lipoprotein profiles, blood pressure, and smoking with CAD among 12,555 men in a metaanalysis of five investigations conducted within the USA from 1959 to 1980 (89). Other studies have noted these correlations as well.

LIPIDS AND LIPOPROTEINS

Tax accountants have marked increases in serum cholesterol levels near deadlines, which regress again within weeks thereafter (90). Theorell and Akerstedt noted that serum cholesterol levels worsened with the advent of shift work in their Swedish subjects (91).

Hazuda and colleagues studied CAD risk among Mexican-American and non-Hispanic white women aged 25 to 64 in San Antonio, Texas. Women working outside the home had more favorable HDL, triglyceride, and HDL/total cholesterol ratios than women working only at home. Better diets among employed women explained some, but not all, of the difference (92).

HYPERTENSION

In a study of blue-collar workers in Pittsburgh, PA, elevated diastolic blood pressure was positively associated with job dissatisfaction, difficulty communicating with co-workers, unsupportive foremen and co-workers, and uncertain job future, and was inversely correlated with participation in decision making and promotion opportunities (93).

Certain occupations appear to be inherently stressful. For example, air traffic controllers have hypertension at an earlier time than would be expected from their demographic characteristics (94).

SMOKING

In the Oslo study, smoking prevalence was inversely correlated with socioeconomic status (95). This relationship holds true in several other study populations, including British men and women (96), men in Switzerland (97), and men and women in the People's Republic of China (98), in the Philippines (99), and in the USA (100).

In Sweden, smoking is more common among lower socioeconomic groups, men with eight years of schooling or less, and single women. It was common among early retired persons as well as those unemployed (101).

MAJOR AND MINOR LIFE EVENTS

Most persons have daily experience with irritating and frustrating elements in their environment. These might include spousal conflict, demands of children or others living in the household, gender role ambiguity and conflicts, and dissention with co-workers (8).

In contrast, some events are less frequent, but exert a major impact on our lives. Holmes and Rahe interviewed persons, asking them to rate 43 different "life events," using 100 points for the death of a spouse (102). Their scale was used extensively, and others developed scales (103) that have been modified to include other events (both positive and negative) and adapted for use in various populations (104, 105). Rahe later cautioned that specific individuals may vary considerably in their rating of the importance of given life events (106).

SOCIAL SUPPORT

Marital and Family Factors

Several studies have documented an increased CAD risk in unmarried persons (107). In a Finnish study of men aged 40 to 64 years, those who were divorced had a risk 1.77 times higher than that of married men. Survival after myocardial infarction (MI) was lowest in divorced and never-married men (27). In a Swedish study, the lower CAD risk after MI in married persons was independent of the size of the MI (108). British investigators found that women had an increased risk of CAD mortality during the first 30 days after being widowed. In men, the elevated risk persisted for a year after they became widowers (109).

In a Pennsylvania study, women were six times more likely to die suddenly during the first six months after the death of a significant other (110). Unmarried women and men in Baltimore had 40 to 50% higher in-hospital fatality rates after MI compared with married persons. During a 10-year follow-up, survival at five years was approximately 50% in unmarried persons and 70% in their married counterparts (111).

The concept of social support may account for some of these differences (112–114). House and Kahn describe social support in four categories: emotional, tangible, informational, and appraisal (115). While it seems reasonable that a spouse would provide appraisal help, tangible services, and informational assistance regarding one's health, two large studies have demonstrated that an educated wife may be hazardous to a man's health. In the Framingham Study, CAD risk in men correlated positively with their wife's educational level (116). Male residents of a southern California community had nearly twice the CAD risk when the wife had college training and the husband did not.

When educational levels were equal, men's rates were 1.5 times higher; minimal risk for men existed when their educational level exceeded that of their wives (117). In the β-Blocker Heart Attack Trial, persons who were both socially isolated and perceived that they were under a high degree of life stress had mortality rates four times higher than persons with neither characteristic (118). While it appears that social support does provide some degree of "stress buffering," there is probably an independent contribution of social support to cardiovascular health and disease (119).

Women appear to maintain more extensive social networks than men, and they may be more aware of the value of the network and the support they derive therefrom (120). They have been described as the "kinship carriers," providing and enhancing social relationships for their family (121). However, attempts at self-change can be either helped or hindered by one's social network. If one's spouse or close friends smoke, attempts to quit will be seriously jeopardized. In one study of women newly abstinent from smoking, "partner facilitation" was the primary predictor of relapse (122). Likewise, attempts to modify exercise or eating habits can be sabotaged by family and friends who don't wish to change themselves. Sallis and co-workers have developed scales to measure social support for diet and exercise habit change (123).

Other Sources of Social Support

Social support may be found outside the family. To assess the measures of such support, comparisons have been made of conceptual frameworks, psychometric properties, and predictive capacities of various instruments (124).

In a nine-year follow-up of Alameda County (California) residents, Berkman and Syme found lower CAD mortality rates among married persons, those with several close family members, friends, or both, and those with church membership or other group affiliations (125). Older persons (particularly white males) in Evans County (Georgia) had increased mortality if they had few social ties (126).

In the Swedish study of men born in 1913 and 1923, mortality was associated with numbers of person per household unit, home activities, and other social activities (127). Orth-Gomer and her colleagues have documented the adverse effects of social isolation in several other Swedish populations (128, 129). In a study of elderly Malmö men, investigators found that CAD mortality was more than doubled in those with low availability of social support, men with low adequacy of social participation, and those living alone (130). Social support resources may vary with time; Kahn and Antonucci have proposed a "convoy" theory, by which they mean the acquisition, maintenance, and relinquishment of friends throughout a lifetime (131).

SPIRITUALITY

Regarding the title of his book *The Meaning of Health,* theologian Paul Tillich wrote "in order to speak of health, one must speak of all dimensions of life" (132). On several occasions, the World Health Organization (WHO) has recognized the spiritual component to health and wellbeing. In May 1984, the World Health Assembly adopted a resolution inviting member states to include in their "Health for All" strategies a spiritual dimension reflecting their social and cultural patterns.

Physiological indicators of CAD risk may vary among adherents to different religious and spiritual views, such as the proscription of smoking by certain groups. Studies of Benedictine, Buddhist, and Trappist monks have documented the relation of diet to blood cholesterol levels (133, 134). Much of the lower risk in Seventh-Day Adventists can be explained by their high prevalence of nonsmoking and consumption of a vegetarian diet (135).

However, there has been considerable reluctance within the medical community to recognize the spiritual dimension involved in emotional and physical diseases. Some mental health workers have postulated an inverse correlation between "religiosity" and emotional health, while others have chosen to ignore any possible relation (136, 137). More recently, some have considered it as only a form of social support, rather than as an independent contributor to coping and adaptation. Sherrill and Larson studied the role of religious views on recovery from burn injuries, noting frequent references by patients to their religious faith or to God (138).

Limiting a better understanding of the spiritual dimension of health is the paucity of indices to measure spirituality or religiosity. Perhaps the most commonly used variable is the frequency of attendance at religious services, but this is, at best, a coarse indicator of a complex concept (139). In her studies, Sherrill modified the Kauffman Religious Life Scale (which contains experiential, ritual, and devotional dimensions of the Christian tradition) to include a historical dimension (140). Little is available in the English literature about scales for traditions other than Christian, although Marty and Vaux have developed a series of monographs entitled "Health/Medicine and the Faith Traditions" in which these issues are explored from the perspective of many of the world's faiths (141, 142).

As Fowler suggests, the impact of religious faith traditions cannot be known solely by utilitarian criteria. In describing faith as the product of a search for meaning in the world, he indicates that our "meaning-making" must "enable us to face tragedy and finitude ... without giving in to despair or morbidity." It has the ability to "link us to communities of shared memory and shared hope with which we join in symbolizing our human condition and in enacting the visions that can animate and give new life" (143).

Despite the lack of epidemiologic clarity, organizations have begun to utilize the place of worship as a place of health promotion. Hypertension screening in rural churches has facilitated reduction of CAD risk (144), and residents of Rhode Island have been trained to serve as volunteer leaders of heart health programs in their churches (145). The Eastern Mediterranean Region of WHO has published booklets in a series called "Health Education Through Religion," such as "The Islamic Ruling on Smoking" in which scholars integrate epidemiologic findings from WHO and religious customs.

SELF-APPRAISAL

Confronted with stressful stimuli, one may make an assessment of one's ability to adapt or cope with the challenge. Attributions, or perceptions of causes, may result from the individual's beliefs about the stimuli; in turn, these attributions will affect behavior (146). When stimuli are repetitive and coping is not completely successful, concepts of self may be eroded, leaving the individual vulnerable to emotional and physical disorders (147).

While self-esteem is considered to be a global concept, the term self-efficacy has been defined as the perception of one's capability to accomplish a certain level of performance in a given task (148). For example, Ewart, Taylor and colleagues have described self-efficacy for walking, running, lifting, and sexual activity in persons at various stages of recovery from myocardial infarction (149).

The concept of "locus of control" is also relevant to self-appraisal. Persons who see their lives as primarily determined by internal considerations appear to be more active in the pursuit and maintenance of optimal health than are persons who largely perceive external causes for their life events (150, 151).

Kobasa and her colleagues have described as "hardiness" the perception of control over one's environment, a strong commitment to one's activities, and an enjoyment and sense of challenge in change. Individuals possessing these characteristics report lower disease rates than those less hardy (152, 153).

Perception of one's health was found to be strongly predictive of subsequent mortality and morbidity in residents of the California counties of Alameda (154) and Los Angeles (155). In the North Karelia, Finland Project, persons in the intervention area reported significantly greater declines in perceived CAD risk and improvements in perceived health status than did those in the reference area (156).

PERSONALITY FACTORS

Although the concept of "coronary-prone" personality typology is perhaps best known among workers in cardiovascular health, other investigators have explored the potential contribution of personality factors to the genesis of CAD and its prevention as part of a broader psychological evaluation. Different characteristics seem to predict the various manifestations of CAD: angina pectoris, the risk of MI, and the probability of surviving after MI (157, 158). Common to these investigations, however, appear to be the characteristics of easily aroused hostility and impatience (159–161).

Modification of coronary-prone (type A) behavior has been demonstrated, but its effect on long-term survival is unclear (162). Assessment methods vary from the structured interview to a 10-item questionnaire used in the Framingham Study (163,

164). In a randomized trial, subjects were allocated to behavioral counseling or cardiology counseling groups at various times following MI. After four and one-half years, the behavioral counseling group had experienced significantly fewer recurrences of MI (165), particularly among those persons with less severe infarctions (166).

In contrast, Ragland and Brand studied patients who survived MI and received no intervention. Those persons classified as type A actually had lower recurrence rates than other subjects (167). The results of the two studies may not be incongruous, however, if type A men randomized to the behavioral counseling group in the first trial successfully eliminated some of their hostility and time-urgent behaviors, while the type A characteristics of subjects in the second study led them to a more ambitious undertaking of health behavior changes such as dietary improvement, regular aerobic exercise, and smoking cessation.

Persons displaying coronary-prone behavior have been noted to suppress expressions of fatigue during exercise (168), allowing them greater activity tolerance, but also making them more vulnerable to exercise-induced ischemia and dysrhythmias.

The concept of John Henryism was developed by James and colleagues in a study of working-class black men residing in the southern United States. Named after the black folk hero, the concept describes a strong personality predisposition to cope actively and control psychosocial environmental stressors through determination and hard work. Men with little education who scored high on this scale had significantly higher diastolic blood pressures than men at the other end of the spectrum (169). While John Henryism was not predictive of blood pressure in whites in the USA (170), it has been correlated with systolic blood pressures in a Dutch population of men, particularly those with less education (171).

The Myers-Briggs Type Indicator inventory, which consists of four bipolar scales, may also be helpful in facilitating heart health improvement. As described by Leiden and colleagues, the Extraversion-Introversion (E-I) scale indicates relative preferences for the external world of people and events or the internal world of concepts and ideas. The Sensing-Intuition (S-I) scale distinguishes between styles of using the five senses to gather information and the use of intuition to determine meanings represented by the facts. The Thinking-Feeling (T-F) scale refers to decision-making styles that reflect emphasis on facts or feelings. The fourth scale, Judging-Perceptive (J-P), reflects preferences for organization and orderliness in relating to the external world versus a more spontaneous, flexible attitude (172).

REFERENCES

1. Havlik RJ, Feinleib M(eds). Proceedings of the conference on the decline in coronary heart disease mortality. Bethesda, MD: National Institutes of Health, 1979. DHEW Publ no. NIH 79-1610.

2. Sprague HB. Emotional factors in coronary heart disease. Circulation 1961;23:648-654.

3. Russek HI. Role of emotional stress in the etiology of clinical coronary heart disease. Dis Chest 1967;52:1-9.

4. Syme SL. Behavioral factors associated with the etiology of physical disease: a social epidemiological approach. Am J Public Health 1974;64:1043-1045.

5. Cassel J. The contribution of the social environment to host resistance. Am J Epidemiol 1976;104:107-123.

6. Manuck SB, Henry JP, Anderson DE, et al. Biobehavioral mechanisms in coronary artery disease. Chronic stress. Circulation 1987;76(suppl 1):I158-I163.

7. Shepherd JT, Dembroski TM, Brody MJ, et al. Biobehavioral mechanisms in coronary artery disease. Acute stress. Circulation 1987;76(suppl 1):I150-I157.

8. Kanner AD, Coyne JC, Schaefer C, Lazarus RS. Comparison of two modes of stress measurement: daily hassles and uplifts versus major life events. J Behav Med 1981;4:1-39.

9. Krantz DS, Raisen SE. Environmental stress, reactivity and ischaemic heart disease. Br J Med Psychol 1988;61:3-16.

10. Trichopoulos D, Katsouyanni K, Zavitsanos X, Tzonou A, Dalla-Vorgia P. Psychological stress and fatal heart attack: the Athens (1981) earthquake natural experiment. Lancet 1983;1:441-444.

11. Lown B, DeSilva RA, Reich P, Murawski BJ. Psychophysiologic factors in sudden cardiac death. Am J Psychiatr 1980;137:1325-1335.

12. Manuck SB, Kaplan JR, Matthews KA. Behavioral antecedents of coronary heart disease and atherosclerosis. Arteriosclerosis 1986;6:2-14.

13. Wolf SG. History of the study of stress and heart disease. In: Beamish RE, Singal PK, Dhalla NS(eds): Stress and heart disease. Boston: Martinus Nijhoff, 1984:3-16.

14. Harvey W. Exercitatio anatomica de motu cordis et sanguinis in animabilus. Frankfurt-am-Main, 1628.

15. Taggart P, Carruthers M. Behaviour patterns and emotional stress in the etiology of coronary heart disease: cardiological and biochemical correlates. In: Wheatley D(ed): Stress and the heart. New York: Raven Press, 1981:25-37.

16. Osler W. The Lumleian lectures on angina pectoris. Lancet 1910;1:839-844.

17. Cassel J, Heyden S, Bartel AG, et al. Incidence of coronary heart disease by ethnic group, social class, and sex. Arch Intern Med 1971;128:901-906.

18. Dobson AJ, Gibberd RW, Leeder SR, O'Connell DL. Occupational differences in ischemic heart disease mortality and risk factors in Australia. Am J Epidemiol 1985;122:283-290.

19. Liberatos P, Link BG, Kelsey JL. The measurement of social class in epidemiology. Epidemiol Rev 1988;10:87-121.

20. Jenkins CD, Tuthill RW, Tannenbaum SI, et al. Social stressors and excess mor-

tality from hypertensive diseases. J Human Stress 1979;5:29–40.

21. Kitagawa EM, Hauser PM. Differential mortality in the United States: a study in socioeconomic epidemiology. Cambridge, MA: Harvard University Press, 1973.

22. Jenkins CD. Recent evidence supporting psychologic and social risk factors for coronary disease. N Engl J Med 1976;294:987–994,1033–1038.

23. Croog SH, Levine S. The heart patient recovers. Social and psychologic factors. New York: Human Services Press, 1978.

24. Marmot MG, Rose G, Shipley M, Hamilton PJ. Employment grade and coronary heart disease in British civil servants. J Epidemiol Community Health 1978;32:244–249.

25. Rose G, Marmot MG. Social class and coronary heart disease. Br Heart J 1981;45:13–19.

26. Pocock SJ, Shaper AG, Cook DG, et al. Social class differences in ischaemic heart disease in British men. Lancet 1987;2:197–201.

27. Koskenvuo M, Kaprio J, Romo M, et al. Incidence and prognosis of ischaemic heart disease with respect to marital status and social class. A national record linkage study. J Epidemiol Community Health 1981;35:192–196.

28. Holme I, Helgeland A, Hjermann I, et al. Four-year mortality by some socioeconomic indicators: the Oslo study. J Epidemiol Community Health 1980;34:48–52.

29. Holme I, Helgeland A, Hjermann I, et al. Socio-economic status as a coronary risk factor: the Oslo study. Acta Med Scand 1982; suppl 660:147–151.

30. Haynes SG, Feinleib M. Women, work and coronary heart disease: prospective findings from the Framingham Heart Study. Am J Public Health 1980;70:133–141.

31. Burr ML, Sweetnam PM. Family size and paternal unemployment in relation to myocardial infarction. J Epidemiol Community Health 1980;34:93–95.

32. Marmot MG, Syme SL, Kagan A, Kato H, Cohen JB, Belsky J. Epidemiologic studies of coronary heart disease and stroke in Japanese men living in Japan, Hawaii and California. Prevalence of coronary and hypertensive heart disease and associated risk factors. Am J Epidemiol 1975;102:514–525.

33. Worth RM, Kato H, Rhoads GG, Kagan A, Syme SL. Epidemiologic studies of coronary heart disease and stroke in Japanese men living in Japan, Hawaii and California. Mortality. Am J Epidemiol 1975;102:481–490.

34. Marmot MG, Syme SL. Acculturation and coronary heart disease in Japanese Americans. Am J Epidemiol 1976;104:225–247.

35. Brenner MH. Economic change, alcohol consumption and heart disease mortality in nine industrialized countries. Soc Sci Med 1987;25:119–132.

36. Moos RH. Work as a human context. In: Pallak MS, Perloff RO(eds): Psychology and work: productivity, change, and employment. Washington: American Psychological Association 1986:9–52.

37. Theorell T, Alfredsson L, Knox S, Perski A, Svensson J, Waller D. On the interplay between socioeconomic factors, personality and work environment in the pathogenesis of cardiovascular disease. Scand J Work Environ Health 1984;10:373–380.

38. Froelicher V, Battler A, McKirnan MD. Physical activity and coronary heart disease. Cardiology 1980;65:153–190.

39. LaPorte RE, Adams LL, Savage DD, Brenes G, Dearwater S, Cook T. The spectrum of physical activity, cardiovascular disease and health: an epidemiologic perspective. Am J Epidemiol 1984;120:507–517.

40. Curfman GD, Thomas GS, Paffenbarger RS Jr. Physical activity and primary prevention of cardiovascular disease. Cardiol Clin 1985;3:203–222.

41. Phelps JR. Physical activity and health maintenance—exactly what is known? West J Med 1987;146:200–206.

42. Powell KE, Thompson PD, Caspersen CJ, Kendrick JS. Physical activity and the incidence of coronary heart disease. Ann Rev Public Health 1987;8:253–287.

43. Morris JN, Heady JA, Raffle PA, Roberts CG, Parks JW. Coronary heart disease and physical activity of work. Lancet 1953;2:1053–1057,1111–1120.

44. Heady JA, Morris JN, Kagan A, Raffle PA. Coronary heart disease in London busmen: a progress report with special reference to physique. Br J Soc Prev Med 1961;15:143–153.

45. Morris JN, Kagan A, Pattison DC, Gardner MJ, Raffle PA. Incidence and prediction of ischaemic heart disease in London busmen. Lancet 1966:553–559.

46. Morris JN, Everitt MG, Pollard R, Chave SP. Vigorous exercise in leisure-time: protection against coronary heart disease. Lancet 1980;2:1207–1210.

47. Paffenbarger RS Jr, Hale WE. Work activity and coronary heart mortality. N Engl J Med 1975;292:545–550.

48. Punsar S, Karvonen MJ. Physical activity and coronary heart disease in populations from east and west Finland. Adv Cardiol 1976;18:196–207.

49. Salonen JT, Slater JS, Tuomilehto J, Raauramaa R. Leisure time and occupational physical activity: risk of death from ischemic heart disease. Am J Epidemiol 1988;127:87–94.

50. Davidson DM. Cardiovascular disease and occupation. Cardiovasc Rev Reports 1984;5:503–517.

51. Sorensen G, Verbrugge LM. Women, work, and health. Annu Rev Public Health 1987;8:235–251.

52. Andren L. Cardiovascular effects of noise. Acta Med Scand 1982;(suppl)657:1–45.

53. El Sharif N, Shahwan L, Sorour AH. The effect of acute thermal stress on general and pulmonary hemodynamics in the cardiac patient. Am Heart J 1970;79:305–317.

54. Bainton D, Moore F, Sweetnam P. Temperature and deaths from ischaemic heart disease. Br J Prev Soc Med 1977;31:49–53.

55. Lund RP, Haggendal J, Johnsson G. Withdrawal symptoms in workers exposed to nitroglycerine. Br J Ind Med 1968;25:136–138.

56. Tolonen M, Hernberg S, Nurminen M, Tiitola K. A follow-up study of coronary heart disease in viscose rayon workers exposed to carbon disulphide. Br J Ind Med 1975;32:1–10.

57. Jappinen P. A mortality study of Finnish pulp and paper workers. Br J Ind Med 1987;44:580–587.

58. Baker DB. The study of stress at work. Annu Rev Public Health 1985;6:367–381.

59. Foster GE, Evans DF, Hardcastle JD. Heart rates of surgeons during operations and other clinical activities and their modification by oxprenolol. Lancet 1978;1:1323–1325.

60. Karasek RA, Baker D, Marxer F, Ahlbom A, Theorell T. Job decision latitude, job demands, and cardiovascular disease: a prospective study of Swedish men. Am J Public Health 1981;71:694–705.

61. Taggart P, Gibbons D, Somerville W. Some effects of motor-car driving on the normal and abnormal heart. Br Med J 1969;4:130–134.

62. Millar-Craig MW, Mann S, Balasubramanian V, Cashman P, Raftery EB. Effects of chronic β-blockade on intra-arterial blood pressure during motor car driving. Br Heart J 1981;45:643–648.

63. Evans GW, Palsane MN, Carrere S. Type A behavior and occupational stress: a cross-cultural study of blue-collar workers. J Pers Soc Psychol 1987;52:1002–1007.

64. Winkleby MA, Ragland DR, Fisher JM, Syme SL. Excess risk of sickness and disease in bus drivers: a review and synthesis of epidemiological studies. Int J Epidemiol 1988;17:255–262.

65. Bellet S, Roman L, Kostis J, Slater A. Continuous electrocardiographic monitoring during automobile driving. Am J Cardiol 1968;22:856–862.

66. Stokols D, Novaco RW, Stokols J, Campbell J. Traffic congestion, type A behavior, and stress. J Appl: Psychol 1978;63:467–480.

67. Russek HI, Russek LG. Behavior patterns and emotional stress in the etiology of coronary heart disease: sociological and occupational aspects. In: Wheatley D(ed): Stress and the heart. New York: Raven Press, 1977:15–32.

68. Herloff B, Jarvholm B. Teachers, stress, and mortality. Lancet 1989;1:159–160.

69. Roberts DE, Berryman HE. Cardiovascular disease and stress in the clergy. Abstracts, Society of Behavioral Medicine Ninth Annual Scientific Sessions 1988; p59.

70. King H, Bailor JC. The health of the clergy: a review of demographic literature. Demography 1969;6:27–43.

71. Ogata M, Ikeda M, Kuratsune M. Mortality among Japanese Zen priests. J Epidemiol Community Health 1984;38:161–166.

72. Kaplan SD. Retrospective cohort mortality study of Roman Catholic priests. Prev Med 1988;17:335–343.

73. Alfredsson L, Karasek R, Theorell T. Myocardial infarction risk and psychosocial work environment: an analysis of the male Swedish working force. Soc Sci Med 1982;16:463–467.

74. Knutsson A, Akerstedt T, Jonsson BG, Orth-Gomer K. Increased risk of ischaemic heart disease in shift workers. Lancet 1986;2:89–92.

75. Orth-Gomer K. Intervention on coronary risk factors by adapting a shift work schedule to biologic rhythmicity. Psychosom Med 1983;45:407–415.

76. Johnson JV, Hall EM. Job strain, work place social support, and cardiovascular disease: a cross-sectional study of random sample of the Swedish working population. Am J Public Health 1988;78:1336–1342.

77. Alfredsson L, Theorell T. Job characteristics of occupations and myocardial infarction risk: effect of possible confounding factors. Soc Sci Med 1983;20:1497–1503.

78. Reed DM, LaCroix AZ, Karasek RA, Miller D, MacLean CA. Occupational strain and the incidence of coronary heart disease. Am J Epidemiol 1989;129:495–502.

79. Magnus K, Matroos AW, Strackee J. The self-employed and the self-driven: two coronary-prone subpopulations from the Zeist study. Am J Epidemiol 1983;118:799–805.

80. Repetti RL. Effects of daily workload on subsequent behavior during marital interaction: the roles of social withdrawal and spouse support. J Pers Soc Psychol 1989;57:651–659.

81. Kaplan BH, Cassel JC, Tyroler HA, Cornoni JC, Kleinbaum DG, Hames CG. Occupational mobility and coronary heart disease. Arch Intern Med 1971;128:938–942.

82. Syme SL, Hyman MM, Enterline PE. Some social and cultural factors associated with the occurrence of coronary heart disease. J Chron Dis 1964;17:277–289.

83. Syme SL, Borhani NO, Buechley RW. Cultural mobility and coronary heart disease in an urban area. Am J Epidemiol 1966;82:334–346.

84. Rees WL. Medical aspects of unemployment. Br Med J 1981;283:1630–1631.

85. Kasl SV, Core S, Cobb S. The experience of losing a job: reported changes in health, symptoms and illness behavior. Psychosom Med 1975;37:106–122.

86. Crombie IK, Kenicer MB, Smith WC, Tunstall-Pedoe HD. Unemployment, socioenvironmental factors, and coronary heart disease in Scotland. Br Heart J 1989;61:172–177.

87. Svensson PG. International social and health policies to prevent ill health in the unemployed: the World Health Organization perspective. Soc Sci Med 1987;25:201–204.

88. Cascelles W, Hennekens CH, Rosner B, DeSilva RA, Lown B. Association of retirement with increased mortality from coronary heart disease. Circulation 1979;59(suppl II):126.

89. Pieper C, LaCroix AZ, Karasek RA. The relation of psychosocial dimensions of work with coronary heart disease risk factors: a meta-analysis of five United States data bases. Am J Epidemiol 1989;129:483–494.

90. Friedman M, Rosenman RH, Carroll V. Changes in the serum cholesterol and blood clotting time in men subjected to cyclic variation of occupational stress. Circulation 1958;17:852–861.

91. Theorell T, Akerstedt T. Day and night work: changes in cholesterol, uric acid, glucose and potassium and in circadian patterns of urinary catecholamine excretion. Acta Med Scand 1976;200:47–53.

92. Hazuda HP, Haffner SM, Stern MP, Knapp JA, Eifler CW, Rosenthal M. Employment status and women's protection against coronary heart disease. Am J Epidemiol 1986;123:623–640.

93. Matthews KA, Cottington EM, Talbott E, Kuller LH, Siegel JM. Stressful work conditions and diastolic blood pressure among blue collar factor workers. Am J Epidemiol 1987;126:280–291.

94. Cobb S, Rose RH. Hypertension, peptic ulcer and diabetes in air traffic controllers. JAMA 1973;224:489–492.

95. Holme I, Helgeland A, Hjermann I, Leren P, Lund-Larsen PG. Coronary risk factors in various occupational groups: the Oslo study. Br J Prev Soc Med 1977;31:96–100.

96. Blaxter M. Evidence on inequality in health from a national survey. Lancet 1987;2:30–33.

97. LaVecchia C, Gutzwiller F, Wietlisbach V. Sociocultural influences on smoking habits in Switzerland. Int J Epidemiol 1987;16:624-626.

98. Weng XZ, Hong ZG, Chen DY. Smoking prevalence in Chinese aged 15 and above. Chinese Med J 1987;100:886-892.

99. Aung-Thwin M. Insecurity hindering Philippine tobacco industry. Tabak J Int 1987;6:399-400,402.

100. Weinkam JJ, Sterling TD. Changes in smoking characteristics by type of employment from 1970 to 1979/1980. Am J Ind Med 1987;11:539-561.

101. Rosen M, Wall S, Hanning M, et al. Smoking habits and their confounding effects among occupational groups in Sweden. Scand J Soc Med 1987;15:233-240.

102. Holmes TH, Rahe RH. The social readjustment rating scale. J Psychosom Res 1967;4:189-194.

103. Sarason IG, Johnson JH, Siegel JM. Assessing the impact of life changes: development of the life experiences survey. J Consult Clin Psychol 1978;46:932-946.

104. Theorell TG. Review of research on life events and cardiovascular illness. Adv Cardiol 1982;29:140-147.

105. Girard DE, Arthur RJ, Reuler JB. Psychosocial events and subsequent illness—a review. West J Med 1985;142:358-363.

106. Rahe RH. Developments of life change measurement. Subjective life change unit scaling. In: Dohrenwend BS, Dohrenwend BP(eds): Stressful life events and their contexts. New Brunswick, NJ: Rutgers University Press, 1984:48-62.

107. Davidson DM. Family and sexual adjustments after cardiac events. Qual Life Cardiovasc Care 1989;5:66-71,77-79.

108. Wiklund I, Oden A, Sanne H, Ulvenstam G, Wilhelmsson C, Wilhelmsen L. Prognostic importance of somatic and psychosocial variables after a first myocardial infarction. Am J Epidemiol 1988;128:786-795.

109. Jones DR. Heart disease mortality following widowhood: some results from the OPCS longitudinal study. J Psychosom Res 1987;31:325-333.

110. Cottington EM, Matthews KA, Talbott E, Kuller LH. Environmental events preceding sudden death in women. Psychosom Med 1980;42:567-574.

111. Chandra V, Szklo M, Goldberg R, Tonascia J. The impact of marital status on survival after an acute myocardial infarction: a population-based study. Am J Epidemiol 1983;117:320-325.

112. Berkman LF. Assessing the physical health effects of social networks and social support. Ann Rev Public Health 1984;5:413-432.

113. Davidson DM, Shumaker SA. Social support and cardiovascular disease. Arteriosclerosis 1987;7:101-104.

114. Ganster DC, Victor B. The impact of social support on mental and physical health. Br J Med Psychol 1988;61:17-36.

115. House JS, Kahn RL. Measures and concepts of social support. In: Cohen S, Syme SL (eds): Social support and health. Orlando, FL: Academic Press, 1985:83-108.

116. Haynes SG, Eaker ED, Feinleib M. Spouse behavior and coronary heart disease in men: prospective results from the Framingham Heart Study. I. Concordance of risk factors and the relationship of psychosocial status to coronary incidence. Am J Epidemiol 1983;118:1-22.

117. Suarez L, Barrett-Connor E. Is an educated wife hazardous to your health? Am J Epidemiol 1984;119:244-249.

118. Ruberman W, Weinblatt E, Goldberg JD, Chaudhary BS. Psychosocial influences on mortality after myocardial infarction. N Engl J Med 1984;311:552-559.

119. Aneshensel CS, Stone JD. Stress and depression. A test of the buffering model of social support. Arch Gen Psychiatr 1982;39:1392-1396.

120. Lowenthal MF, Haven C. Interaction and adaptation. Intimacy as a critical variable. Am Sociol Rev 1968;33:20-30.

121. Kessler RC, McLeod JD, Wethington E. The costs of caring. A perspective on the relationship between sex and psychological distress. In: Saranson IG, Saranson BR(eds): Social support. Theory, research and application. Dordrecht, Netherlands: Martinus Nijhoff, 1985:491-506.

122. Coppotelli HC, Orleans CT. Partner support and other determinants of smoking cessation. Maintenance among women. J Consult Clin Psychol 1985;53:455-460.

123. Sallis JF, Grossman RM, Pinski RB, Patterson TL, Nader PR. The development of scales to measure social support for diet and exercise behaviors. Prev Med 1987;16:825–836.

124. Orth-Gomer K, Unden AL. The measurement of social support in population surveys. Soc Sci Med 1987;24:83–94.

125. Berkman LF, Syme SL. Social networks, host resistance, and mortality. A nine-year follow-up study of Alameda County residents. Am J Epidemiol 1979;109:186–204.

126. Schoenbach VJ, Kaplan BH, Fredman L, Kleinbaum DG. Social ties and mortality in Evans County, Georgia. Am J Epidemiol 1986;123:577–591.

127. Welin I, Tibblin G, Svardsudd K, et al. Prospective study of social influences on mortality. The study of men born in 1913 and 1923. Lancet 1985;1:915–928.

128. Orth-Gomer K, Johnson JV. Social network interaction and mortality. J Chron Dis 1987;40:949–957.

129. Orth-Gomer K, Unden AL, Edwards ME. Social isolation and mortality in ischemic heart disease. Acta Med Scand 1988;224:205–215.

130. Hanson BS, Isacsson SO, Janzon L, Lindell SE. Social network and social support influence mortality in elderly men. The prospective population of "men born in 1914," Malmo, Sweden. Am J Epidemiol 1989;130:100–111.

131. Kahn RL, Antonucci TC. Convoys over the life course. Attachment roles and social support. In: Baltes PB, Brim OG(eds): Lifespan development and behavior. New York: Academic Press, 1980:253–286.

132. Tillich P. The meaning of health. The relation of religion and health. Richmond, CA: North Atlantic Books, 1981.

133. Groen JJ, Tijong KB, Koster M, Willebrands AF, Verdonck G, Pierloot M. The influence of nutrition and ways of life on blood cholesterol and the prevalence of hypertension and coronary heart disease among Trappist and Benedictine monks. Am J Clin Nutr 1962;10:456–470.

134. Ogata M, Ikeda M, Kuratsune M. Mortality among Japanese Zen Priests. J Epidemiol Community Health 1984;38:161–166.

135. Fraser GE. Determinants of ischemic heart disease in Seventh-Day Adventists: a review. Am J Clin Nutr 1988;48:833–836.

136. Kung H. Freud and the problem of God. New Haven: Yale University Press, 1984.

137. Larson DB, Pattison EM, Blazer DG, et al. Systematic analysis of research on religious variables in four major psychiatric journals, 1978–1982. Am J Psychiatry 1986;143:329–334.

138. Sherrill KA, Larson DB. Adult burn patients: the role of religion in recovery. Southern Med J 1988;81:821–825.

139. Levin JS, Vanderpool HY. Is frequent religious attendance really conducive to better health? Toward an epidemiology of religion. Soc Sci Med 1987;24:589–600.

140. Sherrill KA. The role of religion in recovery from burn injury. M.P.H. thesis, Chapel Hill: University of North Carolina, 1989.

141. Marty ME. Health and medicine in the Lutheran tradition. Being well. New York: Crossroad Publishing, 1986.

142. Vaux KL. Health and medicine in the Reformed tradition. Promise, providence, and care. New York: Crossroad Publishing, 1986.

143. Fowler JW. Stages of faith. The psychology of human development and the quest for meaning. San Francisco: Harper & Row, 1981.

144. Strogatz DS, James SA, Elliott D, Ramsey D, Cutchin LM, Ibrahim MA. Community coverage in a rural, church-based, hypertension screening program in Edgecombe County, North Carolina. Am J Public Health 1985;75:401–402.

145. DePue JD, Wells BL, Lasater TM, Carleton RA. Training volunteers to conduct heart health programs in churches. Am J Prev Med 1987;3:51–57.

146. Kelley HH, Michela JL. Attribution theory and research. Annu Rev Psychol 1980;31:457–501.

147. Pearlin LI, Menaghan EG, Lieberman MA, Mullan JT. The stress process. J Health Soc Behav 1981;22:337–356.

148. Bandura A. Social foundations of thought and action. A social cognitive theory. Englewood Cliffs, NJ: Prentice-Hall, 1986.

149. Ewart CK, Taylor CB, Reese LB, DeBusk RF. Effects of early postmyocardial infarction exercise testing of self-perception and subsequent physical activity. Am J Cardiol 1983;51:1076–1080.

150. Rotter JB. Some problems and misconceptions related to the construct of internal versus external control of reinforcement. J Consult Clin Psychol 1975;43:56–67.

151. Wallston BS, Wallston KA, Kaplan GD, Maides SA. Development and validation of the Health Locus of Control (HLC) Scale. J Consult Clin Psychol 1976;44:580–585.

152. Kobasa SC. Stressful life events, personality, and health: an inquiry into hardiness. J Pers Soc Psychol 1979;37:1–11.

153. Kobasa SC, Maddi SR, Puccetti MC, Zola MA. Effectiveness of hardiness, exercise and social support as resources against illness. Psychosom Res 1985;29:525–533.

154. Kaplan GA, Camacho T. Perceived health and mortality: a nine-year follow-up of the Human Population Laboratory cohort. Am J Epidemiol 1983;117:292–304.

155. Goldstein MS, Siegel JM, Boyer R. Predicting changes in perceived health status. Am J Public Health 1984;74:611–614.

156. Kottke TE, Puska P, Salonen JT, Tuomilehto J, Nissinen A. Changes in perceived heart disease risk and health during a community-based heart disease prevention program: the North Karelia Project. Am J Public Health 1984;74:1404–1405.

157. Appels A, Mulder P. Type A behavior and myocardial infarction. A 9.5 year follow-up of a small cohort. Int J Cardiol 1985;8:465–470.

158. Matthews KA, Haynes SG. Type A behavior pattern and coronary disease risk. Am J Epidemiol 1986;123:923–960.

159. van Doornen LP. The coronary risk personality: psychological and psychophysiological aspects. Psychother Psychosom 1980;34:204–215.

160. Chesney MA. Anger and hostility: future implications for behavioral medicine. In: Chesney MA, Rosenman RH(eds): Anger and hostility in cardiovascular and behavioral disorders. Washington: Hemisphere Publishing, 1985:277–290.

161. Hecker MH, Chesney MA, Black GW, Frautschi N. Coronary-prone behaviors in the Western Collaborative Group Study. Psychosom Med 1988;50:153–164.

162. Dimsdale JE. A perspective on type A behavior and coronary disease. N Engl J Med 1988;318:110–112.

163. Haynes SG, Levine S, Scotch N, Feinleib M, Kannel WB. The relationship of psychosocial factors to coronary heart disease in the Framingham Study. I. Methods and risk factors. Am J Epidemiol 1978;107:362–383.

164. Siegel JM. Type A behavior: epidemiologic foundations and public health implications. Annu Rev Public Health 1984;5:343–367.

165. Friedman M, Thoresen CE, Gill JJ, et al. Alteration of type A behavior and its effect on cardiac recurrences in post-myocardial infarction patients. Summary results of the Recurrent Coronary Prevention Project. Am Heart J 1986;112:653–665.

166. Powell LH, Thoresen CE. Effects of type A behavior counseling and severity of prior myocardial infarction on survival. Am J Cardiol 1988;62:1159–1163.

167. Ragland DR, Brand RJ. Type A behavior and mortality from coronary heart disease. N Engl J Med 1988;318:65–69.

168. Carver CS, Coleman AE, Glass DC. The coronary-prone behavior pattern and the suppression of fatigue on a treadmill test. J Pers Soc Psychol 1976;33:460–466.

169. James SA, Hartnett SA, Kalsbeek WD. John Henryism and blood pressure differences among black men. J Behav Med 1983;6:259–278.

170. James SA, Strogatz DS, Wing SB, Ramsey DL. Socioeconomic status, John Henryism, and hypertension in blacks and whites. Am J Epidemiol 1987;126:664–673.

171. Duijkers TJ, Drijver M, Kromhout D, James SA. "John Henryism" and blood pressure in a Dutch population. Psychosom Med 1988;50:353–359.

172. Leiden LI, Veach TL, Herring MW. Comparison of the abbreviated and original versions of the Myers-Briggs Type Indicator Personality Inventory. J Med Educ 1986;61:319–321.

11

gender and hormonal factors

Coronary artery disease (CAD), the leading cause of death in North American women, becomes manifest in women at least a decade later than in men. At any given age in mid-adulthood, the incidence of myocardial infarction in women is half that of men (1). While this disparity may result from differences in the prevalence of risk indicators discussed in earlier chapters, there is a growing body of evidence suggesting a protective effect from estrogens in women.

This chapter focuses on the hormonal changes that a woman experiences as she encounters menarche, contraceptive choices, pregnancy, menopause, and decisions regarding hormonal replacement. It concludes with a brief discussion of the roles of male and female hormones in the development of CAD in men.

WOMEN

Differences between genders in levels of CAD physiological risk indicators begin to appear at the time of puberty. Physiological changes in these indicators also occur during the menstrual cycle and throughout pregnancy, but symptomatic CAD usually does not occur until the fourth decade. Natural or surgical menopause is accompanied by a worsening of

CAD risk, but appropriate dosages of hormonal replacement can minimize these adverse changes.

Puberty

In contrast to boys, whose HDL-cholesterol (HDL-C) levels drop considerably while their plasma testosterone levels rise (2, 3), puberty does not adversely affect the lipid and lipoprotein levels in girls.

However, oral contraceptive use by adolescent girls can reverse this natural advantage by increasing LDL-C and triglyceride levels, while decreasing HDL-C (4).

Menses

Throughout the menstrual cycle, HDL-cholesterol (HDL-C) and triglyceride levels are largely unchanged. In contrast, LDL-cholesterol (LDL-C) begins to decline at the onset of the follicular phase and remains lower throughout the luteal phase. Concomitant decreases in apolipoprotein B have been documented, with a return to baseline values in the luteal phase (5).

Oral Contraceptives

The oral contraceptive (OC) was introduced in the early 1960s in North America, and by the middle of the next decade, more than eight million women were using OCs. Worldwide, the number of women using OCs was estimated to exceed 150 million (6). Ten years later, more than 13 million women in North America were using OCs (7). Almost immediately, cardiovascular complications were reported (8), including venous and arterial thromboembolic events (9–15).

In women under age 45 who had been hospitalized for myocardial infarction (MI) in Edinburgh between 1964 and 1972, Oliver noted that 52% had been taking OCs. After examining the prevalence of other major CAD risk indicators, he concluded that OCs only increase MI risk when a woman is otherwise at risk (16).

Mann and colleagues interviewed women discharged with a diagnosis of MI from major hospitals in England and Wales from 1968 to 1972. They found that, during their fourth decade, OC use triples a woman's risk of nonfatal MI; during the subsequent five years, the relative risk increases to five. When other indicators of CAD risk were also present, MI risk rose exponentially (17, 18). These studies, done in the mid-1970s, involved women using OCs with much higher estrogen doses than are currently employed. Early attention focused on the potential for estrogen to enhance thrombogenesis at the site of arteriosclerotic injury (19).

Ethinyl estradiol (EE) and mestranol are the only estrogens currently used in OCs; mestranol is biologically converted into EE. Compared to other estrogens, EE is particularly effective in suppressing gonadotropin secretion by the pituitary gland, so it can be used at much lower doses than other estrogens for this purpose. Most of an orally administered dose is extracted during its first pass through the enterohepatic circulation, leading to considerable variation in bioavailability from patient to patient (20).

Two major forms of progestogens are used in North America. Norethindrone is the active substance in the first category; related compounds (norethynodrel, norethindrone mono- and diacetates) are biologically converted to norethindrone. Between 25 and 50% of norethindrone is removed on the first pass through the liver, resulting in considerable interindividual variability from a given oral dose.

Norgestrel is the other major substance; only its levo- form is biologically active, although it is available in both l- and dl- forms. Because levonorgestrel is not subject to first-pass extraction in the liver, it has 100% bioavailability after oral ingestion and displays less variation in plasma steroid concentrations (20). Newer progestogens are currently available in Europe; gestodene and norgestimate are active in their parent forms. Desogestrel requires two metabolic steps for conversion into norgestrel (21).

In a study of more than 120,000 nurses in the USA who responded to mailed questionnaires, 156 reported MI before menopause (23 were using OCs at the time of MI). Relative risk for OC use was 1.8 (22).

In a case-control study of young women in the USA who were hospitalized for acute MI, Slone and colleagues noted an increased relative risk even in past users of OCs. For those who had used OCs for 5 to 9 years, relative risk was 1.6; this value increased to 2.5 for women whose duration of use was 10 years or more. Relative risk for current users aged 25 to 49 was 3.5 (23). In contrast, in the USA Nurses' Health Study, investigators found no increase in risk from past OC use, regardless of duration (24).

Further analysis of early studies (which included patients no longer eligible for OCs and the use of higher estrogen doses) suggests that the older woman who is healthy and a nonsmoker is at high risk only if she also has other CAD risk indicators (25). However, indications of increased risk for older OC users are compounded by the observation that women 35 to 39 years of age are twice as likely as women 15 to 19 to be receiving OC preparations containing more than 50 μg of estrogen (26).

CAD RISK INDICATORS

Lipids

In the Lipid Research Clinics study of 10 North American centers, serum total cholesterol, LDL-C, and triglycerides were higher in OC users than in women of similar age not using oral contraceptives; levels were positively associated with the estrogen dose in the OC preparations (27). Using the 95th percentile as a threshold, OC users 20 to 24 years old were up to three times more likely to have elevated total cholesterol levels and up to five times more likely to be hypertriglyceridemic (28). Similarly, women less than 20 years of age taking OCs had significantly higher cholesterol and triglyceride levels than nonusers (29). Estrogens in OCs can decrease postheparin lipoprotein and increase the turnover rate of triglycerides, while progestogens counteract these effects (30).

Several investigators have demonstrated the HDL-C lowering effect of oral contraceptives, regardless of smoking status and age (31, 32).

After widespread employment of low-dose estrogen OCs, differences in CAD risk indicators in women were noted between those taking OCs with the progestogens norethindrone acetate and levonorgesterol. HDL_2 concentrations were lower in women taking levonorgestrel or dl-norgestrel than in those using norethindrone (33, 34). Other studies revealed that CAD rates correlated with the dose of norethindrone acetate in the OC preparation (35, 36). These and other observations have led to the

testing and use of OC preparations with lower doses of progestogens.

Marz and colleagues compared OCs containing triphasic levonorgestrel and EE with those composed of monophasic desogestrel and EE. HDL-C was higher in the latter group, and HDL_2 was lower in the levonorgestrel treated group (37). Differences in HDL_2 concentrations were also noted when the two formulations were examined by Kloosterboer and colleagues. HDL_2 levels were markedly decreased in the levonorgestrel group, while HDL_3 concentrations were elevated in both groups (38). Subsequent studies in the Netherlands of seven OC preparations confirmed that HDL_2 was depressed much more by monophasic levonorgestrel, while treatment with monophasic cyproterone acetate and biphasic desogestrel produced the smallest declines. The authors concluded that these observations are consistent with the intrinsic androgenicity of the various progestogens tested (39). Wynn and colleagues point out that the reduced androgenicity of the newer progestogens may expose women to an increased prevalence of estrogen-induced hypertriglyceridemia (40), but this consequence will have a much smaller influence on CAD risk than the improvement in HDL-C.

Preparations containing norethindrone appear to cause less of a rise in blood total cholesterol (41) and less of a decline in HDL-C (42) and HDL_2 (43) than do levonorgestrel OCs. In one study, norethindrol diacetate (also called ethynodiol diacetate) had no significant effect on HDL-C and increased LDL-C less than did norethindrone and levonorgestrel preparations (44). In a USA study of three popular OCs, the preparation containing 50 μg ethinyl estradiol and 0.5 mg dl-norgestrel significantly raised LDL-C and lowered HDL-C and HDL_2, while the other two agents (containing EE and either ethynodiol acetate or norethindrone acetate) displayed no significant changes in those parameters (45).

Welch and colleagues reviewed the records of 1000 consecutive women under age 50 whom they had studied by coronary angiography. Only 10% of women with blood total cholesterol under 200 mg/dl had arterial lumen narrowing of 50% or more; in women whose level exceeded 275 mg/dl, 44% had disease of that severity (46).

Blood Pressure

Early studies noted a definite linkage of hypertension to OC use, but these investigations used different estrogen preparations and doses, methods for blood pressure measurement, age of subjects, and criteria for hypertension. In a prospective study of more than 11,000 women, OC users were six times more likely to develop hypertension (47). In the Walnut Creek Oral Contraceptive Study, 1500 black women and 5000 white women were studied. In both races, mean blood pressure (BP) was approximately 2 mm Hg higher in OC users, an important difference from the public health point of view (48). Similar results were obtained from a prospective study in Glasgow, Scotland. Weir found that the increased BP generally occurred within two years. Longer duration of use was associated with a higher prevalence and a greater severity of hypertension. From 5 to 15% of women who used OCs for five years or more increased their diastolic BP by 10 mm Hg or more, giving them a relative risk of 2.6 compared with nonusers (49).

In the Lipid Research Clinics Prevalence Study, investigators also found a 2 to 3 mm Hg higher SBP in OC users; concurrent alcohol intake elevated this difference even more (50).

Some studies have shown that approximately half of women who developed OC-related hypertension had some contraindication to the original prescription of the contraceptive. These factors included age, obesity, antecedent individual or family history of hypertension, and urologic or nephrologic abnormalities (48). Women with a history of transient hypertension during pregnancy had a fourfold risk of BP increase during subsequent OC use (51).

Several studies have documented a direct relation between the progestogen dose (norethindrone acetate or norgestrel) and hypertension, but additional studies are indicated to examine the effects of OCs containing lower doses of both estrogen and progestogen (36).

Women who develop high BP while taking OCs should have the medication withdrawn immediately. BP typically returns to normal within four months, but if OCs are reinstated, hypertension often recurs.

Smoking

Smoking and OC use appear to synergistically increase the risk of CAD in young women, in part due to coronary artery spasm (52). A collaborative study based in Boston reviewed the cases of 107 women with MI at age 45 or less; 26 were found to be otherwise healthy and capable of childbearing. Of the 26, 20 (77%) had been taking OCs just prior to admission; 24 of the 26 were cigarette smokers (53). In another Boston study, 234 premenopausal women with MI were compared to 1742 women hospitalized for other reasons. Although the selection of hospitalized persons for "controls" represents suboptimal study design, findings were similar to earlier reports. Women who both smoked and used OCs had a relative risk of MI of 39 (54).

In the absence of OC use, smoking has a dose-response relation to MI. Slone and co-workers found that non–OC users who smoked 35 or more cigarettes daily had a relative risk of MI more than 20 times that of never-smokers (55). In a random population sample of women from eastern Finland, concurrent OC and cigarette use conferred a relative risk of 7.2 compared with those who neither smoked nor used OCs (56).

In a study of more than 23,000 women in the state of Maryland in 1963, smoking status was recorded. Later, this information was compared with death from a variety of causes. After adjustment for marital status and education, women younger than 65 who smoked 20 or more cigarettes per day were more likely to have died from CAD. For women 25 to 44 initially, the relative risk was 3.6; for women from 45 to 64, it was 2.2. For sudden cardiac death, the relative risks were 6.5 and 2.7 for the two age groups, respectively (57).

A highly visible group of women smokers is found in the nursing profession. The prevalence of smoking among female nurses is double that of physicians, and smoking nurses have maintained attitudes that potentially reduce their effectiveness in helping patients stop smoking (58).

Hematologic Factors

Estrogens in OCs accelerate platelet aggregation (59) and decrease antithrombin III activity (60). They also decrease the plasminogen-activator content of endothelium (61), which enhances the formation and accumulation of fibrin. Plasma fibrinogen levels and the activity of factors VII and X are increased (62). It appears that the risk of thromboembolism in OC users is limited to current use and is unrelated to the duration of use (63).

Diabetes

Diminished glucose tolerance has been noted with all OC preparations (64), regardless of estrogen dose (although early pills with 75 μg or more produced the greatest impairment) (65). This effect is greater with levonorgestrel-containing compounds than with those with norethindrone and may be dose dependent (66). Studies using plasma C-peptide concentrations to monitor insulin secretion have confirmed the adverse effect of levonorgestrel OC combinations. Studies are in progress on the effects of triphasic preparations on carbohydrate metabolism (40).

Contraceptive Implants

Subdermal implants of levonorgestrel capsules are being used in more than 10 countries and are undergoing trials in 30 other nations. Through the silicone capsule, approximately 30 μg of levonorgestel diffuses each day, which provides effective contraception for three to five years (67). In a study of 11 women receiving such implants, mean blood total cholesterol decreased by 10%, LDL-C decreased 7%, while HDL-C dropped 15% (68).

Pregnancy

Postpartum MI is a rare event whose immediate causes include coronary artery spasm, thromboembolic disease, and coronary artery dissection. During pregnancy, clotting is more likely, spontaneous thrombolytic activity is diminished, and arterial walls have reduced structural integrity (69). These events may be superimposed on atherosclerotic disease, which may be present in the pregnant woman, depending on the status of her CAD risk indicators (70).

LIPIDS

Concentrations of plasma triglycerides often rise dramatically during gestation, and plasma total cholesterol rises throughout pregnancy (71). By the time of delivery, LDL-C increases by some 50% over prepregnancy levels. HDL-C rises in similar proportion during the first 20 weeks of gestation, but then decreases during the remainder of pregnancy to a level approximately 15% above baseline (72). Increases in HDL_2 account for most of the rise and subsequent decline in HDL-C (73, 74).

Maternal increases in LDL-C and HDL_2 support placental endocrine steroidogenesis; half of the fetal cholesterol supply comes from the maternal circulation, and this transfer may be mediated by HDL-C (75).

Because of the elevations in LDL-C and triglycerides during pregnancy, one might hypothesize that the number of pregnancies might correlate with the development of CAD, but this appears to not be the case (76).

BLOOD PRESSURE

Blood pressures are often measured during prenatal visits, but the accuracy and reliability of these observations have been appropriately questioned. Increased attention to the many sources of bias (e.g., digit preference, too rapid deflation of cuff) can enhance the usefulness of BP data from the obstetric clinic (77).

Some investigators consider that gestational hypertension and preeclampsia are diseases with etiological differences. For example, the finding that cigarette smoking reduces the risk of preeclampsia and gestational hypertension, but to different degrees, has led Marcoux et al. to make such a suggestion. Despite this minor benefit, she and her coauthors point out the many risks of maternal smoking. These include the risk of intrauterine growth retardation, premature rupture of membranes and birth, low birth weight, and fetal death (78). Further, the perinatal death rate due to preeclampsia is higher in smokers than in nonsmokers (79). The American College of Obstetricians and Gynecologists suggested four categories of hypertensive disorders of gestation. These include (a) preeclampsia and eclampsia, (b) chronic

hypertension of any etiology, (c) chronic hypertension with superimposed preeclampsia, and (d) late or transient hypertension (80).

Preeclampsia is a disorder whose etiology is being actively pursued. Recent work has investigated such possibilities as prostacyclin and thromboxane imbalance (81), endothelial cell dysfunction, and lipid peroxidation (82). If the woman is near term, induction is the treatment of choice. If not, treatment with methyldopa, β-blockers, and hydralazine have proved effective and safe. Converting-enzyme inhibitors, diuretics, ganglion-blocking agents, and nitroprusside should not be used (80).

SMOKING

For the reasons mentioned above (78), women should stop smoking during pregnancy. Efforts as simple as a serialized set of printed materials mailed to pregnant women over an eight-week period can significantly improve quitting rates (83).

DIABETES

Gestational diabetes mellitus is the most common medical complication of pregnancy. Since sulfonylurea agents are contraindicated in this setting, and insulin is simply palliative, Jovanovic-Peterson and colleagues considered exercise as therapy for this disorder. Noting that fetal bradycardia has been associated with stationary bicycle ergometric training, they designed arm ergometric exercises for 19 untrained women with gestational diabetes. They found that such therapy added to diet modification to produce improved glycosylated hemoglobin and fasting and one-hour plasma glucose concentrations in their exercising subjects (84).

CARDIOVASCULAR DRUGS

While the calcium-channel blockers nifedipine and nicardipine are of great use as vasodilators in the treatment of hypertension and CAD, they have been documented to significantly alter fetal cardiorespiratory status and placental function in animal studies (85).

Menopause

Several studies have documented a higher CAD risk (86) and all-cause mortality (87) in women following menopause. Because the onset of menopause and the development of symptomatic CAD are both positively correlated with age, it is preferable to review studies that have examined women at the exact same age. However, further adjustment must be made for smoking status, since cigarette smokers develop menopausal symptoms at an earlier age (88). MacMahon et al. have suggested that this might result from a lowered estrogen stimulus in smokers (89). Other proposed mechanisms await definitive testing (90). In the Nurses' Health Study carried out in the USA, never-smoking women had a median age at menopause of 52.4 years; as the number of cigarettes per day increased, median age decreased. Women who smoked 35 or more cigarettes daily, reached menopause two years earlier than never-smokers (91). Distinctions between bilateral and unilateral oophorectomy (OOP), hysterectomy alone, and natural menopause are also important in evaluating the effect of menopause on CAD events. Definitions of CAD events differ by investigation. Because angina pectoris is both more common and less predictive of coronary atherosclerosis in women, care must be taken in evaluating end-points used in different studies. Because studies of persons coming to coronary angiography do not make a random selection from the community, biases can also occur when comparing persons with and without "significant" coronary obstructions as determined by angiography.

These methodologic concerns are illustrated by results from early studies. In 1958, Robinson and colleagues reported a twofold risk for developing angina or MI in women with bilateral OOP compared with women with unilateral OOP or hysterectomy alone, but no significant differences when MI alone was considered as the outcome (92). The following year, Oliver and Boyd reported CAD incidence rates in women who were under age 35 at the time of bilateral or unilateral OOP. In the former group, 25% developed CAD during the subsequent 20 years, while the incidence was only 3% in women with unilateral OOP (93). In 1963, Ritterband et al. defined CAD as nonfatal MI, a positive exercise test, or clinically diagnosed angina and found no relation to ovarian status. They did note a CAD relative risk of 1.4 for women with bilateral OOP compared with women who had hysterectomy only (94). Manchester and associates studied women referred for coronary angiography who were under age 41 at oophorectomy and under age 61 at the time of angiography. They noted significant coronary artery obstructions in a smaller percentage of postmenopausal women than in age-matched premenopausal women (95).

The association of menopause with increased CAD risk became clearer as studies were completed that had a larger sample size and clearer CAD end-points. In the Nurses' Health Study, more than 121,700 women from 11 states in the USA completed mail questionnaires in 1976. During the next six years, the follow-up rate was 98.3% for mortality and 95.4% for nonfatal events (96).

Before consideration of replacement estrogen status, MI rates were considerably lower in premenopausal women (Table 11.1).

Women with hysterectomies, particularly those with bilateral OOP, are more likely to receive replacement hormonal therapy, so the data in Table 11.1 must be

Table 11.1. Myocardial Infarction Rate (per 10,000 Women-Years)

Status	Fatal	Nonfatal	Total
Premenopausal	0.74	3.45	4.19
Hysterectomy (H) only	0	5.37	5.37
Natural menopause	2.04	7.60	9.64
Unilateral OOP[a] + H	1.08	9.68	10.76
Bilateral OOP + H	1.84	6.45	8.29

[a]OOP = oophorectomy.

further examined for replacement estrogen (RE) status (which is done in the next section).

LIPIDS

In the longitudinal study of women in Göteborg, Sweden, investigators noted an increase in blood total cholesterol and triglycerides during the transition through menopause. In women who were exactly 50 years old, the number of years spent in menopause before age 50 was positively correlated with blood total cholesterol (97).

Matthews and colleagues completed a 2.5-year follow-up of 541 healthy, initially premenopausal women 42 to 50 years of age. Of the 69 women who had spontaneously stopped menstruating for at least 12 months at study end, 37 had not started REs. Their mean LDL-C increased 12 mg/dl, while their HDL-C dropped 3.5 mg/dl (98).

Earlier, Hallberg and Svanborg had examined plasma lipids in women exactly 50 years old, noting increased levels of total cholesterol, LDL-C, and triglycerides in those who had reached menopause (99). Paterson and colleagues compared 35 postmenopausal women with 35 premenopausal women of the same age and height. The former group had higher serum total cholesterol levels initially, but the differences between groups disappeared after the former were placed on sequential mestranol and norethisterone for two months.

Serum triglycerides were not different initially, but they rose significantly after the onset of therapy (100).

In the Evans County (Georgia) study, Baird and her co-workers noted a higher mean serum total cholesterol in postmenopausal white women compared to premenopausal white women, but no differences in black women (101).

Studies of Japanese women have indicated similar rises in total cholesterol and LDL-C as a consequence of menopause (102). In 65 Pima Indian women, however, no total cholesterol changes were noted when they were examined before menopause and at a mean interval of six years later. In this population of native Americans, diabetes is very prevalent, but it did not appear to influence the lipid changes in women passing through menopause. Total cholesterol levels in the Pima population show no age-related rise (103).

In female cynomolgus monkeys fed an atherogenic diet for 30 months, atherosclerosis was 2 to 10 times as extensive in coronary, carotid, and iliacofemoral arteries of the oophorectomized monkeys. While the investigators attributed this in part to 15 to 20% increases in LDL-C, they also noted that socially submissive monkeys (with intact ovaries) were also susceptible to advanced atherosclerosis. They hypothesized that adrenal and ovarian dysfunction in this latter group may be related independently to atherogenesis (104).

Several investigators have documented the positive association of sex hormone–binding globulin (SHBG) to HDL-C in premenopausal (105) and postmenopausal women (106). It appears that the adverse effects of progestogens and natural progesterone on HDL-C are dose related (107). In almost all women, observation of the bleeding pattern will obviate the necessity for endometrial biopsy in determining the optimal dosage of progestin (108).

Other considerations dictate a careful search for this optimal dose (109).

FAMILY HISTORY

In the USA study of nurses, subjects upon entry reported if either parent had experienced MI before the age of 61. During the next four years, more than 100 had MI themselves. The age-adjusted MI risk for women with parental MI before age 61 was 2.8; in women without parental MI before that age, the relative risk was 1.0. In comparison with women without parental history of CAD, fatal heart disease was five times more common in nurses with parental MI before age 61 and 2.6 times as likely if parental MI occurred after the age of 60 (110). In their study of a retirement community in southern California, Khaw and Barrett-Connor did not find a family history of CAD predictive of the development of CAD in their female subjects (111), but a history of paternal stroke did identify women at high risk for stroke themselves (112). Age of parental cardiovascular events was not elicited, suggesting that risk of subjects with early parental MI may not have been detectable with their methods.

Austin and colleagues studied 434 adult female twin pairs, finding that levels of LDL-C, HDL-C, and relative weight may explain in part observations of family resemblance in CAD risk (113).

BLOOD PRESSURE, GLUCOSE INTOLERANCE, AND WEIGHT

Most authors agree that there are no significant changes in systolic or diastolic blood pressure, glucose tolerance, or body weight during the transition through menopause (97, 98, 114). However, mean body weight and systolic blood pressure in 50-year-old premenopausal women are each greater than in their postmenopausal contemporaries (115). Because obese women are both more likely to be hyper-tensive and premenopausal, these effects might nullify a potential increase in blood pressure as a consequence of menopause. When newly diagnosed postmenopausal hypertensive women are adequately treated, their risk of CAD events is reduced to that of normotensive women (116).

In their seven-year prospective study of a geographically defined population in southern California, investigators noted that diabetic women had a relative risk of CAD death of 3.4 before adjustment for other CAD risk indicators, and 3.5 thereafter (117).

Replacement Estrogens

By the end of this century, more than 700 million of the world's population will be women age 45 and older (118). More than 50 million of these women will reside in Canada and the USA (119), where replacement estrogen and progestin therapy has changed dramatically in the past two decades (120). During the 1970s, replacement estrogen (RE) use declined in the USA because of concerns about endometrial carcinoma (121, 122). During the 1980s, combinations of estrogen and progestin were widely prescribed, and it is expected that the use of these two agents in combination will continue throughout the 1990s (123).

REPLACEMENT ESTROGENS AND CAD EVENTS

More than 30 years ago, Robinson, Cohen, and Higano suggested that CAD risk in postmenopausal women was lower in those taking REs (92, 124).

During the past two decades, some controversy has surrounded the acceptance of a definite association between the use of REs and CAD events. Methodologic considerations discussed earlier also apply in this area. In addition, the population of women who take REs is probably qualitatively different from the population of women who do not. Because they all have access to medical care, they are likely to be healthier than postmenopausal women who are not taking REs (125). The prevalence of other CAD risk indicators may differ in the two populations as well (126).

Despite these limitations, the preponderance of evidence from several prospective studies (96, 125–132) as well as case-control and cross-sectional investigations (133–138) supports the hypothesis that postmenopausal RE administration reduces CAD risk (72, 139). One investigation, using a decision-analysis model, considered the many effects of REs, including quality-of-life considerations. The authors concluded that estrogen therapy provides a significant gain in quality-adjusted life expectancy (140).

In the Nurses' Health Study, a definite risk was established for bilateral OOP and absence of replacement estrogen (RE) therapy. In that subset of women, relative risk was 2.2. In contrast, women with natural menopause and no REs had a relative risk of 1.2. Women taking REs fared much better; their relative risks were 0.8 and 0.9 for those having natural menopause and bilateral OOP, respectively (96).

The Framingham Heart Study was thought for some years to show an adverse effect of REs on CAD risk, but recent analysis indicates that risk was reduced in women age 50 to 60 who were using REs. In older women, risk was increased only in those who smoked (141).

Investigators from the Lipid Research Clinics (LRC) Program Follow-up Study found that the 593 RE users had only one-third the CAD risk of the 1677 women not using estrogen replacement after menopause. This marked difference in risk persisted after adjustment for age, systolic BP, and smoking status, and was

true for women at all educational levels (126).

LIPIDS

Several investigative teams have reported reduction in LDL-C and increased levels of HDL-C after RE administration (142–144). Hirvonen and colleagues treated three groups of six women each with estradiol valerate for three weeks, then a different progestogen was added to each group's regimen. HDL-C decreased approximately 20% in the two groups receiving androgenic progesterones (norethindrone acetate and norgestrel), but there was no change in HDL-C in those receiving medroxyprogesterone, a hydroxyprogesterone derivative (145).

Farish et al. compared two groups both taking conjugated equine estrogens (0.625 mg/day); the second group also received norgestrel (0.15 mg) on each of the last 12 days of a 28-day cycle. By 24 weeks, LDL-C was more than 15% lower in the second group, and triglycerides were approximately 5% lower. However, HDL-C was also approximately 15% lower (146).

LRC investigators noted that more than half of the beneficial effect in CAD mortality reduction enjoyed by their subjects using REs could be explained by more favorable levels in LDL-C and HDL-C (126).

Among 585 women using REs and 1093 others who did not, investigators in the Walnut Creek study found a dose-response pattern between conjugated estrogen and LDL-C and HDL-C, but the maximal intergroup difference in LDL-C was noted at 1.25 mg/day. The difference between the groups in HDL-C was maximal (8 to 10 mg/dl) at that dose. The enhancement in lipid profile afforded by RE administration was partially offset by smoking (147).

In the study by Matthews et al. cited

earlier, RE therapy further differentiated the lipid and lipoprotein values of healthy women in their fifth decade. In contrast to women taking REs, nonusers had increased LDL-C and lower HDL-C levels. In RE users, apoA-I and apoA-II levels rose significantly. This favorable picture was marred only by higher serum triglycerides (by 37 mg/dl) in users (98).

Transdermal estradiol applied twice weekly, while eliciting many of the beneficial actions of estrogen, has a less beneficial effect on LDL-C and HDL-C than do oral estrogens (148).

Treatment of postmenopausal women with suboptimal lipid and lipoprotein profiles includes hygienic (nutrition and exercise) methods along with consideration of RE prescription for this purpose. In a study of 28 postmenopausal women aged 45 to 64 who participated in a 24-day residential cardiovascular risk-reduction program, daily exercise and a diet low in saturated fat and cholesterol reduced LDL-C from 129.4 mg/dl to 118.8 mg/dl in women taking REs, and from 154.0 mg/dl to 126.5 mg/dl in women of comparable age, weight, and alcohol use who were not using these agents. Similarly, serum triglycerides decreased from 125.4 mg/dl to 101.2 mg/dl in RE users compared with a reduction from 113.4 mg/dl to 97.6 mg/dl in nonusers (149). In a Finnish study of 29 postmenopausal women aged 35 to 60 who had type II dyslipidemia (elevated LDL-C), 12 months of estradiol valerate therapy lowered LDL-C by 22%. HDL-C rose 21%, while there was little change in serum triglycerides (150).

BLOOD PRESSURE

Several studies have confirmed that REs have no detrimental effect on systolic or diastolic blood pressures (151). In one, women aged 55 to 74 taking REs had lower BPs than nonusers (152). In some prospective investigations, BP declined after RE initiation (153), and the incidence of newly diagnosed hypertension was lower in women taking REs (130). In an Australian study, BP changes depended upon the type of estrogen (154).

OTHER CONSIDERATIONS

Increases in thromboembolic phenomena during OC administration prompted careful hematologic studies of chronic RE use, but none have found changes in coagulation, fibrinolysis, platelet count, or function (130, 155). Estrogen can directly influence arterial wall metabolism, and estrogen receptors within the arterial wall have been documented (156).

In one LRC center, women 55 to 64 years of age who were taking REs had lower fasting blood glucose than nonusers, but this effect was not seen in older women. Values were adjusted for obesity (152).

NONCARDIOVASCULAR CONSIDERATIONS

While it is quite clear that CAD risk is minimized by lowering progestin dose and increasing estrogen dose (144), other considerations may dictate prescription for individual women. The risk of endometrial cancer is increased with estrogen administration (157), although its magnitude may have been overestimated in early studies (158). In contrast, increasing progestin doses will decrease this risk (159). Estrogen may also increase slightly the risk of breast cancer, an association that is not diminished by progestin addition (160). In contrast, estrogen offers a clear benefit in reducing osteoporosis, being more effective than calcium supplementation in early postmenopausal bone loss (161, 162). Conjugated estrogen dosages of less than 0.625 mg are probably ineffective in preventing bone loss; conversely, dosages higher than that level are no more effective (163).

In a retrospective study of 2873 women in the Framingham Heart Study, investigators noted that the risk of hip fracture was decreased by one-third in women who had taken REs at any time, and was reduced by two-thirds in women who had taken estrogens in the previous two years (164).

MEN

The Coronary Drug Project in the USA initially assigned one group to treatment with conjugated equine estrogens. Significant elevations in CAD morbidity and mortality caused investigators to terminate early that part of the study (165). At approximately the same time, cancer researchers noted an increase in CAD mortality in men receiving diethylstilbesterol for prostatic cancer (166, 167).

Phillips found significantly higher levels of serum estradiol and estrone in 15 men below the age of 43 who survived MI, compared with age-matched controls (168). Phillips joined Framingham investigators to examine this relation in men aged 61 to 88 in their prospective study. Matching 61 CAD patients with 61 control men, they found that serum estradiol levels were significantly higher in their subjects with CAD (169).

A study of young male Scots recovering from MI noted that, compared with age-matched men without MI, 34 of 35 men had higher estradiol concentrations and 29 of the 35 had higher estrone levels (170). However, Heller and colleagues found no significant differences between men with MI and control men in estrone or testosterone levels (171). Taggart et al. noted no difference in estradiol or testosterone levels between men who survived a stroke and control men (172). Nordoy and colleagues noted a direct relationship between severe concentrations of testosterone and HDL-C (173).

Studies examining the relation of vasectomy to CAD risk have found no association between the operation and incidence of MI, even among men predisposed to MI because of smoking, dyslipidemia, hypertension, or angina (174).

Barrett-Connor, Khaw, and colleagues found an inverse relation between dehydroepiandrosterone sulfate (DHEAS) and cardiovascular mortality in more than 700 men (175, 176). In examining thawed plasma from 1009 white men initially 40 to 79 years of age, the same investigators found no association of cardiovascular disease at baseline, or during a 12-year surveillance with plasma testosterone, androstenedione, estrone, or estradiol. Similarly, no association was noted with sex hormone–binding globulin levels. They did note an inverse relation of plasma testosterone with blood pressure, fasting plasma glucose and triglyceride levels, and body-mass index. Plasma estrone correlated positively with plasma levels of total cholesterol, triglycerides, and glucose (177).

In recent years, there has been a dramatic increase in the number of persons using anabolic steroids for competitive advantage in sports and body-building. Dramatic drops in HDL-C and HDL_2 concentrations have been documented (178), associated with reduced survival of HDL proteins in plasma and marked increases in hepatic triglyceride lipase activity and HDL catabolism. Thompson and colleagues studied 11 male weight lifters in a crossover-design study of oral stanozol and intramuscular testosterone. With stanozol, HDL-C and HDL_2 concentrations dropped 33 and 71%, respectively, compared with drops of 9 and 7% in those receiving supraphysiological doses of testosterone intramuscularly. LDL-C concentrations increased 29% with stanazol, but decreased 16% with testosterone administration.

Postheparin hepatic triglyceride lipase activity was increased by 123 and 25% in the stanazol and testosterone groups (179).

REFERENCES

1. Lerner DJ, Kannel WB. Patterns of coronary heart disease morbidity and mortality in the sexes: a 26-year follow-up of the Framingham population. Am Heart J 1986;111:383–390.

2. Laskarzewski PM, Morrison JA, Gutai J, Orchard T, Khoury PR, Glueck CJ. High and low density lipoprotein cholesterols in adolescent boys: relationships with endogenous testosterone, estradiol, and quetelet index. Metabolism 1983;32:262–271.

3. Kirkland RT, Keenan BS, Probstfield JL, et al. Decrease in plasma high-density lipoprotein cholesterol levels at puberty in boys with delayed adolescence. JAMA 1987;257:502–507.

4. Voors AW, Srinivasan SR, Hunter SM, Webber LS, Sklov MC, Berenson GS. Smoking, oral contraceptives, and serum lipid and lipoprotein levels in youths. Prev Med 1982;11:1–12.

5. Kim HJ, Kalkhoff RK. Changes in lipoprotein composition during the menstrual cycle. Metabolism 1979;28:663–668.

6. Russell-Briefel R, Ezzati T, Perlman J. Prevalence and trends in oral contraceptive use in premenopausal females ages 12–54 years, United States, 1971–80. Am J Public Health 1985;75:1173–1176.

7. Mishell DR Jr. Contraception. N Engl J Med 1989;320:777–787.

8. Jordan WM. Pulmonary embolism. Lancet 1961;2:1146–1147.

9. Inman WH, Vessey MP. Investigation of deaths from pulmonary, coronary, and cerebral thrombosis and embolism in women in child-bearing age. Br Med J 1968;2:193–199.

10. Inman WH, Vessey MP, Westerhold B. Thromboembolic disease and the steroidal content of oral contraceptives: a report to the Committee on Safety of Drugs. Br Med J 1970;2:203–209.

11. Hoover R, Bain C, Cole P, MacMahon B. Oral contraceptive use: association with frequency of hospitalization and chronic disease risk indicators. Am J Public Health 1978; 68:335–341.

12. Vessey MP, Mann JI. Female sex hormones and thrombosis. Epidemiological aspects. Br Med Bull 1978;34:157–162.

13. Shapiro S, Slone D, Rosenberg L, Kaufman DW, Stolley PD, Miettinen OS. Oral contraceptive use in relation to myocardial infarction. Lancet 1979;1:743–747.

14. Stadel BV. Oral contraceptives and cardiovascular disease. N Engl J Med 1981; 305:612–618, 672–677.

15. Sartwell PE, Stolley PD. Oral contraceptives and vascular disease. Epidemiol Rev 1982;4:95–109.

16. Oliver MF. Ischemic heart disease in young women. Br Med J 1974;4:253–259.

17. Mann JI, Vessey MP, Thorogood M, et al. Myocardial infarction in young women with special reference to oral contraceptive practice. Br Med J 1975;2:241–245.

18. Mann JI, Inman WH. Oral contraceptives and death from myocardial infarction. Br Med J 1975;2:245–248.

19. Engel HJ, Engel E, Lichtlen PR. Coronary atherosclerosis and myocardial infarction in young women: role of oral contraceptives. Eur Heart J 1983;4:1–6.

20. Goldzieher JW. Pharmacology of contraceptive steroids: a brief review. Am J Obstet Gynecol 1989;160:1260–1264.

21. Chez RA. Clinical aspects of three new progestogens: desogestrel, gestodene, and norgestimate. Am J Obstet Gynecol 1989;160:1296–1300.

22. Rosenberg L, Hennekens CH, Rosner B, Belanger C, Rothman KJ, Speizer FE. Oral contraceptive use in relation to nonfatal myocardial infarction. Am J Epidemiol 1980;111:59–66.

23. Slone D, Shapiro S, Kaufman DW, Rosenberg L, Miettinen OS, Stolley PD. Risk of myocardial infarction in relation to current and discontinued use of oral contraceptives. N Engl J Med 1981;305:420–424.

24. Stampfer MJ, Willett WC, Colditz GA, Speizer FE, Hennekens CH. A prospective study of past use of oral contraceptive agents and risk of cardiovascular diseases. N Engl J Med 1988;319:1313–1317.

25. Mishell DR Jr. Use of oral contraceptives in women of older reproductive age. Am J Obstet Gynecol 1988;158:1652–1657.

26. van de Carr SW, Kennedy DL, Rosa FW, Anello C, Jones JK. Relationship of oral contraceptive estrogen dose to age. Am J Epidemiol 1983;117:153–159.

27. Wallace RB, Hoover J, Barrett-Connor E, et al. Altered plasma lipid and lipoprotein levels associated with oral contraceptives and oestrogen use. Lancet 1979;2:112–115.

28. Wallace RB, Hoover J, Sandler D, Rifkind BM, Tyroler HA. Altered plasma-lipids associated with oral contraceptive or oestrogen consumption. The Lipid Research Clinic Program. Lancet 1977;2:11–14.

29. Wallace RB, Tamir I, Heiss G, Rifkind BM, Christensen B, Glueck CJ. Plasma lipids, lipoproteins, and blood pressure in female adolescents using oral contraceptives. J Pediatr 1979;95:1055–1059.

30. Rossner SH, Larsson-Cohn U, Carlson LA, Boberg J. Effects of an oral contraceptive agent on plasma lipids, plasma lipoproteins, the intravenous fat tolerance and the post-heparin lipoprotein lipase activity. Acta Med Scand 1971;190:301–305.

31. Arntzenius AC, van Gent CM, van der Voort H, Stegerhoek CI, Styblo K. Reduced high density lipoprotein in women aged 40–41 using oral contraceptives. Lancet 1978;1:1221–1223.

32. Bradley DD, Wingerd J, Petitti DB, Krauss RM, Ramcharan S. Serum high density lipoprotein cholesterol in women using oral contraceptives, estrogens and progestins. N Engl J Med 1978;299:17–20.

33. Wynn V, Niththyananthan R. The effects of progestins in combined oral contraceptives on serum lipids with special reference to high-density lipoproteins. Am J Obstet Gynecol 1982;142:766–772.

34. Krauss RM, Roy S, Mishell DR Jr, Casagrande J, Pike MC. Effects of two low-dose oral contraceptives on serum lipids and lipoproteins: differential changes in high-density lipoprotein subclasses. Am J Obstet Gynecol 1983;145:446–452.

35. Kay CR. Progestogens and arterial disease—evidence from the Royal College of General Practitioners' study. Am J Obstet Gynecol 1982;142:762–765.

36. Meade TW. Risks and mechanisms of cardiovascular events in users of oral contraceptives. Am J Obstet Gynecol 1988;158:1646–1652.

37. Marz W, Gross W, Gahn G, Romberg G, Taubert HD, Kuhl H. A randomized crossover comparison of two low-dose contraceptives: effects on serum lipids and lipoproteins. Am J Obstet Gynecol 1985;153:287–293.

38. Kloosterboer HJ, Van Wayjen RG, Van den Ende A. Comparative effects of monophasic desogestrel plus ethinyloestradiol and triphasic levonorgestrel plus ethinyloestradiol on lipid metabolism. Contraception 1986;34:135–144.

39. van der Vange N, Kloosterboer HJ, Haspels AA. Effects of seven low dose combined oral contraceptives on high density lipoprotein subfractions. Br J Obstet Gynecol 1987;94:559–567.

40. Crook D, Godsland IF, Wynn V. Oral contraceptives and coronary heart disease: modulation of glucose tolerance and plasma lipid risk factors by progestins. Am J Obstet Gynecol 1988;158:1612–1620.

41. Notelovitz M, Feldman EB, Gillespy M, Gudat J. Lipid and lipoprotein changes in women taking low-dose, triphasic oral contraceptives: a controlled, comparative, 12-month clinical trial. Am J Obstet Gynecol 1989;160:1269–1280.

42. Percival-Smith RK, Morrison BJ, Sizto R, Abercrombie B. The effects of triphasic and biphasic oral contraceptive preparations on HDL cholesterol and LDL cholesterol in young women. Contraception 1987;35:179–187.

43. Capitanio GL, Bertolini S, Croce S, de Cecco L. Lipidemic changes induced by two different oral contraceptive formulations. Adv Contracept 1985;1:238–239.

44. Burkman R, Robinson JC, Kruszon-Moran D, Kimball AW, Kwiterovich P, Burford RG. Lipid and lipoprotein changes associated with oral contraceptive use: a randomized clinical trial. Obstet Gynecol 1988;71:33–38.

45. LaRosa JC. The varying effects of progestins on lipid levels and cardiovascular disease. Am J Obstet Gynecol 1988;158:1621–1629.

46. Welch CC, Proudfit WL, Sheldon WC. Coronary arteriographic findings in 1,000 women under age 50. Am J Cardiol 1975; 35:211–215.

47. Ramcharan S, Pellegrin FA, Hoag E. The occurrence and course of hypertensive disease in users and nonusers of oral contraceptive drugs. In: Fregly MJ, Fregly MS (eds): Oral contraceptives and high blood pressure. Gainesville, FL: Dolphin Press, 1974:1–16.

48. Fisch IR, Frank J. Oral contraceptives and blood pressure. JAMA 1977;237:2499–2503.

49. Weir RJ. Blood pressure in women taking oral contraceptives. Am Heart J 1976;92:119–120.

50. Wallace RB, Barrett-Connor E, Criqui M, et al. Alteration in blood pressures associated with combined alcohol and oral contraceptive use—the Lipid Research Clinics Prevalence Study. J Chron Dis 1982;35:251–257.

51. Kaplan NM. Cardiovascular complications of oral contraceptives. Annu Rev Med 1978;29:31–40.

52. Jugdutt BI, Stevens GF, Zacks DJ, Lee SJ, Taylor RF. Myocardial infarction, oral contraception, cigarette smoking, and coronary artery spasm in young women. Am Heart J 1983;106:757–761.

53. Jick H, Dinan B, Rothman KJ. Oral contraceptives and nonfatal myocardial infarction. JAMA 1978;239:1403–1406.

54. Shapiro S, Slone D, Rosenberg L, et al. Oral contraceptive use in relation to myocardial infarction. Lancet 1979;1:743–747.

55. Slone D, Shapiro S, Rosenberg L, et al. Relation of cigarette smoking to myocardial infarction in young women. N Engl J Med 1978;298:1273–1276.

56. Salonen JT. Oral contraceptives, smoking and risk of myocardial infarction in young women. Acta Med Scand 1982;212:141–144.

57. Bush TL, Comstock GW. Smoking and cardiovascular mortality in women. Am J Epidemiol 1983;118:480–488.

58. Becker DM, Myers AH, Sacci M, et al. Smoking behavior and attitudes toward smoking among hospital nurses. Am J Public Health 1986;76:1449–1451.

59. Poller L. Oral contraceptives, blood clotting and thrombosis. Br Med Bull 1978;34:151–156.

60. Leff B, Henriksen RA, Owen WG. Effect of oral contraceptive use on platelet prothrombin converting (platelet factor 3) activity. Thromb Res 1979;15:631–638.

61. Conard J, Samama M, Horellou MH, Zorn JR, Neau C. Antithrombin III and oral contraception with progestagen-only preparation. Lancet 1979;2:471.

62. Bonnar J. Coagulation effects of oral contraception. Am J Obstet Gynecol 1987; 157:1042–1048.

63. Vessey M, Mant D, Smith A, Yeates D. Oral contraceptives and venous thromboembolism: findings in a large prospective study. Br Med J 1986;292:526.

64. Wynn V, Doar JW. Some effects of oral contraceptives on carbohydrate metabolism. Lancet 1969;2:761–766.

65. Wynn V. Effect of duration of low-dose oral contraceptive administration on carbohydrate metabolism. Am J Obstet Gynecol 1982;142:739–746.

66. Spellacy WN. Carbohydrate metabolism during treatment with estrogen, progestogen, and low-dose oral contraceptives. Am J Obstet Gynecol 1982;142:732–734.

67. Shoupe D, Mishell DR. Norplant: subdermal implant system for long-term contraception. Am J Obstet Gynecol 1989;160:1286–1292.

68. Roy S, Mishell DR, Robertson DN, Krauss RM, LaCarra M, Duda MJ. Long term reversible contraception with levonorgestrel-releasing silastic rods. Am J Obstet Gynecol 1984;148:1006–1013.

69. Giudici MC, Artis AK, Webel RR, Alpert MA. Postpartum myocardial infarction treated with percutaneous transluminal coronary angioplasty. Am Heart J 1989;118:614–616.

70. Beary JF, Summer WR, Bulkley BH. Postpartum myocardial infarction: a rare occurrence of uncertain etiology. Am J Cardiol 1979;43:158–161.

71. Punnonen R. The relationship between serum oestradiol levels and serum triglyceride, cholesterol and phospholipid levels

in normal human pregnancy. Br J Obstet Gynaecol 1977;84:838–845.

72. Knopp RH. Cardiovascular effects of endogenous and exogenous sex hormones over a woman's lifetime. Am J Obstet Gynecol 1988;158:1630–1643.

73. Fahraeus L, Larsson-Cohn U, Wallentin L. Plasma lipoproteins including high density lipoprotein subfractions during normal pregnancy. Obstet Gynecol 1985;66:468–472.

74. Desoye G, Schweditsch M, Pfieffer KP, Zechner R, Kostner GH. Correlation of hormones with lipid and lipoprotein levels during normal pregnancy and postpartum. J Clin Endocrinol Metab 1987;64:704–712.

75. Knopp RH, Warth MR, Charles D, et al. Lipoprotein metabolism in pregnancy, fat transport to the fetus, and the effects of diabetes. Biol Neonate 1986;50:297–317.

76. Bengtsson C, Rybo G, Westerberg H. Number of pregnancies, use of oral contraceptives and menopausal age in women with ischaemic heart disease, compared to a population sample of women. Acta Med Scand 1973;549(suppl):75–81.

77. Villar J, Repke J, Markush L, Calvert W, Rhoads G. The measuring of blood pressure during pregnancy. Am J Obstet Gynecol 1989;161:1019–1024.

78. Marcoux S, Brisson J, Fabia J. The effect of cigarette smoking on the risk of preeclampsia and gestational hypertension. Am J Epidemiol 1989;130:950–957.

79. Duffus GM, MacGillivray I. The incidence of pre-eclamptic toxaemia in smokers and non-smokers. Lancet 1968;1:994–995.

80. Lindheimer MD, Katz AI. Hypertension in pregnancy. N Engl J Med 1985;313:675–680.

81. Walsh SW. Pre-eclampsia: an imbalance in placental prostacyclin and thromboxane production. Am J Obstet Gynecol 1985;152:335–340.

82. Hubel CA, Roberts JM, Taylor RN, Musci TJ, Rogers GM, McLaughlin MK. Lipid peroxidation in pregnancy: new perspectives on preeclampsia. Am J Obstet Gynecol 1989;161:1025–1034.

83. Ershoff DH, Mullen PD, Quinn VP. A randomized trial of a serialized self-help smoking cessation program for pregnant women in an HMO. Am J Public Health 1989;79:182–187.

84. Jovanovic-Peterson L, Durak EP, Peterson CM. Randomized trial of diet versus diet plus cardiovascular conditioning on glucose levels in gestational diabetes. Am J Obstet Gynecol 1989;161:415–419.

85. Parisi VM, Salinas J, Stockmar EJ. Fetal vascular responses to maternal nicardipine administration in the hypertensive ewe. Am j Obstet Gynecol 1989;161:1035–1039.

86. Witteman JC, Grobbee DE, Kok FJ, et al. Increased risk of atherosclerosis in women after the menopause. Br Med J 1989;298:642–644.

87. Snowdon DA, Kane RL, Beeson WL. Is early natural menopause a biologic marker of health and aging? Am J Public Health 1989;79:709–714.

88. Jick H, Porter J, Morrison AS. Relation between smoking and age of natural menopause. Lancet 1977;1:1354–1355.

89. MacMahon B, Trichopoulos D, Cole P, Brown J. Cigarette smoking and urinary estrogens. N Engl J Med 1982;307:1062–1065.

90. Baron JA. Smoking and estrogen-related disease. Am J Epidemiol 1984;119:9–22.

91. Willet W, Stampfer MJ, Bain C, et al. Cigarette smoking, relative weight, and menopause. Am J Epidemiol 1983;117:651–658.

92. Robinson RW, Cohen WD, Higano N. Estrogen replacement therapy in women with coronary atherosclerosis. Ann Intern Med 1958;48:95–101.

93. Oliver MF, Boyd GS. Effect of bilateral ovariectomy on coronary artery disease and serum lipid levels. Lancet 1959;2:690–694.

94. Ritterband AB, Jaffe IA, Densen PM, Magagna JF, Reed E. Gonadal function and the development of coronary heart disease. Circulation 1963;27:237–251.

95. Manchester JH, Herman MV, Gorlin R. Premenopausal castration and documented coronary atherosclerosis. Am J Cardiol 1971;28:33–37.

96. Colditz GA, Willett WC, Stampfer MJ, Rosner B, Speizer FE, Hennekens CH. Menopause and the risk of coronary heart disease in women. N Engl J Med 1987;316:1105–1110.

97. Bengtsson C, Lapidus L, Lindquist O. Association between menopause and risk factors for ischaemic heart disease. In: Oliver MF, Vedin A, Wilhelmsson C (eds): Myocardial infarction in women. Edinburgh: Churchill Livingstone; 1986:93–100.

98. Matthews KA, Meilahn E, Kuller LH, Kelsey SF, Caggiula AW, Wing RR. Menopause and risk factors for coronary heart disease. N Engl J Med 1989;321:641–646.

99. Hallberg L, Svanborg A. Cholesterol, phospholipids, and triglycerides in plasma in 50-year old women: influence of menopause, body weight, skinfold thickness, weight gain, and diet in a random population sample. Acta Med Scand 1967;181:185–194.

100. Paterson ME, Sturdee DW, Moore B, Whitehead TP. The effect of menopausal status and sequential mestranol and norethisterone on serum cholesterol, triglyceride and electrophoretic lipoprotein patterns. Br J Obstet Gynecol 1979;86:810–815.

101. Baird DD, Tyroler HA, Heiss G, Chambless LE, Hames CG. Menopausal change in serum cholesterol: black/white differences in Evans County, Georgia. Am J Epidemiol 1985;122:982–993.

102. Shibata H, Matsuzaki T, Hatano S. Relationship of relevant factors of atherosclerosis to menopause in Japanese women. Am J Epidemiol 1979;109:420–424.

103. Hamman RF, Bennett PH, Miller M. The effect of menopause on serum cholesterol in American (Pima) Indian women. Am J Epidemiol 1975;102:164–169.

104. Adams MR, Kaplan JR, Clarkson TB, Koritnik DR. Ovariectomy, social status, and atherosclerosis in cynomolgus monkeys. Arteriosclerosis 1985;5:192–200.

105. Haffner SM, Katz MS, Stern MP, Dunn JF. Association of decreased sex hormone binding globulin and cardiovascular risk factors. Arteriosclerosis 1989;9:136–143.

106. Masarei JR, Armstrong BK, Skinner MW, et al. HDL-cholesterol and sex hormone status. Lancet 1980;1:208.

107. Ottosson UB, Johannson BG, von Schoultz B. Subfractions of high-density lipoprotein cholesterol during estrogen replacement therapy: a comparison between progestogens and natural progesterone. Am J Obstet Gynecol 1985;151:746–750.

108. Padwick ML, Pryse-Davies J, Whitehead MI. A simple method for determining the optimal dosage of progestin in postmenopausal women receiving estrogens. N Engl J Med 1986;315:930–934.

109. Whitehead M, Lobo RA. Progestagen use in postmenopausal women. Lancet 1988;2:1243–1244.

110. Colditz GA, Stampfer MJ, Willett WC, Rosner B, Speizer FE, Hennekens CH. A prospective study of parental history of myocardial infarction and coronary heart disease in women. Am J Epidemiol 1986;123:48–58.

111. Barrett-Connor E, Khaw KT. Family history of heart attack as an independent predictor of death due to cardiovascular disease. Circulation 1984;69:1065–1069.

112. Khaw KT, Barrett-Connor E. Family history of stroke as an independent predictor of ischemic heart disease in men and stroke in women. Am J Epidemiol 1986;123:59–66.

113. Austin MA, King MC, Bawol RD, Hulley SB, Friedman GD. Risk factors for coronary heart disease in adult female twins. Genetic heritability and shared environmental influences. Am J Epidemiol 1987;125:308–318.

114. Hjortland MC, McNamara PM, Kannel WB. Some atherogenic concomitants of menopause: the Framingham study. Am J Epidemiol 1976;103:304–311.

115. Lindquist O, Bengtsson C. Serum lipids, arterial blood pressure and body weight in relation to the menopause: results from a population study of women in Goteborg, Sweden. Scand J Clin Lab Invest 1980;40:629–636.

116. Sigurdsson JA, Bengtsson C, Lapidus L, Lindquist O, Rafnsson V. Morbidity and mortality in relation to blood pressure and antihypertensive treatment. A 12-year follow-up study of a populations sample of Swedish women. Acta Med Scand 1984;215:313–322.

117. Barrett-Connor E, Wingard DL. Sex differential in ischemic heart disease mortality in diabetics: a prospective population-based study. Am J Epidemiol 1983;118:489–496.

118. Diczfalusy F. Menopause, developing countries and the 21st century. Acta Obstet Gynecol Scand Suppl 1986;134:45–57.

119. Statistical Abstract of the United States, ed 108. Washington, DC: US Bureau of the Census, 1987.

120. Ferguson KJ, Hoegh C, Johnson S. Estrogen replacement therapy. A survey of women's knowledge and attitudes. Arch Intern Med 1989;149:133–136.

121. Ziel HK, Finkle WD. Increased risk of endometrial carcinoma among users of conjugated estrogens. N Engl J Med 1975;293:1167–1170.

122. Mack TM, Pike MC, Henderson BE, et al. Estrogens and endometrial cancer in a retirement community. N Engl J Med 1976;294:1262–1267.

123. Hemminki E, Kennedy DL, Baum C, McKinlay SM. Prescribing of noncontraceptive estrogens and progestins in the United States, 1974–86. Am J Public Health 1988;78:1478–1481.

124. Higano N, Robinson RW, Cohen WD. Increased incidence of cardiovascular disease in castrated women. Two-year followup studies. N Engl J Med 1963;268:1123–1125.

125. Petitti DB, Perlman JA, Sidney S. Postmenopausal estrogen use and heart disease. N Engl J Med 1986;315:131–132.

126. Bush TL, Barrett-Connor E, Cowan LD, et al. Cardiovascular mortality and non-contraceptive use of estrogen in women: results from the Lipid Research Clinics Program Follow-up Study. Circulation 1987;75:1102–1109.

127. Burch JC, Byrd BF Jr, Vaughn WK. The effects of long-term estrogen on hysterectomized women. Am J Obstet Gynecol 1974;118:778–782.

128. MacMahon B. Cardiovascular disease and noncontraceptive oestrogen therapy. In: Oliver MF (ed): Coronary heart disease in young women. New York: Churchill Livingstone, 1978:197–207.

129. Nachtigall LE, Nachtigall RH, Nachtigall RD, Beckman EM. Estrogen replacement therapy. II. A prospective study in the relationship to carcinoma and cardiovascular and metabolic problems. Obstet Gynecol 1979;54:74–79.

130. Hammond CB, Jelovsek FR, Lee KL, Creasman WT, Parker RT. Effects of long term estrogen replacement therapy. I. Metabolic. Am J Obstet Gynecol 1979;133:525–536.

131. Lafferty FW, Helmuth DO. Postmenopausal estrogen replacement: the prevention of osteoporosis and systemic effects. Maturitas 1985;7:147–159.

132. Ross RK, Paganini-Hill A, Mack TM, Henderson BE. Cardiovascular benefits of estrogen replacement therapy. Am J Obstet Gynecol 1989;160:1301–1306.

133. Rosenberg L, Armstrong B, Jick H. Myocardial infarction and estrogen therapy in postmenopausal women. N Engl J Med 1976;294:1256–1259.

134. Talbott E, Kuller LH, Detre K. Biologic and psychosocial risk factors of sudden death from coronary disease in white women. Am J Cardiol 1977;39:858–864.

135. Pfeffer RI, Whipper GH, Kurosaki TT, Chapman JM. Coronary risk and estrogen use in postmenopausal women. Am J Epidemiol 1978;107:479–487.

136. Adam S, Williams V, Vessey MP. Cardiovascular disease and hormone replacement treatment: a pilot case-control study. Br Med J 1981;282:1277–1278.

137. Ross RK, Paganini-Hill A, Mack TM, Arthur M, Henderson BE. Menopausal estrogen therapy and protection from death from ischaemic heart disease. Lancet 1981;1:858–860.

138. Szklo M, Tonascia J, Gordis L, Bloom I. Estrogen use and myocardial infarction risk: a case-control study. Prev Med 1984;13:510–516.

139. Ernster VL, Bush TL, Huggins GR, Hulka BS, Kelsey JL, Schottenfeld D. Benefits and risk of menopausal estrogen and/or progestin hormone use. Prev Med 1988;17:201–223.

140. Hillner BE, Hollenberg JP, Pauker SG. Postmenopausal estrogens in the prevention of osteoporosis. Benefit virtually without risk if cardiovascular effects are considered. Am J Med 1986;80:1115–1127.

141. Eaker ED, Castelli WP. Coronary heart disease and its risk factors among women in the Framingham Study. In: Eaker ED, Packard B, Wenger NK, Clarkson TB, Tyroler HH (eds): Coronary heart disease in women. New York: Haymarket, 1987:122–130.

142. Tikkanen MJ, Nikkila EA, Vartiainen E. Natural oestrogen as an effective treat-

ment for type II hyperlipoproteinemia in post-menopausal women. Lancet 1978;2:490–491.

143. Fahraeus L, Wallentin L. High-density lipoprotein subfractions during oral and cutaneous administration of 17-estradiol to menopausal women. J Clin Endocrinol Metab 1983;56:797–801.

144. Barrett-Connor E, Wingard DL, Criqui MH. Postmenopausal estrogen use and heart disease risk factors in the 1980s. JAMA 1989;261:2095–2100.

145. Hirvonen E, Malkonen M, Manninen V. Effects of different progestogens on lipoproteins during postmenopausal replacement therapy. N Engl J Med 1981;304:560–563.

146. Farish E, Fletcher CD, Hart DM. The effects of conjugated equine oestrogens with and without a cyclical progestogen on lipoproteins and HDL subfractions in post-menopausal women. Acta Endocrinol 1986;113:123–127.

147. Krauss RM, Perlman JA, Ray R, Petitti D. Effects of estrogen dose and smoking on lipid and lipoprotein levels in postmenopausal women. Am J Obstet Gynecol 1988;158:1606–1611.

148. Chetkowski RJ, Meldrum DR, Steingold KA, et al. Biologic effects of transdermal estradiol. N Engl J Med 1986;314:1615–1620.

149. Davidson DM. Cardiovascular risk reduction in postmenopausal women. J Nutr Elderly 1986;5(4):3–10.

150. Tikkanen MJ, Kussi T, Vartiainen N, Nikilla E. Treatment of postmenopausal hypercholesterolemia with estradiol. Acta Obstet Gynecol Scand 1979;88:83–88.

151. Pfeffer RI, Kurosaki TT, Charlton SK. Estrogen use and blood pressure in later life. Am J Epidemiol 1979;110:469–478.

152. Barrett-Connor E, Brown V, Turner J, et al. Heart disease risk factors and hormone use in postmenopausal women. JAMA 1978;241:2167–2169.

153. Lind T, Cameron FC, Hunter FM, et al. A prospective controlled trial of six forms of hormone replacement therapy given to post-menopausal women. Br J Obstet Gynaecol 1979;86:(Suppl 3):1–29.

154. Wren BG, Routledge DA. Blood pressure changes. Oestrogens in climacteric women. Med J Austral 1981;2:528–531.

155. Varma TR, Patel RH, Rosenberg D. Effect of hormone replacement therapy on anti-thrombin III activity in postmenopausal women. Int J Gynaecol Obstet 1986;24:69–73.

156. Adams MR, Kaplan JR, Koritnik PR, Clarkson TB. Pregnancy associated inhibition of coronary artery atherosclerosis in monkeys. Arteriosclerosis 1987;7:378–384.

157. Shapiro S, Kelly JP, Rosenberg L, et al. Risk of localized and widespread endometrial cancer in relation to recent and discontinued use of conjugated estrogens. N Engl J Med 1985;313:969–972.

158. Horwitz RI, Feinstein AR. Estrogens and endometrial cancer. Am J Med 1986;81:503–507.

159. Whitehead MI, Townsend PT, Pryse-Davies J, et al. Effects of estrogens and progestins on the biochemistry and morphology of the postmenopausal endometrium. N Engl J Med 1981;305:1599–1605.

160. Bergkvist L, Adami HO, Persson I, Hoover R, Schairer C. The risk of breast cancer after estrogen and estrogen-progestin replacement. N Engl J Med 1989;321:293–297.

161. Riis B, Thomsen K, Christiansen C. Does calcium supplementation prevent postmenopausal bone loss? N Engl J Med 1987;316:173–177.

162. Thorneycroft IH. The role of estrogen replacement therapy in the prevention of osteoporosis. Am J Obstet Gynecol 1989;160:1306–1310.

163. Lindsay R, Hart DM, Clark DM. The minimum effective dose of estrogen for prevention of postmenopausal bone loss. Obstet Gynecol 1984;63:759–763.

164. Kiel DP, Felson DT, Anderson JJ, Wilson PW, Moskowitz MA. Hip fracture and the use of estrogens in postmenopausal women. N Engl J Med 1987;317:1169–1174.

165. Coronary Drug Project Research Group. The Coronary Drug Project: findings leading to discontinuation of the 2.5 mg/day estrogen group. JAMA 1973;226:652–657.

166. Blackard CE, Doe RP, Mellinger GT, Byar DP. Incidence of cardiovascular disease and death in patients receiving diethylstilbesterol for carcinoma of the prostate. Cancer 1970;26:249–256.

167. Byar DP. The Veterans Administration Cooperative Urological Group's studies of cancer of the prostate. Cancer 1973;32:1126–1130.

168. Phillips GB. Evidence for hyperoestrogenaemia as a risk factor for myocardial infarction in men. Lancet 1976;2:14–18.

169. Phillips GB, Castelli WP, Abbott RD, McNamara PM. Association of hyperestrogenemia and coronary heart disease in men in the Framingham cohort. Am J Med 1983;74:863–869.

170. Entrican JH, Beach C, Carroll D, Klopper A, Mackie M, Douglas AS. Raised plasma oestradiol and estrone levels in young survivors of myocardial infarction. Lancet 1978;2:487–490.

171. Heller RF, Jacobs HS, Vermeulen A, Deslypere JP: Androgens, oestrogens, and coronary heart disease. Br Med J 1981;282:438–439.

172. Taggart H, Sheridan B, Stout RW. Sex hormone levels in younger male stroke survivors. Atherosclerosis 1980;35:123–125.

173. Nordoy A, Aakvaag A, Thelle D: Sex hormones and high density lipoproteins in healthy males. Atherosclerosis 1979;34:431–436.

174. Rosenberg L, Schwingl PJ, Kaufman DW, Helmrich SP, Palmer JR, Shapiro S. The risk of myocardial infarction 10 or more years after vasectomy in men under 55 years of age. Am J Epidemiol 1986;123:1049–1056.

175. Barrett-Connor E, Khaw KT, Yen SS. A prospective study of dehydroepiandrosterone sulfate, mortality, and cardiovascular disease. N Engl J Med 1986;315:1519–1524.

176. Barrett-Connor E, Khaw KT. Absence of an inverse relation of dehydroepiandrosterone sulfate with cardiovascular mortality in postmenopausal women. N Engl J Med 1987;317:711.

177. Barrett-Connor E, Khaw KT. Endogenous sex hormones and cardiovascular disease in men. A prospective population-based study. Circulation 1988;78:539–545.

178. Hurley BF, Seals DR, Hagberg JM, et al. High-density-lipoprotein cholesterol in bodybuilders v powerlifters. JAMA 1984;252:507–513.

179. Thompson PD, Cullinane EM, Sady SP, et al. Contrasting effects of testosterone and stanozol on serum lipoprotein levels. JAMA 1989;261:1165–1168.

12

hematologic considerations

In the normal coronary artery, endo-thelial integrity allows for smooth laminar flow of blood. With the development of atherosclerotic plaques, which are often eccentric, flow becomes turbulent. This can lead to further endothelial damage and progression of coronary artery narrowing. When flow is sufficiently impaired by plaque or spasm, thrombosis is more likely.

These processes are mediated by the components of the coagulation cascade, in-cluding fibrinogen, as well as platelet and prostaglandin factors. These concepts, along with current interventions, are dis-cussed in this chapter.

RHEOLOGY

Optimal myocardial metabolism de-pends upon adequate extraction of oxygen from coronary artery blood flow. Along with arterial and arteriolar caliber and pressures, physical characteristics of the blood, such as hematocrit, hemoglobin type, and viscosity, are important deter-minants of oxygen delivery to myocardial tissue.

Cardiac output can be affected at both ends of the hematocrit spectrum, ane-mia and polycythemia. In severe anemia, blood viscosity is lowered, while heart rate and cardiac output increase, raising the myocardial oxygen demand. When anemia is associated with hematologic abnormali-ties that increase viscosity, there may be no change in cardiac output. Cases of myo-cardial infarction secondary to sickle-cell anemia have been reported (1). Polycythe-mia, which is more common in cigarette smokers, increases plasma viscosity and may result in sludging of myocardial blood flow (2). In a study of 6151 urban Puerto Rican men, the risk of myocardial infarc-tion and coronary heart disease risk was more than doubled in men with hemato-crits of 50 or greater, compared to those with hematocrits less than 42. This rela-tionship remained significant after adjust-ment for the standard CAD risk indicators, such as smoking, hypertension, and body weight (3).

In patients with chronic, stable an-gina, Rainer and colleagues noted several rheologic abnormalities compared with controls. These included increased levels of hematocrit, plasma viscosity, whole blood viscosity, red cell aggregation, and fi-brinogen concentration (4). Neumann and colleagues noted even higher values in per-sons with unstable angina (5).

Persons with dyslipidemias also dis-play increased plasma viscosity. This ef-fect is most marked in hypertriglyceridemia, but is significantly present in persons with elevated blood total cholesterol as well. Habitual exercise is associated with decreased plasma viscosity, presumably through reduced fibrinogen levels. Additionally, fibrinogen also acts adversely on coronary blood flow through its role in coagulation (6).

FIBRINOGEN AND FIBRINOLYSIS

During the tenth biennial examination of the Framingham Study subjects, fibrinogen was measured. Twelve years later, investigators found a positive correlation of baseline fibrinogen levels with new cases of coronary heart disease and stroke. They also noted significant correlations of fibrinogen level with hypertension, glucose intolerance, and cigarette smoking in both genders and with hematocrit in women, but the correlation of fibrinogen and CAD events was independent of these standard risk indicators (7). In the Northwick Park Heart Study, Meade and colleagues noted a strong correlation of both factor VII and fibrinogen with the incidence of ischemic heart disease, particularly during the first five years of follow-up. Risk of death was doubled for men in the upper tertile of fibrinogen concentration; nonfatal MIs in that tertile were more than three times those in the lowest tertile (8). The association of fibrinogen level with MI and stroke incidence was also noted in the Göteborg Study. The association with stroke persisted even after blood pressure, serum total cholesterol, and smoking were taken into account (9).

Hamsten et al. studied plasma fibrinogen concentration in 85 families containing a proband with early MI and 85 control families. More than half of the variance in fibrinogen levels was attributable to genetic heritability (10).

Fibrinogen is converted to fibrin, which is often found within atherosclerotic plaque. Fibrin may stimulate cell proliferation, and fibrin degradation products can stimulate mitogenesis and collagen synthesis. Fibrin may also be involved in the binding of LDL and the accumulation of lipid in advanced plaques (11).

Fibrin is cleaved by plasmin in the fibrinolytic sequence. Francis and co-workers studied 99 CAD patients, noting increased fibrinogen levels and higher levels of plasminogen-activator inhibitor, which impaired fibrinolysis in these patients (12). Hamsten and colleagues found that increased levels of plasminogen activator inhibitor was associated with the risk of reinfarction in young subjects (13). Williams et al. demonstrated enhanced fibrinolytic activity at rest and after stimulation by venous occlusion after a 10-week physical conditioning program (14). Meade and colleagues have demonstrated lower concentrations of fibrinogen and increased fibrinolytic activity in alcohol consumers (15). It has also been shown that fibrinolytic activity appears to be lower on Fridays, which correlated with an increased incidence of myocardial infarction on Saturdays, Sundays, and Mondays (16).

PLATELETS AND PROSTAGLANDINS

In addition to rheologic and thrombotic considerations, CAD risk is influenced by platelets and prostaglandins. Recent developments have led to consideration of platelet-active agents at all levels of CAD and even in its primary prevention.

Platelet and Prostaglandin Physiology

Figure 12.1 illustrates current thinking about the relationship of platelets, prostaglandins, and atherosclerosis. Tra-

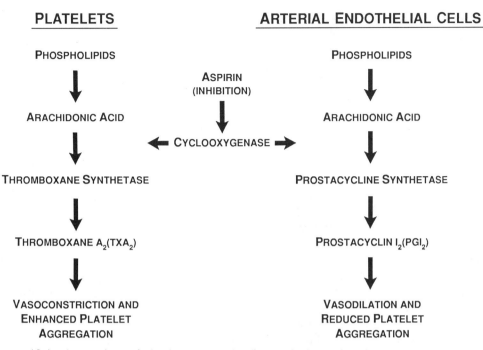

Figure 12.1. Interactions of platelets, prostaglandins, and atherosclerosis.

ditional risk indicators such as hypertension, smoking, diabetes, and hyperbetalipoproteinemia (elevated LDL-cholesterol) may result in endothelial damage, increased platelet adherence, and increased susceptibility to platelet activation. The latter event produces thromboxane $A_2(TXA_2)$, which can lead to arterial spasm and induces platelet aggregation. Prostacyclin $I_2(PGI_2)$ induces vasodilation and inhibits platelet aggregation, making it desirable to find an agent and dose that could differentially affect one but not the other.

Aspirin (ASA) irreversibly inhibits cyclooxygenase, through which cyclic endoperoxides (*a*) convert arachidonic acid to TXA_2 in the platelet, and (*b*) convert arachidonic acid to PGI_2 in the vessel wall. After a single 325-mg aspirin, platelet TXA_2 is completely inhibited for 48 hours. After 5 to 6 days, approximately 50% of platelets function normally. While an ASA

dose of 1000 mg/day will completely inhibit both TXA_2 synthesis and PGI_2 synthesis, it is currently under investigation whether a dose much less than 325 mg/day will have a differential effect on TXA_2 and PGI_2 (17).

Investigators in a study on Myocardial Infarction Limitation (MILIS) noted a preponderance of acute MIs in the morning hours between 8 and 11, coinciding with increased platelet aggregation responses, especially after assuming the upright posture (18).

Primary Prevention of CAD

The Physicians' Health Study followed 22,071 male physicians in the United States for an average of 5 years after randomization to 325 mg ASA or placebo tablet every other day. There was a 44% reduction in MI risk in the ASA group, but there was no reduction in mortality from all cardiovascular causes and a doubling of risk for hemorrhagic stroke. The MI risk reduction was present only in men 50 years of age and older, but appeared at all levels of blood total cholesterol. Conclusions were limited by the cardiovascular event rate among physician participants, which was only 15% of that expected in a general population of white men of the same age (19).

A similar, but smaller trial was conducted in British male physicians, using 500 mg ASA daily, and a single blind design. Participants had a lower compliance rate than in the US study. There was no appreciable difference between ASA and placebo groups in MI incidence, but nonfatal cerebral transient ischemic attacks were more frequent in the ASA group (20).

Fuster and colleagues, in an editorial accompanying the final report of the American trial, conclude that aspirin appears to be beneficial in the prevention of a first MI in men over 50, particularly those with other CAD risk indicators that are uncontrolled. They discourage its use in patients with diabetic retinopathy or poorly controlled hypertension (21). One might add the relative contraindication of a family history of hemorrhagic stroke as well.

Treatment of Unstable Angina Pectoris

Recent arteriographic evidence suggests that platelet activation and thrombin generation may result in thrombi, which partly occlude arteries in unstable angina pectoris (22–24). Three major trials have examined the effectiveness of aspirin in improving the prognosis in persons with unstable angina (Table 12.1.)

After a 12-month follow-up of 1266 men in the Veterans Administration Cooperative Study, those taking 324 mg ASA daily had a lower incidence of each cardiovascular event outcome measure than the control group. There were 52% fewer nonfatal MIs, 83% fewer fatal MIs, and a 40% reduction in other deaths, resulting in a 52% lower rate of persons experiencing death or nonfatal MI (25). In the Canadian Multicenter Trial, 406 men and 149 women admitted to a coronary care unit were randomized to aspirin (325 q.i.d.), sulfinpyrazone (200 mg q.i.d.), both, or neither. After a mean follow-up of 19 months, there was no significant difference in nonfatal MI rates, but fatal MIs occurred less than half as often in those taking aspirin. Sulfinpyrazone had no effect (26). Another

Table 12.1. Antiplatelet Agents in Unstable Angina Pectoris

Study	Year	Drug/Dose (mg/day)	n	NFMI[a]	FMI	Other Death	All Death	Death or NFMI
VA Coop (25)	1983	ASA 325	625	21	1	9	10	31
		Placebo	641	44	6	15	21	65
Canadian Multicenter (26)	1985	ASA 1300	139	9	7	2	9	18
		Sulf 800	140	7	14	1	15	22
		ASA + Sulf	137	8	5	2	7	15
		Placebo	139	7	13	0	13	20
Theroux (27)	1988	ASA*	121	4	0	0	0	4
		Heparin#	118	1	0	0	0	1
		ASA + Hep#	122	2	0	0	0	2
		Placebo	118	12	2	0	0	14

[a]Abbreviations: NFMI = nonfatal myocardial infarction, FMI = fatal MI, ASA = aspirin, Sulf = sulfinpyrazone, Hep = heparin,
* = 650 mg ASA immediately then daily, # = 5000 units heparin as bolus, then 1000 units per hour infusion.

Canadian team enrolled 341 men and 138 women in a double-blind trial, randomizing their participants to aspirin, heparin, both, or neither on admission for unstable angina. Aspirin was given 650 mg stat and 325 mg b.i.d.; sulfinpyrazone was administered 5000 units stat and 1000 units per hour thereafter. After a mean of 6 days, all treatment groups had significantly better outcomes than the placebo group (Table 12.1). Angina was refractory in 20 ASA patients, 10 heparin patients, 13 combined-treatment subjects, and in 27 of the placebo group (27).

Treatment of Acute MI

Aspirin is also useful in the setting of an acute MI. During the Second International Study of Infarct Survival (ISIS-2), streptokinase, aspirin, both, or neither, were administered to 17,187 individuals entering the hospital with suspected acute

MI. After five weeks of follow-up, those receiving aspirin had a 9.4% mortality compared to 11.8% in the placebo group, a 23% reduction. Streptokinase alone resulted in a similar reduction; together the two agents produced an 8.0% mortality. Aspirin significantly reduced reinfarction (1.0% vs. 2.0%) and nonfatal stroke (0.3% vs. 0.6%) without a significant increase in cerebral hemorrhage or other bleeding requiring transfusion. After 15 months of follow-up, the significant differences in vascular and all-cause mortality persisted (28).

Long-term Treatment after Myocardial Infarction

Several large trials have tested aspirin and other platelet-active agents on cardiovascular morbidity and mortality during the months following MI (Table 12.2). Seven of the eight studies listed (29–36)

Table 12.2.   Antiplatelet Trials after Myocardial Infarction

Study (Mean F/U)[a]	Year	Drug/Dose (mg/day)	n	NFMI	Cardiac Death	Other Death	All Death	Death or NFMI
So Wales I	1974	ASA 300	566	—	—	—	—	—
(12 mos) (29)		Placebo	560	—	—	—	—	
Cor Drug	1976	ASA 972	727	3.8	5.6	0.4	6.0	9.9
Project		Placebo	744	4.3	8.1	0.5	8.6	12.9
(22 mos) (30)								
So Wales II	1979	ASA 900	832	3.7	—	—	12.2	16.0
(12 mos) (31)		Placebo	850	7.4	—	—	14.8	22.2
Austro-German	1980	ASA 1500	231	4.8	5.6	6.1	11.7	16.4
(24 mos) (32)		Placebo	215	7.0	10.2	4.7	14.9	21.9
AMIS	1980	ASA 1000	2267	5.4	8.7	2.1	10.8	16.2
(38 mos) (33)		Placebo	2257	6.8	8.0	1.7	9.7	16.5
PARIS I	1980	ASA 972	810	6.9	9.1	1.3	10.5	17.4
(41 mos) (34)		ASA + DP	810	7.9	9.0	1.7	10.7	18.6
		Placebo	406	9.9	11.1	1.7	12.8	22.7
Anturane	1980	Sulf 800	580	—	7.4	0.2	7.6	—
Reinfarction		Placebo	563	—	11.1	0.0	11.0	—
(24 mos) (35)								
PARIS II	1986	DP + ASA 972	1563	4.5	4.9	2.2	7.1	9.0
(23 mos) (36)		Placebo	1563	7.1	5.2	2.1	7.3	11.8

[a]Abbreviations: F/U = follow-up; NFMI = nonfatal myocardial infarction; ASA = aspirin; DP = dipyridamole; Sulf = sulfinpyrazone.

showed all-cause mortality was reduced from 3 to 30% during follow-up periods from 12 to 41 months. Because time from MI to study entry varied as well as study protocol differences existed, the mortality reduction was not significant in any of the seven individual trials. However, a metaanalysis did show statistical significance when data from these trials were pooled (37). In the Aspirin Myocardial Infarction Study, overall mortality was not decreased, but the incidence of nonfatal MI was significantly lower in the aspirin group (33).

Treatment after Coronary Angioplasty

Successful angioplasty produces a controlled injury of the intima, media, and adventitia of the coronary artery segment dilated. Platelet aggregation at the site of the endothelial injury results in growth-factor production, leading to proliferation of smooth-muscle cells. This neointimal proliferation and subsequent thrombus formation can be reduced by pretreatment with antiplatelet agents (38). Aspirin in doses ranging from 65 to 975 mg/day is sometimes combined with either dipyridamole or sulfinpyrazone; such treatment reduces acute vessel closure from 10% (when untreated) to 2%. In contrast, most trials of these medications have failed to show improvement in long-term patency of the dilated artery segments (39). Mehta and Conti speculate that this failure may reflect the intense platelet deposition and platelet-vessel wall interactions that occur after angioplasty (40).

Dehmer et al. tested the efficacy of adding an omega-3 fatty acid dietary supplement consisting of 18 capsules (3.2 g of eicosapentanoic acid and 2.2 g of docoshex-anoic acid) daily for the week before and six months after angioplasty in 82 men. Subjects received this or placebo in addition to a regimen of 325 mg ASA and di-

pyridamole, 75 mg t.i.d. Those randomized to the n-3 fatty acid group had a 77% lower rate of restenosis (41).

Treatment after Coronary Artery Bypass Surgery

Mayo Clinic investigators reported in 1984 improvement in short- and long-term vein graft patency after (*a*) dipyridamole (75 mg t.i.d.) started two days before surgery, given on the morning of, and one hour after surgery, and (*b*) aspirin (325 mg t.i.d.), begun seven hours after surgery (42). Subsequent studies of that combination of drugs or aspirin alone (as low as 100 mg/day) (43) yielded improved graft patency (typically 90% patency versus 75% with placebo) (40).

SUMMARY

Hematologic considerations in the prevention of coronary artery disease include rheology, fibrinogen, fibrinolysis, prostaglandin, and platelet physiology (44, 45). Atherosclerotic plaque produces turbulent flow and raises the hematocrit, which increases plasma viscosity.

Impaired fibrinolysis is seen in CAD, increases the risk of reinfarction, and can be improved with regular, vigorous exercise. Aspirin can decrease platelet aggregability and has been successfully tested in the primary prevention of CAD, the acute treatment of unstable angina pectoris and myocardial infarction, and in long-term treatment after coronary angioplasty and coronary artery bypass surgery (46).

REFERENCES

1. Martin CR, Cobb C, Tatter D, Johnson C, Haywood LJ. Acute myocardial infarction in sickle cell anemia. Arch Intern Med 1983;143:830–831.

2. Baker IA, Sweetnam PM, Yarnell JW, Bainton D, Elwood PC. Haemostatic and other risk factors for ischaemic heart disease and so-

cial class: evidence from the Caerphilly and Speedwell Studies. Int J Epidemiol 1988;17:759-765.

3. Sorlie PD, Garcia-Palmieri MR, Costas R Jr, Havlik RJ. Hematocrit and risk of coronary heart disease: the Puerto Rican Heart Health Program. Am Heart J 1981;101:456-461.

4. Rainer C, Kawanishi DT, Chandraratna AN, et al. Changes in blood rheology in patients with stable angina pectoris as a result of coronary artery disease. Circulation 1987;76:15-20.

5. Neumann FJ, Tillmanns H, Roebruck P, Zimmerman R, Haupt HM, Kubler W. Haemorrheological abnormalities in unstable angina pectoris: a relation independent of risk factor profile and angiographic severity. Br Heart J 1989;62:421-428.

6. Letcher RL, Pickering TG, Chien S, Laragh JH. Effects of exercise on plasma viscosity in athletes and sedentary normal subjects. Clin Cardiol 1981;4:172-179.

7. Kannel WB, Wolf PA, Castelli WP, D'Agostino RB. Fibrinogen and risk of cardiovascular disease. JAMA 1987;258:1183-1186.

8. Meade TW, Mellows S, Brozovic M, Miller GJ, Cakrabarti RR, North WR, et al. Haemostatic function and ischemic heart disease: principal results of the Northwich Park Heart Study. Lancet 1986;2:533-537.

9. Wilhelmsen L, Svardsudd K, Korsan-Bengtsen K, et al. Fibrinogen as a risk factor for stroke and myocardial infarction. N Engl J Med 1984;311:501-505.

10. Hamsten A, Iselius L, de Faire U, Blomback M. Genetic and cultural inheritance of plasma fibrinogen concentration. Lancet 1987;2:988-991.

11. Smith EB. Fibrinogen, fibrin and fibrin degradation products in relation to atherosclerosis. Clin Haemotol 1986;15:355-370.

12. Francis RB Jr, Kawanishi D, Baruch T, Mahrer P, Rahimtoola S, Feinstein DI. Impaired fibrinolysis in coronary artery disease. Am Heart J 1988;115:776-780.

13. Hamsten A, de Faire U, Walldius G, et al. Plasminogen activator inhibitor in the blood of patients with coronary artery disease. Lancet 1987;2:3-9.

14. Williams RS, Logue EE, Lewis JL, et al. Physical conditioning augments the fibrinolytic response to venous occlusion in healthy adults. N Engl J Med 1980;302:987-991.

15. Meade TW, Chakrabarti R, Haines AP, North WR, Stirling Y. Characteristics affecting fibrinolytic activity and plasma fibrinogen concentrations. Br Med J 1979;1:153-156.

16. Imeson JD, Meade TW, Stewart GM. Day-by-day variation in fibrinolytic activity and in mortality from ischemic heart disease. Int J Epidemiol 1987;16:626-627.

17. Hirsh J, Salzman EW, Harker L, et al. Aspirin and other platelet active drugs. Relationship among dose, effectiveness and side effects. Chest 1989;95:(suppl):128-188.

18. Anonymous. Diurnal variation in platelet aggregation responses. Lancet 1988; 2:1405-1406.

19. The Steering Committee of the Physicians' Health Study and Research Group. Final report on the aspirin component of the ongoing Physicians' Health Study. N Engl J Med 1989;321:129-135.

20. Peto R, Gray R, Collins R, et al. Randomised trial of prophylactic daily aspirin in British male doctors. Br Med J 1988;296:313-316.

21. Fuster V, Cohen M, Halperin J. Aspirin in the prevention of coronary artery disease. N Engl J Med 1989;321:183-185.

22. Ambrose JA, Hjemdahl-Monsen CE. Arteriographic anatomy and mechanisms of myocardial ischemia in unstable angina. J Am Coll Cardiol 1987;9:1397-1402.

23. Kruskal JB, Commerford PJ, Franks JJ, Kirsch RE. Fibrin and fibrinogen-related antigens in patients with stable and unstable coronary artery disease. N Engl J Med 1987;317:1361-1365.

24. Fitzgerald DJ, Roy L, Catella F, FitzGerald GA. Platelet activation in unstable coronary disease. N Engl J Med 1986;315:983-989.

25. Lewis HD, Davids JW, Archibald DG, et al. Protective effects of aspirin against acute myocardial infarction and death in men with unstable angina. N Engl J Med 1983;309:396-403.

26. Cairns JA, Gent M, Singer J, et al. Aspirin, sulfinpyrazone or both in unstable angina. Results of a Canadian Multicenter Trial. N Engl J Med 1985;313:1369-1375.

27. Theroux P, Quimet H, McCans J. Aspirin, heparin or both to treat acute unstable angina. N Engl J Med 1988;319:1105–1111.

28. ISIS-2 (Second International Study of Infarct Survival) Collaborative Group. Randomised trial of intravenous streptokinase, oral aspirin, both or neither among 17,187 cases of suspected acute myocardial infarction: ISIS-2. Lancet 1988;2:349–360.

29. Elwood PC, Cochrane AL, Burr ML, et al. A randomized controlled trial of acetylsalicylic acid in the secondary prevention of mortality from myocardial infarction. Br Med J 1974;1:436–440.

30. Coronary Drug Project Research Group. Aspirin in coronary heart disease. J Chron Dis 1976;29:625–642.

31. Elwood PC, Sweetnam PM. Aspirin and secondary mortality after myocardial infarction. Lancet 1979;2:1313–1315.

32. Breddin K, Loew D, Lechner K, Ueberla K, Walter E. Secondary prevention of myocardial reinfarction: a comparison of acetylsalicylic acid, placebo and phenprocoumon. Haemostasis 1982;9:325–344.

33. Aspirin Myocardial Infarction Study Research Group. A randomized, controlled trial of aspirin in persons recovered from myocardial infarction. JAMA 1980;243:661–669.

34. Persantin-Aspirin Reinfarction Study Research Group. Persantine and aspirin in coronary heart disease. Circulation 1980;62:449–461.

35. Anturane Reinfarction Trial Research Group. Sulfinpyrazone in the prevention of sudden death after myocardial infarction. N Engl J Med 1980;302:250–256.

36. Klimt CR, Knatterud GL, Stamler J, Meier P. Persantine-aspirin reinfarction with persantine and aspirin. J Am Coll Cardiol 1986;7:251–269.

37. Antiplatelet Trialists' Collaboration. Secondary prevention of vascular disease by prolonged antiplatelet treatment. Br Med J 1988;296:320–331.

38. McBride W, Lange RA, Hillis LD. Restenosis after successful coronary angioplasty. Pathophysiology and prevention. N Engl J Med 1988;318:1734–1737.

39. Popma JJ, Dehmer GJ. Care of the patient after coronary angioplasty. Ann Intern Med 1989;110:547–559.

40. Mehta JL, Conti CR. Aspirin in myocardial ischemia: why, when and how much? Clin Cardiol 1989;12:179–184.

41. Dehmer GJ, Popma JJ, van den Berg EK, et al. Reduction in the rate of early restenosis after coronary angioplasty by a diet supplemented with n-3 fatty acids. N Engl J Med 1988;319:733–740.

42. Chesebro JH, Fuster V, Elveback LR, et al. Effect of dipyridamole and aspirin on late vein-graft patency after coronary bypass operations. N Engl J Med 1984;310:209–214.

43. Lorenz RL, Weber M, Kotzur J, et al. Improved aortocoronary bypass patency by low-dose aspirin (100 mg daily). Lancet 1984;1:1261–1264.

44. Oates JA, FitzGerald GA, Branch RA, Jackson EK, Knapp HR, Roberts LJ. Clinical implications of prostaglandin and thromboxane A_2 formation. N Engl J Med 1988;319:689–698.

45. Coller BS. Platelets and antithrombotic therapy. N Engl J Med 1990;322:33–42.

46. Stein B, Fuster V, Halperin JL, Chesebro JH. Antithrombotic therapy in cardiac disease. Circulation 1989;80:1501–1513.

Section III

Primary Prevention

13

CAD risk assessment and modification in children

It has become quite clear that the process of atherosclerosis begins early in life (1). Autopsy studies of men killed in the Korean War (2, 3), and the Vietnam War (4) documented significant atheromatous lesions. In the earlier study, more than three-quarters of male soldiers (mean age 22) had fibrous plaques in their coronary arteries; in the latter investigation of men somewhat younger, nearly half had coronary lesions. Autopsies in Louisiana indicated that, even in the absence of the stress of combat, atherosclerosis lesions are found in adolescents and young adults. Fatty streaks have been noted in children as young as three years of age (5-7). Fatty streaks and intimal thickenings have been found in most Finnish and American children (8), leading some to question their importance. However, the extent of arterial fatty streaking in children has been directly correlated with systolic blood pressure and levels of blood total and LDL cholesterol determined earlier in childhood (9). Further, progression of these lesions to fibrous plaques has been demonstrated (10). Although white adults have more extensive aortic surface involvement with fibrous plaques than do blacks, ado-

lescent blacks have more fatty streaks than their white contemporaries (11).

Several longitudinal studies of children were designed to assess characteristics that are indicative of coronary artery disease (CAD) in adults. Within North America, large-scale investigations have been carried out in Bogalusa, Louisiana (12), Cincinnati, Ohio (13), and Muscatine, Iowa (14). The Bogalusa study, which began in 1973, has followed cohorts of black and white children from birth to 17 years of age. It described "tracking" of height, weight, blood pressure and lipid and lipoprotein values, indicating that children tend to remain in the same relative ranking through their young adult years (15-17). Similar findings have been reported by Muscatine and Cincinnati investigators (18, 19).

Given that atherosclerosis begins early in life and assuming that children with high levels of CAD risk indicators will continue to be at higher risk during their adulthood, one might question whether alteration of the increased risk will be clinically and economically effective. A 1987 report by Nader et al. of their survey of pediatricians in the USA revealed that few feel confident in their ability to change children's health habits, that a relatively low level of dietary advice is provided, and that most pediatricians do not routinely measure blood cholesterol levels (20). In the remainder of this chapter, each of the major CAD risk indicators are considered, and recommendations about CAD risk intervention in children are provided.

NUTRIENT INTAKE, LIPIDS, AND LIPOPROTEINS

DIETARY INTAKE

Dietary patterns have been extensively studied in the large-scale studies, with differences noted by age, race, and gender (21).

Among 10-year-old children in Bogalusa, girls and boys, black and white, had nearly identical values for nutrient intake; total fat represented 37 to 39% of all calories (22, 23), with 16% of total calories coming from saturated fat (24). Snacks represented approximately one-fourth of total caloric intake, with approximately 37% of snack calories coming from fat. School lunches in Louisiana in 1977 contained 38% of calories from fat (22). From 1973 to 1982, total fat intake of Bogalusa 10-year-old children remained at 38% of calories, but the proportions of fatty acids shifted in the healthy direction. Dietary cholesterol decreased 16% from 1978 to 1982 (25). These trends reflected food market trends of increased use of vegetable fats (26).

The USA National Health and Nutrition Examination Survey (NHANES) series studied children 9 to 11 years of age in the late 1970s, finding that fat constituted 36 to 39% of calories. The Nationwide Food Consumption Survey had similar results (23).

In the Princeton School study done in Cincinnati during the same period, boys and girls consumed 36 to 38% of calories as

fat; approximately 15% of caloric intake came from saturated fat. Dietary cholesterol was nearly identical in girls and boys aged 6 to 9 years (238 to 275 mg/day), but in the 10 to 12-year-old age group, boys consumed nearly 30% more cholesterol (in mg/day) than girls (27).

Six of the Lipid Research Clinics (five in USA, one in Canada) pooled information on nutrient intake in children ages 6 to 19 years. Approximately 38% of calories came from fat; 15% were derived from saturated fat. Fat intake increased with age in both genders. Dietary cholesterol intake averaged approximately 145 mg/ 1000 kcal consumed (28).

In other studies, dietary information was accurately obtained from parents or even from children themselves (29, 30). By 1987, 8-year-old Australian children had reduced fat intake to less than 35% of calories, with a 14% contribution from saturated fats, 11% from monounsaturated fats, and 6% from polyunsaturated fats (31), reflecting the movement of food consumption patterns toward recommended guidelines during the previous two decades (32).

In 1980, Finnish children consumed 38% of their total energy intake as fat, with a higher polyunsaturated to saturated fat ratio than was noted previously. In 1981, the Ministry of Social Affairs and Health in Finland published diet recommendations that included a limitation of 30 to 35% of calories coming from fat (33).

Taste preferences probably develop in infancy and are further modified during infancy and childhood by familiarity and social influences, including those of parents (34) and other children. Food can be used by parents to manipulate a child's behavior, which may alter the child's food preferences. During adolescence, food choices will be further affected by preoccupation with body image (35).

LIPID AND LIPOPROTEIN LEVELS

Tables and grids relating age to lipid and lipoprotein values have been published by investigators from several centers (36). Values show the most dramatic change during the first year of life (37), remain stable during childhood, but change significantly during adolescence and sexual maturation. Levels are similar in boys and girls until puberty, at which time HDL-C drops abruptly in boys (38–41). Differences in these values in Finnish youth are correlated with regional differences in CAD prevalence (42).

In 1972, serum cholesterol levels in rural children from Mexico and Wisconsin were reported; for those aged 5 to 14 years, total cholesterol levels were nearly twice as high in the Wisconsin children (187 vs. 100 mg/dl) (43).

Within the United States, differences between black, white, and Hispanic children in lipoprotein and apolipoprotein concentrations have been noted (44–47).

The Pima Indian children of North America have relatively low levels of serum cholesterol; in a study of those ages 5 to 16, values were found to be approximately 20 to 30 mg/dl lower than those of Caucasian children of the same ages in the United States (48).

EFFECTS OF DIETARY INTAKE ON BLOOD LIPIDS AND LIPOPROTEINS

Studies of the effect of dietary fat and cholesterol on lipids and lipoproteins have started as early as the neonatal period (49, 50). One study followed 172 women from infancy to the age of 32; those who had been breast-fed had significantly lower mean plasma cholesterol levels than those who had been bottle-fed (51).

In the Bogalusa Study, infants who were fed soy formula had significantly lower serum total cholesterol values at one year of age than those fed cow's milk or milk formula. The investigators concluded that serum lipid and lipoprotein levels in infants are responsive to the dietary intake of fat and cholesterol (52). Among 10-year-old children in Bogalusa, those in the lowest quartile of serum cholesterol distribution had significantly lower total and saturated fat intake in their diet than other children (53). While the Lipid Research Clinics Program Prevalence Study focused on adults, sufficient sampling of children was done to allow preparation of percentile tables for children (54), and nutrient data from several of the clinics have been compared to lipid and lipoprotein levels (55). Results from the NHANES II study showed that children aged 1 to 2 consume more than 300 mg of dietary cholesterol per day. For those aged 2 to 18 years, mean intake was approximately 280 mg/day, with 34% exceeding the adult recommended intake of 300 mg cholesterol daily. Surveys conducted by the USA National Center for Health Statistics revealed that approximately one-third of children aged 1 to 18 years in the USA receive more than 40% of their calories from fat; approximately 80% consume more than 10% of their calories in the form of saturated fat (56).

In 12-year-old Finnish children, those in the highest quartile of plasma cholesterol distribution had a significantly higher intake of saturated fats than those in the lowest plasma cholesterol quartile (57). Differences have been seen by geographical area and socioeconomic circumstances of the Finnish children (58).

In a study of Arab and Jewish schoolchildren ages 6 to 8 years in Jerusalem, Arab children had significantly lower serum total cholesterol (153 vs. 170 mg/dl) and LDL-cholesterol (91 vs. 109 mg/dl), but there were no significant differences between consumption levels of foods high in saturated fats or cholesterol between the two groups (59).

SCREENING OF CHILDREN FOR DYSLIPIDEMIAS

In 1980, Berwick, Cretin, and Keeler published their analysis of alternatives regarding children, cholesterol, and heart disease. They considered various proposed approaches to screening and intervention, using existing prevalence rates for childrens' cholesterol levels and incidence rates of adult MI within the USA. Allowing for variations in the discount rate (which recognizes that investment in screening occurs now while savings in hospital cost must be realized some decades later), they concluded that a one-time screening of school-age children would be cost-effective (60).

However, the following year, the Nutrition Committee of the Canadian Paediatric Society recommended cholesterol screening only in those children with (a) a family history of myocardial infarction (MI) before the age of 50, (b) abnormal parental serum lipid concentrations, or (c) obesity, hypertension, or both in the child (61).

In 1989, the American Academy of Pediatrics reiterated their opposition to screening of all children for total blood cholesterol, reserving screening for only those children with "a family history (parent, sibling, grandparent, uncle, aunt) of hyperlipidemia or early myocardial infarction (<50 years of age in men, <60 years of age in women)" (62). They cited a lack of confidence in existing instrumentation and testing procedures and a concern that a single cholesterol measurement will not reflect true values over time and could lead to "unwarranted diet or treatment (which) could be deleterious to growth and development" (62).

Several studies have indicated an association between lipid, lipoprotein, and apolipoprotein levels in children and a parental history of myocardial infarction or angiographically diagnosed CAD (63, 64). Similarly, children with a blood total cholesterol level in the upper 5% for their age have a higher probability of first-degree relatives with dyslipidemias (65–67). In a study of 102 adolescent twin pairs, children with a family history of early CAD death had lower levels of HDL_2 than those without such a history (68).

The policies mentioned above may lead to a failure to detect the majority of children with dyslipidemias; approximately 10 to 20% of children have blood total cholesterol levels of 200 mg/dl or above (69, 70). Considering that such levels should be considered as undesirable in children as they are in adult patients, Davidson and colleagues studied 118 children ages 9 and 10 whose parents provided parental and grandparental history of cardiovascular disease events and risk indicators. Of 157 children with blood total cholesterol of 200 mg/dl or above, only 39% had a family history of early MI or hyperlipidemia. The prevalence of a positive family history ranged from 2.8% in Vietnamese-American children, to 38.5% in Spanish-surnamed students, to 52.6% in white children. The authors concluded that capillary blood testing in schools is safe, well-accepted by students and parents, and necessary to detect cases of dyslipidemias in children without knowledge of family history or without sufficient family financial resources to afford testing of adult relatives (71). Blood cholesterol screening can also be efficiently conducted in the physician's office (72), given the reliability and convenience of desktop analyzers (73).

In a Cleveland (Ohio) study, 6500 children (mean age 6.4 years) had a blood total cholesterol measurement done during a two-year period. Approximately 9% had levels of 200 mg/dl or more; of 487 who had a lipid profile accomplished, 76% had LDL-cholesterol levels exceeding 130 mg/dl. In the latter group, only half had a family history of MI before 55 years of age or known dyslipidemia. The authors recommended that a random, nonfasting cholesterol test be done in all children (74). When the value exceeds 200 mg/dl, a lipid profile should be done. Of course, confirmation of initial elevated readings should precede consideration of treatment (dietary or drug) by clinicians. If confirmation is obtained, and the elevated total cholesterol is not due solely to elevated HDL-cholesterol, nutritional advice is in order.

DIET MODIFICATION

The American Heart Association recommends a diet low in saturated fat and cholesterol for all persons older than age 2 years (75).

Although they have not recommended universal screening of children for blood total cholesterol, the American Academy of Pediatrics does recommend a diet identical to the American Heart Association recommendations (76) and to step 1 of the National Cholesterol Education Program Expert Panel guidelines for any child with a value greater than 175 mg/dl. As indicated in Chapter 3, total fat intake in this diet is limited to 30% of the total calories, with 10% or less from saturated fat. Total dietary cholesterol intake should be less than 100 mg/1000 calories/day, not to exceed 300 mg/day (62, 77). Several authors have reported reductions of 10 to 15% in total cholesterol in children by using a low-fat, low-cholesterol diet (78).

It is important that families avoid restriction of dietary cholesterol and fat in children under two years of age, so that normal growth and development will not be inhibited. Although a few cases have been reported of overzealous parents who fed their young children a very low fat diet

(79), most studies have indicated that parents can safely institute a heart-healthy diet for their children after detection of hypercholesterolemia (80). Adherence to a diet containing 30% fat results in no impairment of growth and development in children after the first two years of life (81). Parents should also understand that occasional splurging by children or other family members will not appreciably affect the individual's lipid and lipoprotein levels (82). Family-based education programs have proved very effective, particularly when the families are psychologically healthy (83, 84).

In a Finnish study of children ages 8 to 18 years, reduction of dietary fat percentage from 35 to 24% resulted in a 15% decrease in mean serum total cholesterol (85). In the USA, the Dietary Intervention Study in Children (DISC) is underway to assess the efficacy and safety of diet intervention in families of children with elevated LDL-C levels. They attend 14 sessions over a 5-month period (86).

Bogalusa investigators developed the "Heart Smart" program to test the relative advantages of a population-based risk reduction strategy and one focusing on children considered to be at high risk. Their specific objective regarding blood cholesterol is to lower a child's total fat intake to 30% or less, and saturated fat consumption to 10% or less of total calories. Intervention components include teacher training, classroom instruction, heart-healthy lunches, parent education, and blood cholesterol screening (87).

A number of school-based programs have been based on the social-learning-theory principles of modeling, behavioral rehearsal, goal specification, feedback, and reinforcement for behavior change (88). In 1979, the "Know Your Body" program was introduced to determine the feasibility and effectiveness of a school-based primary chronic disease prevention program (89).

After one year of follow-up of 2283 New York elementary school children, total cholesterol had decreased in the intervention group and risen in the control group (90). After five years of follow-up of 1769 children from demographically dissimilar areas in and around New York City, the investigators found small but statistically significant decreases in total cholesterol, along with favorable trends in dietary intake and health knowledge (91). The program has also been implemented in black schoolchildren, in whom total cholesterol values are inversely related to socioeconomic status (92, 93).

The USA National Institutes of Health have actively supported a number of investigations (94) in the promotion of cardiovascular health. Particularly important in such studies is a rigorous evaluation (95).

Among recent efforts is a program by Coates and colleagues that produced significant changes in the eating behavior of elementary students and their parents (96), and another by the same team attempted to modify the snacking habits of inner-city high-school students (97).

The Hearty Heart curriculum was designed by Perry and her colleagues in the Minnesota Heart Health Program for elementary school students. The 20-session program resulted in self-reported, favorable eating-behavior changes in approximately half of the targeted foods (98). In a subsequent study, this school-based curriculum was compared with a home-based program, the Hearty Heart Home Team, which involved a five-week correspondence course for students, requiring the participation of their parents. Students who participated in the home program had greater changes in dietary fat consumption (99).

In the San Diego Family Health Project, Hispanic and Anglo families with a fifth or sixth grader (ages 10 to 12 years)

met for 12 weekly sessions and 6 maintenance sessions designed to transmit knowledge and build skills for long-term changes in diet and physical-activity habits. Favorable changes in these parameters were noted in both children and adults (100).

The Go for Health program combines social learning theory and organizational change principles to promote physical activity and healthier eating behaviors (101). After one year of the program in two schools, school lunch meals contained 28 to 42% less fat than at baseline (102). Ellison and colleagues worked with school food service workers to reduce saturated fat intake by students by 20% (without specific intervention with the children) (103).

In North Karelia, Finland, the addition of a school-based program to community education efforts in intervention communities resulted in a significant decrease in fat intake in adolescents (37 to 32% of calories). Margarine replaced butter, skim milk was used in place of whole milk, egg yolks were avoided, and fish, poultry, vegetables, and salads were promoted. Serum cholesterol was lowered by 20 mg/dl in boys and 17 mg/dl in girls (104). In another North Karelia study, 16 adolescents were part of a 30-family study population. Mean serum cholesterol in the young persons dropped 28 mg/dl as a result of family-based counseling and subsequent changes in home meals (105).

If early efforts at office-based counseling are not sufficient, an appointment should be scheduled with a registered dietitian skilled in working with children and their families.

REFERRAL FOR DRUG TREATMENT

If the best combined efforts of clinician, office staff, consultant dietitian, family, and child do not result in an acceptable improvement of the child's lipid values, referral to a pediatric cardiologist is appropriate. Pediatric preventive cardiology clinics are now available in each region of North America, and their number is growing rapidly (106).

Familial hypercholesterolemia (FH) occurs in the heterozygous form in 1 in 500 persons; such individuals have too few LDL receptors, and LDL is cleared from plasma at a reduced rate. Homozygous FH occurs when two heterozygotes mate, resulting in one case per million persons.

When pharmacologic treatment is indicated, the bile acid sequestrants (cholestyramine, colestipol) are the first choice; they may lower total and LDL-cholesterol as much as 20 to 30%. In one family with four homozygous children, two received no treatment and died at ages 9 and 10 years. A third sibling died at age 3 years despite treatment with diet and thyroxine, but with no change in the plasma cholesterol level of 888 mg/dl. However, a fourth sibling was started on diet, cholestyramine, clofibrate, and nicotinic acid at the age of one year. At age 15, coronary arteriography was essentially normal (107). As in adults, careful assessment of liver function must be undertaken before and during treatment. To date, children with severe familial hypercholesterolemia have been treated with nicotinic acid or HMG-CoA reductase inhibitors only under investigational protocols (108, 109).

An Expert Panel on Blood Cholesterol Levels in Children and Adolescents has been convened by the USA National Cholesterol Education Program to address the issues discussed above and to provide recommendations for screening and treatment.

BLOOD PRESSURE

Systolic and diastolic blood pressures rise throughout childhood and adolescence. A random sample survey of pediatricians in the USA in 1985 revealed that almost all primary care pediatricians routinely assess BP after infancy, but approximately 20% of respondents did not recognize high values as being abnormal in children younger than 9 years of age (20). Early recognition is important because Bogalusa investigators found that fibrous plaques in coronary arteries of autopsied youth were related even more strongly to systolic blood pressure than to serum cholesterol (9), and researchers in Muscatine noted that school children in the upper quintile of the blood pressure distribution already display signs of left ventricular hypertrophy (110).

The Task Force on Blood Pressure Control in Children was commissioned by the USA National Heart, Lung, and Blood Institute to identify proper measurement techniques, prepare blood pressure (BP) distribution curves by age, recommend classifications of BPs in children, identify appropriate diagnostic algorithms, and delineate hygienic and drug treatment strategies. Ten years after their first report, the task force published their revised findings in 1987 (111). These topics are reviewed in this section.

Several studies, including those in Bogalusa (15, 112) and Muscatine (18, 113), have documented tracking (persistence within BP ranks) into young adulthood (114). A study of 17,130 children living in Cuba, the German Democratic Republic, Hungary, and the Soviet Union also found patterns of BP persistence (115). BP-age prevalence charts have been prepared by Finnish investigators from their studies of five areas (116), similar to those developed by the Bogalusa Heart Study team (12).

Within the USA, several cross-sectional (prevalence) studies of children of different races and ethnic groups have examined BP. In some studies, black children had higher BP levels, but adjustment for size reduced this disparity (117, 118). In the Bogalusa and Cincinnati studies, however, no significant BP differences were seen in black and white children (119, 120). In one study, children of Asian ethnicity had higher BPs (118), while in another, Mexican-American children in Texas displayed lower BPs than Anglo children (121). A Venezuelan study showed no differences among mestizo, white, and black children (122), while a British study showed significant BP differences among children in nine towns, which correlated with cardiovascular mortality in adults in the respective regions (123).

Measurement Methods

Potential sources of error in BP measurement in children include physiologic variability, variability among multiple determinations, equipment differences, and patterns of bias by individual observers. In the Bogalusa Heart Study, considerable effort was expended to standardize BP measurement. This included frequent training sessions, use of dual stethoscopes and sphygmomanometers, audiometric testing, and careful evaluation of a variety of instruments. Random resampling of children added further credence to the reliability of measurements. For more details, the reader is referred to their

publications (12, 124) and to the report of the Task Force on Blood Pressure Control in Children (111). These documents describe the selection of proper compression-cuff size, preparation and positioning of the child, inflation and deflation rates, and choice of Korotkoff sounds for diastolic BP measurement (phase IV for infants and children, phase V for adolescents). Correlations of measurements by an oscillometric device and conventional auscultatory equipment with direct radial-artery pressure were high, with the former method being more accurate (125).

The task force defined normal BP as systolic and diastolic BPs less than the 90th percentile for age and gender. The term "high normal BP" is attached to values between the 90th and 95th percentiles. "Hypertension" is diagnosed if values exceed the 95th percentile; as shown in Table 13.1, this category is further divided into significant and severe hypertension.

Measurements above the 90th percentile should be repeated during subsequent visits; if it continues between the 90th and 95th percentiles and the high BP cannot be attributed to elevated height and weight, BP should be monitored at least every six months.

If BP persists at the 95th percentile or above in an obese child, a weight-control

Table 13.1. Classification of Hypertension in Children and Adolescents

Age	Significant Hypertension (mm Hg)		Severe Hypertension (mm Hg)	
	SBP	DBP	SBP	DBP
Newborn to 7 days	> 95		> 105	
Neonates (8 days to 30 days)	> 104		> 109	
Infant (less than 2 years)	> 111	> 73	> 117	> 82
Children				
(3–5 years)	> 115	> 75	> 123	> 83
(6–9 years)	> 121	> 78	> 129	> 85
(10–12 years)	> 125	> 81	> 133	>89
Adolescents				
(13–15 years)	> 135	> 86	> 143	> 91
(16–18 years)	> 141	> 91	> 149	> 97

program should be instituted. If weight is normal, or if reduction of the child's weight to an ideal level does not reduce BP, non-pharmacologic treatment is indicated. Should these interventions be ineffective, drug therapy can be considered.

In children over the age of six, primary hypertension is the most common cause of milder diastolic hypertension. In younger children, aortic coarctation and renal and renal artery disorders are the major causes of chronic, sustained hypertension. Persistent isolated systolic hypertension is not normal in the young, but its long-term significance is less clear than in adults (111).

Influence of Other Factors

EFFECTS OF WEIGHT AND HEIGHT

Blood pressure levels in children are related to both their height and weight; for a given height, BP correlates directly with body weight and fatness (126). Among 4196 Bogalusa children examined between 1981 and 1983, there was a strong positive association of weight/height^3 and blood pressure (127).

In the Muscatine Study of 2925 children, ponderosity and blood pressures were measured at least once between ages 6 and 15 years and again between ages 15 and 18 years. Changes in blood pressure were positively correlated with changes in ponderosity (128). A majority of children with elevated blood pressure were obese (relative weight more than 120% of ideal); those who lowered their weight substantially after dietary counseling normalized their blood pressure (129).

DIETARY FACTORS

Evidence from experimental and population studies suggests a relation between sodium intake and blood pressure. In infants fed one gram of sodium per day from birth, BPs were significantly lower at six months of age than in control infants (130). In a Dutch study, BP in schoolchildren was related to high sodium levels in drinking water (131). A Chicago study indicated a relation between individual sodium excretion and BP, independent of height, weight, age, and race (132), and in the Bogalusa Heart Study, an association between sodium intake and BP was suggested (133). Their Heart Smart Program recommends a maximum of 5 g/day of sodium intake, asking the children to choose low-sodium snacks, increase aerobic exercise time, and maintain body weight at an ideal level (134). Within families in the USA, a majority of the sodium ingested comes from processed foods (135).

While fat intake does not appear to be associated with BP in children (85), one Australian study found a negative correlation between diastolic BP and fiber intake in 9-year-old children (136).

FAMILY INFLUENCES

Twin and adoptive studies have clarified the role of genetics and environment in hypertension in children (137); familial aggregation of blood pressure can be detected as early as infancy (138). In the Muscatine Study, this aggregation was particularly prominent in families of children with labile, high-systolic BP (139). A family history of hypertension predicted BP in Bogalusa children after 8 years of surveillance (140), although parental diastolic BP was a poor predictor of children's values (67). BP aggregation is seen in Mexican-American as well as Anglo families in the USA (141), and in families in Cuba, Eastern Europe, and the Soviet Union (115).

EMOTIONAL STRESS AND REACTIVITY

In the Bogalusa Heart Study, children displaying higher levels of diastolic BP reactivity to orthostatic, handgrip, and cold pressor tasks had significantly higher diastolic BP levels four years later (142). In a study of adolescents, BP was higher in individuals displaying life dissatisfaction, impatience, anger, and hostility (143). Progressive muscle relaxation reduced BP in adolescents while it was practiced, but failed to achieve long-term BP reduction (144).

PHYSICAL FITNESS AND TRAINING

In general, BPs are lower in children with higher levels of physical fitness (145). Systolic BP responses to exercise appear to be relatively stable with time (146). Adolescents with BP persistently above the 95th percentile can significantly lower their BP with aerobic exercise training (147).

BP Detection and Evaluation

If the hypertensive child is obese or has a family history of primary hypertension, a urinalysis is indicated initially. In nonobese children, urine culture, a complete blood count, and blood urea, creatinine, and electrolyte determinations are indicated as well. Beyond these evaluations, the level of BP will direct further evaluation (148).

Treatment

HYGIENIC

Given the factors described above, hygienic treatment of high BP in children and adolescents involves an integrated program of weight reduction, increased physical activity, and a trial of sodium intake limitation. In addition, adolescent girls with hypertension should avoid oral contraceptives if possible.

Successful programs of sodium reduction have been developed for school lunch programs (102), and snacking (97), especially when parental involvement is emphasized (104). Using the "Know Your Body" curriculum with black students, blood pressure reduction from a comprehensive hygienic approach was associated with decreased obesity and increased physical fitness (92).

PHARMACOLOGIC

The Task Force on Blood Pressure Control in Children Report lists blood pressure medications and dosages suitable for use in children. Even when it is necessary to initiate drug treatment, efforts should continue to maintain dietary, exercise, and weight modification (149). If the blood pressure responds well to medication, "step-down" treatment should be considered (111).

SMOKING

Smoking adoption is closely related to smoking by parents, older siblings, and close friends. Children perceive smoking as a way to appear mature, relax, and release anger, as well as to enhance their appeal to the opposite gender (150). In Bogalusa, half of children starting to smoke before age 12 years smoked their first cigarettes with a family member or older friend. Black children showed a greater sibling and peer effect, while whites were more influenced by their parents' smoking habits. Smoking habits were well established by age 14 (151, 152). In Muscatine, half of the variance in adolescent cigarette smoking was explained by friends who smoked and by social disaffection with school and family (153). In Finnish children, the smoking behavior of the adolescent's best friend was the best predictor (154). Bogalusa children smoking three or more packs weekly displayed greater increases in LDL-cholesterol and triglyceride levels and greater reductions in HDL-cholesterol than nonsmokers (155). Although cigarette smoking decreased among Bogalusa children between the mid-1970s and the 1980s, smokeless tobacco use increased (156).

Intervention programs based in the home, school, and community have been effective in reducing the rate of smoking adoption. The Preschool Health Education Program in Galveston, Texas demonstrated less smoking adoption by the intervention group (157). The Oslo Youth Study based their successful antismoking efforts in the schools (158), as did the North Karelia Youth Program, which showed significant results after four years of follow-up (159). Children from 22 schools participating in the First Waterloo School Smoking Prevention Trial were followed for six years; smoking at age 11 years predicted smoking at 17. Children who had left school were smoking at twice the rate of those who were still in school at the latter age (160).

Although most adolescents are aware of long-term dangers when they start smoking, they do not respond to antismoking efforts featuring these hazards. Discussions emphasizing short-term effects such as appearance, breath, clothing odor, and impaired athletic ability may be more persuasive (150).

PHYSICAL ACTIVITY

Although most Finnish children are active in their leisure time (161), most children in the USA are not. In the Second National Children and Youth Fitness Study in that country, investigators found declining levels of physical activity and fitness.

Methods are available for field-testing of children (162), and statements have been issued by the American Academy of Pediatrics and the American Heart Association on the importance of physical activity for risk factor modification (163).

Physical activity levels have been correlated positively with HDL-cholesterol and inversely with body mass index (164) and systolic blood pressure (165).

OBESITY

In the Muscatine Study, children in the highest quintile of relative weight on three surveys had higher levels of systolic BP and lower levels of HDL-cholesterol. Investigators estimated that half of the variance in childhood obesity is familial (both genetic and environmental) (166). In overweight Bogalusa children, other CAD risk indicators were clustered (127). Height and weight tracked closely in Bogalusa children, with prevalence of overweight increasing from 15 to 24% between ages 5 and 14 years (167).

Although most pediatricians do not feel confident in designing and implementing weight-loss programs for children (168), behavioral treatment of childhood obesity is effective (169), particularly when parents are actively involved (170).

REFERENCES

1. Berenson GS, Srinivasan SR, Freedman DS, Radhakrishnamurthy B, Dalferes ER Jr. Atherosclerosis and its evolution in childhood. Am J Med Sci 1987;294:429–440.

2. Enos WR, Holmes RH, Beyer J. Coronary artery disease among United States soldiers killed in action in Korea. JAMA 1953; 152:1090–1093.

3. Enos WF, Beyer JC, Holmes R. Pathogenesis of coronary disease in soldiers killed in Korea. JAMA 1955;148:912–914.

4. McNamara JJ, Molot MA, Stremple JF, Cutting RT. Coronary artery disease in combat casualties in Vietnam. JAMA 1971; 216:1185–1187.

5. Strong JP, McGill HC Jr. The natural history of coronary atherosclerosis. Am J Pathol 1962;40:37–49.

6. Strong JP, McGill HC. The pediatric aspects of atherosclerosis. J Atherosclerosis Res 1969;9:251–265.

7. Stary HC. Evolution and progression of atherosclerotic lesions in coronary arteries of

children and young adults. Arteriosclerosis 1989;9(suppl I): I19–I32.

8. Hirvonen J, Yla-Herttuala S, Laaksonen H, et al. Coronary intimal thickenings and lipids in Finnish children who died suddenly. Acta Paediatr Scand 1985;318(suppl):221–224.

9. Newman WP III, Freedman DS, Voors AW, et al. Relation of serum lipoprotein levels and systolic blood pressure to early atherosclerosis: the Bogalusa Study. N Engl J Med 1986;314:138–144.

10. McGill HC Jr. Persistent problems in the pathogenesis of atherosclerosis. Arteriosclerosis 1984;4:443–451.

11. Freedman DS, Newman WP III, Tracy RE, et al. Black-white differences in aortic fatty streaks in adolescence and early adulthood: the Bogalusa Heart Study. Circulation 1988;77:856–864.

12. Berenson GS, McMahan CA, Voors AW, et al. Cardiovascular risk factors in children. The early natural history of atherosclerosis and essential hypertension. New York: Oxford University Press, 1980.

13. Khoury PJ, Morrison JA, Kelly K, et al. Clustering and interrelationships of coronary heart disease risk factors in schoolchildren, ages 6–19. Am J Epidemiol 1980;112:524–538.

14. Lauer RM, Connor WE, Leaverton PE, Reiter MA, Clarke WR. Coronary heart disease risk factors in children. J Pediatr 1975;86:697–706.

15. Webber LS, Cresanta JL, Voors AW, Berenson GS. Tracking of cardiovascular risk factor variables in school aged children. J Chron Dis 1983;36:647–660.

16. Webber LS, Cresanta JL, Croft JB, Srinivasan SR, Berenson GS. Transitions of cardiovascular risk from adolescence to young adulthood—the Bogalusa Heart Study. II. Alterations in anthropometric blood pressure and serum lipoprotein values. J Chron Dis 1986;39:91–103.

17. Berenson GS, Srinivisan SR, Nicklas TA, Webber LS. Cardiovascular risk factors in children and early prevention of heart disease. Clin Chem 1988;34:B115–B122.

18. Clarke WR, Schrott HG, Leaverton PE, Connor WE, Lauer RM. Tracking of lipids and blood pressure in school age children: The Muscatine Study. Circulation 1978;58:626–634.

19. Laskarzewski P, Morrison JA, deGroot I, et al. Lipid and lipoprotein tracking in 108 children over a four-year period. Pediatrics 1979;64:584–591.

20. Nader PR, Taras HL, Sallis JF, Patterson TL. Adult heart disease prevention in childhood: a national survey of pediatricians' practices and attitudes. Pediatrics 1987;79:843–850.

21. Nicklas TA, Farris RP, Major C, et al. Dietary intakes. Pediatrics 1987;80(suppl):797–806.

22. Frank GC, Voors AW, Schilling PE, Berenson GS. Dietary studies of rural school children in a cardiovascular survey. J Am Diet Assoc 1977;71:31–35.

23. Farris RP, Cresanta JL, Croft JB, Webber LS, Frank GC, Berenson GS. Macronutrient intakes of 10-year-old children, 1973 to 1982. J Am Diet Assoc 1986;86:765–770.

24. Frank GC, Farris RP, Cresanta JL, Webber LS, Berenson GS. Dietary trends of 10- and 13-year-old children in a biracial community—the Bogalusa Heart Study. Prev Med 1985;14:123–139.

25. Cresanta JL, Farris RP, Croft JB, Webber LS, Frank GC, Berenson GS. Trends in fatty acid intakes of 10-year-old children, 1973 to 1982. J Am Diet Assoc 1988;88:178–184.

26. Farris RP, Cresanta JL, Frank GC, Webber LS, Berenson GS. Dietary studies of children from a biracial population: intakes of fat and fatty acids in 10- and 13-year olds. Am J Clin Nutr 1984;39:114–128.

27. Morrison JA, Larsen R, Glatfelter L, et al. Nutrient intake: relationships with lipids and lipoproteins in 6–19 year-old children—the Princeton School District Study. Metabolism 1980;29:133–140.

28. Salz KM, Tamir I, Ernst E, et al. Selected nutrient intakes of free-living white children ages 6–19 years. The Lipid Research Clinics Program Prevalence Study. Pediatr Res 1983;17:124–130.

29. Baranowski T, Dworkin R, Henske J, et al. The accuracy of childrens' self-reports of diet: Family Health Project. J Am Diet Assoc 1986;86:1381–1385.

30. Farris RP, Frank GC, Webber LS, Berenson GS. A group method for obtaining dietary recalls for children. J Am Diet Assoc 1985;85:1315-1320.

31. Magarey A, Boulton TJ. Food intake during childhood: percentiles of food energy, macronutrient and selected micronutrients from infancy to eight years of age. Med J Austral 1987;147:124-127.

32. Gracey M. What children eat: food for the future. Med J Austral 1987;147:111-112.

33. Rasanen L, Ahola M, Kara R, Uhari M. Atherosclerosis precursors in Finnish children and adolescents. VIII. Food consumption and nutrient intakes. Acta Paediatr Scand Suppl 1985;318:135-153.

34. Laskarzewski P, Morrison JA, Khoury P, et al. Parent-child nutrient intake interrelationships in school children ages 6 to 19: the Princeton School District Study. Am J Clin Nutr 1980;33:2350-2355.

35. Rolls BJ. Food beliefs and food choices in adolescents. Med J Austral 1988; 148:S9-S13.

36. Cresanta JL, Srinivasan SR, Webber LS, Berenson GS. Serum lipid and lipoprotein cholesterol grids for cardiovascular risk screening of children. Am J Dis Child 1984;138:379-387.

37. Berenson GS, Blonde CV, Farris RP, et al. Cardiovascular risk factor variables during the first year of life. Am J Dis Child 1979;133:1049-1057.

38. Berenson GS, Srinivasan SR, Cresanta JL, Foster TA, Webber LS. Dynamic changes of serum lipoproteins in children during adolescence and sexual maturation. Am J Epidemiol 1981;113:157-170.

39. Freedman DS, Srinivasan SR, Webber LS, Burke GL, Berenson GS. Black-white differences in serum lipoproteins during sexual maturation: the Bogalusa Heart Study. J Chron Dis 1987;40:309-318.

40. Tell GS, Mittelmark MB, Vellar OD. Cholesterol, high density lipoprotein cholesterol and triglycerides during puberty: the Oslo Youth Study. Am J Epidemiol 1985;122:750-761.

41. Viikari J, Akerblom HK, Nikkari T, et al. Atherosclerosis precursors in Finnish children and adolescents. IV. Serum lipids in newborns, children and adolescents. Acta Paediatr Scand Suppl 1985;318:103-109.

42. Solakivi-Jaakkola T, Nikkari T, Viikari J, et al. Atherosclerosis precursors in Finnish children and adolescents. VI. Serum apolipoproteins A-I and B. Acta Paediatr Scand Suppl 1985;318:119-125.

43. Golubjatnikov R, Paskey T, Inhorn SL. Serum cholesterol levels of Mexican and Wisconsin school children. Am J Epidemiol 1972;96:36-39.

44. Webber LS, Harsha DW, Phillips G, Simpson J, Srinivasan SR, Berenson GS. A contrast of serum lipids and lipoproteins in hispanic, anglo, and black children—Brooks County and Bogalusa Heart studies. Circulation 1986;74(suppl II):II—382.

45. Srinivasan SR, Freedman DS, Sharma C, Webber LS, Berenson GS. Serum apolipoproteins A-1 and B in 2,854 children from a biracial community: Bogalusa Heart Study. Pediatrics 1986;78:189-200.

46. Srinivasan SR, Freedman DS, Webber LS, Berenson GS. Black-white differences in cholesterol levels of serum high-density lipoprotein subclasses among children: the Bogalusa Heart Study. Circulation 1987;76:272-279.

47. Walter HJ, Hofman A. Socioeconomic status, ethnic origin, and risk factors for coronary heart disease in children. Am Heart J 1987;113:812-818.

48. Savage PJ, Hamman RF, Bartha G, et al. Serum cholesterol levels in American (Pima) Indian children and adolescents. Pediatrics 1976;58:274-282.

49. Hodgson PA, Ellefson RD, Elveback LR, Harris LE, Nelson RA, Weidman WH. Comparison of serum cholesterol in children fed high, moderate, or low cholesterol milk diets during neonatal period. Metabolism 1976;25:739-746.

50. Weidman WH, Elveback LR, Nelson RA, Hodgson PA, Ellefson RD. Nutrient intake and serum cholesterol level in normal children 6 to 16 years of age. Pediatrics 1978;61:354-359.

51. Marmot MG, Page CM, Atkins E, Douglas JW. Effect of breast-feeding on plasma

cholesterol and weight in young adults. J'Epidemiol Comm Health 1980;34:164–167.

52. Farris RP, Frank GC, Webber LS, Srinivasan SR, Berenson GS. Influence of milk source on serum lipids and lipoproteins during the first year of life, Bogalusa Heart Study. Am J Clin Nutr 1982;35:42–49.

53. Frank GC, Berenson GS, Webber LS. Dietary studies and the relationship of diet to cardiovascular disease risk factor variables in 10-year-old children—the Bogalusa Heart Study. Am J Clin Nutr 1978;31:328–340.

54. LaRosa JC, Chambless LE, Criqui MH, et al. Patterns of dyslipoproteinemia in selected North American populations. Circulation 1986;73(suppl I):I12–I29.

55. Prewitt TE, Haynes SG, Graves K, Haines PS, Tyroler HA. Nutrient intake, lipids, and lipoprotein cholesterols in black and white children. Prev Med 1988;17:247–262.

56. Carroll MD, Abraham S, Dresser CM. Dietary intake source data: United States 1976–1980. Vital Statistics, Series 11, No. 231. Washington: US Department of Health and Human Services; 1983. DHHS Publication no. (PHS) 83–1681.

57. Akerblom HK, Viikari J, Uhari M, et al. A study of cardiovascular risk factors and their determinants in Finnish children. Ann Clin Res 1984;16:23–33.

58. Akerblom HK, Viikari J, Kouvalainen K. Cardiovascular risk factors in Finnish children and adolescents. Acta Paediatr Scand Suppl 1985;318:5–6.

59. Tamir D, Edelstein P, Reshef A, Halfon ST, Palti H. Serum cholesterol, triglyceride levels, and fat consumption among Jerusalem Arab and Jewish schoolchildren. Prev Med 1987;16:752–760.

60. Berwick DM, Cretin S, Keeler EB. Cholesterol, children, and heart disease: an analysis of alternatives. New York: Oxford University Press, 1980.

61. Nutrition Committee of the Canadian Paediatric Society. Children's diets and atherosclerosis. Canad Med Assoc J 1981;124:1545–1548.

62. American Academy of Pediatrics Committee on Nutrition. Indications for cholesterol testing in children. Pediatrics 1989;83:141–142.

63. Glueck CJ, Fallat RW, Tsang R, Buncher CR. Hyperlipemia in progeny of parents with myocardial infarction before age 50. Am J Dis Child 1974;127:70–75.

64. Lee J, Lauer RM, Clarke WR. Lipoproteins in the progeny of young men with coronary artery disease: children with increased risk. Pediatrics 1986;78:330–337.

65. Schrott HG, Clarke WR, Wiebe DA, Connor WE, Lauer RM. Increased coronary mortality in relatives of hypercholesterolemic school children: the Muscatine Study. Circulation 1979;59:320–326.

66. Freedman DS, Srinivasan SR, Shear CL, Franklin FA, Webber LS, Berenson GS. The relation of apolipoproteins A-1 and B in children to parental myocardial infarction. N Engl J Med 1986;315:721–726.

67. Rosenbaum PA, Elston RC, Srinivasan SR, Webber LS, Berenson GS. Predictive value of parental measures in determining cardiovascular risk factor variables in early life. Pediatrics 1987;80(suppl):807–816.

68. Bodurtha JN, Schieken R, Segrest J, Nance WE. High-density lipoprotein-cholesterol subfractions in adolescent twins. Pediatrics 1987;79:181–189.

69. Berenson GS, Epstein FH. Conference on blood lipids in children: optimal levels for early prevention of coronary artery disease. Prev Med. 1983;12:741–797.

70. deGroot I, Morrison JA, Kelly KA, et al. Lipids in schoolchildren 6 to 17 years of age: upper normal limits. Pediatrics 1977;60:437–443.

71. Davidson DM, Iftner CA, Bradley BJ, Landry SM, Rose MY, Wong ND. Family history predictors of high blood cholesterol levels in 4th grade school children. J Am Coll Cardiol 1989;13:36A.

72. Davidson DM, Smith RM, Qaqundah PY. Cholesterol screening in children during office visits. J Pediatr Health Care 1990:4:11–17.

73. Burke JJ II, Fischer PM. A clinician's guide to the office measurement of cholesterol. JAMA 1988;259:3444–3448.

74. Garcia RE, Moodie DS. Routine cholesterol surveillance in childhood. Pediatrics 1989;84:751–755.

75. Weidman W, Kwiterovich P Jr, Jesse MJ, Nugent E. Diet in the healthy child: Amer-

ican Heart Association Nutrition Committee Report. Circulation 1983;67:1411A–1414A.

76. American Heart Association. Diagnosis and treatment of primary hyperlipidemia in childhood. Circulation 1986;74:1181A–1188A.

77. National Cholesterol Education Program Expert Panel. Report of the National Cholesterol Education Program Expert Panel on detection, evaluation, and treatment of high blood cholesterol in adults. Arch Intern Med 1988;148:36–39.

78. Widhalm K. Paediatric guidelines for lipid reduction. Eur Heart J 1987;8(suppl E):65–70.

79. Pugliese MT, Weyman-Daum M, Moses N, Lifshitz F. Parental health beliefs as a cause of nonorganic failure to thrive. Pediatrics 1987;80:175–182.

80. Dobrin BE, Starc TJ, Belamarich PF, et al. Unsupervised parental implementation of cholesterol lowering diets in hyperlipidemic children. Pediatr Res 1989;25:98A.

81. Budow L, Beseler L, Arden M, et al. The effect of dietary therapy on growth in hyperlipidemic children and adolescents: a prospective clinical trial. Pediatr Res 1989;25:22A.

82. Denke MA, Breslow JL. The effect of low fat diets with and without splurging on lipid, lipoprotein and apolipoprotein levels. Circulation 1987;76(suppl IV):IV-531.

83. Kirks BA, Hughes C. Long-term behavioral effects of parent involvement in nutrition education. J Nut Educ 1986;18:203–206.

84. Laundy KC, Whittemore R. Family psychosocial functioning and compliance with treatment for familial hyperlipidemia. Pediatr Res 1989;25:27A.

85. Vartiainen E, Puska P, Pietinen P, Nissinen A, Leino U, Uusitalo U. Effects of dietary fat modifications on serum lipids and blood pressure in children. Acta Paediatr Scand 1986;75:396–401.

86. DISC Research Group. Dietary Intervention Study in Children (DISC): a randomized clinical trial. Pediatr Res 1989;25:101A.

87. Downey AM, Butcher AH, Frank GC, Webber LS, Miner MH, Berenson GS. Development of implementation of a school health promotion program for reduction of cardiovascular risk factors in children: "Heart Smart". In: Hetzel B, Berenson GS (eds): Cardiovascular risk factors in childhood: epidemiology and prevention. New York: Elsevier, 1987:103–121.

88. Bandura A. Social foundations of thought and action. A social cognitive theory. Englewood Cliffs, NJ: Prentice-Hall, 1986.

89. Williams CL, Carter BJ, Arnold CB, Wynder EL. Chronic disease risk factors among children. The "Know Your Body" study. Prev Med 1979;32:505–511.

90. Walter HJ, Hofman A, Connelly PA, Barrett LT, Kost KL. Primary prevention of chronic disease in childhood: changes in risk factors after one year of intervention. Am J Epidemiol 1985;122:772–781.

91. Walter HJ, Hofman A, Vaughn RD, Wynder EL. Modification of risk factors for coronary heart disease. Five-year results of a school-based intervention trial. N Engl J Med 1988;318:1093–1100.

92. Bush PJ, Zuckerman AE, Theiss PK, et al. Cardiovascular risk factor prevention in black schoolchildren: two-year results of the "Know Your Body" program. Am J Epidemiol 1989;129:466–482.

93. Zuckerman AE, Olevsky-Peleg E, Bush PJ, et al. Cardiovascular risk factors among black schoolchildren: comparisons among four Know Your Body studies. Prev Med 1989;18:113–132.

94. Stone EJ, Perry CL, Luepker RV. Synthesis of cardiovascular behavioral research for youth health promotion. Health Educ Quart 1989;16:155–169.

95. Evans RI, Raines BE, Owen AE. Formative evaluation in school-based health promotion investigations. Prev Med 1989;18:229–234.

96. Coates TJ, Jeffrey RW, Slinkard LA. Heart healthy eating and exercise: introducing and maintaining changes in health behaviors. Am J Public Health 1981;71:15–23.

97. Coates TJ, Barofsky I, Saylor KE, et al. Modifying the snack food consumption patterns of inner city high school students: the Great Sensations Study. Prev Med 1975; 14:234–247.

98. Perry CL, Mullis RM, Maile MC. Modifying the eating behavior of young children. J School Health 1985;55:399–402.

99. Perry CL, Luepker RV, Murray DM, et al. Parent involvement with children's health

promotion: a one-year follow-up of the Minnesota Home Team. Health Educ Quart 1989;16:171-180.

100. Nader PR, Sallis JF, Patterson TL, et al. A family approach to cardiovascular risk reduction: results from the San Diego Family Health Project. Health Educ Quart 1989;16:229-244.

101. Parcel GS, Simons-Morton BG, O'Hara NM, Baranowski T, Kolbe LJ, Bee DE. School promotion of healthful diet and exercise behavior: an integration of organizational change and social learning theory interventions. J School Health 1987;57:150-156.

102. Simons-Morton BG, Parcel GS, O'Hara NM. Implementing organizational changes to promote healthful diet and physical activity at school. Health Educ Quart 1989; 15:115-130.

103. Ellison RC, Capper AL, Goldberg RJ, Witschi JC, Stare FJ. The environmental component: changing school food service to promote cardiovascular health. Health Educ Quart 1989;16:285-297.

104. Puska P, Vartiainen E, Pallonen U, et al. The North Karelia Youth Project: evaluation of two years of intervention on health behavior and CVD risk factors among 13-15 year old children. Prev Med 1982;11:550-570.

105. Ehnholm C, Huttunen JK, Pietinen P, et al. Effect of diet on serum lipoproteins in a population with a high risk of coronary heart disease. N Engl J Med 1982;307:850-855.

106. Bricker JT, Schieken RM, Strong WB. Pediatric preventive cardiology clinics. Am J Dis Child 1989;142:953-956.

107. West R, Gibson P, Lloyd J. Treatment of homozygous familial hypercholesterolemia: an informative sibship. Br Med J 1985;291:1079-1080.

108. Illingworth DR, Bacon S. Treatment of heterozygous familial hypercholesterolemia with lipid-lowering drugs. Arteriosclerosis 1989;9(suppl I):I121-I124.

109. Stein EA. Treatment of familial hypercholesterolemia with drugs in children. Arteriosclerosis. 1989;9(suppl I):I145-I151.

110. Schieken RM, Clarke WR, Lauer RM. Left ventricular hypertrophy in children with blood pressures in the upper quintile of the distribution. The Muscatine Study. Hypertension 1981;3:669-675.

111. Task Force on Blood Pressure Control in Children. Report of the Second Task Force on Blood Pressure Control in Children—1987. Pediatrics 1987;79:1-25.

112. Voors AW, Webber LS, Berenson GS. Time course studies of blood pressure in children—the Bogalusa Heart Study. Am J Epidemiol 1979;109:320-334.

113. Lauer RM, Clarke WR, Beaglehole R. Level, trend, and variability of blood pressure during childhood: the Muscatine study. Circulation 1984;69:242-249.

114. Hait HI, Lemeshow S, Rosenman KD. A longitudinal study of blood pressure in a national survey of children. Am J Public Health 1982;72:1285-1287.

115. Gyarfas I. Blood pressure in childhood and adolescence. Results from an international collaborative study on juvenile hypertension. Acta Paediatr Scand Suppl 1985; 318:11-22.

116. Dahl M, Uhari M, Viikari J, et al. Atherosclerosis precursors in Finnish children and adolescents. III. Blood pressure. Acta Paediatr Scand Suppl 1985;318:89-102.

117. Gutgesell M, Terrell G, Labarthe D. Pediatric blood pressure: ethnic comparisons in a primary care center. Hypertension 1981;3:39-47.

118. Levinson S, Liu K, Stamler J, et al. Ethnic differences in blood pressure and heart rate of Chicago school children. Am J Epidemiol 1985;122:366-377.

119. Berenson GS, Cresanta JL, Webber LS. High blood pressure in the young. Ann Rev Med 1984;5:535-560.

120. Morrison JA, Khoury P, Kelly K, et al. Studies of blood pressure in schoolchildren (ages 6-19) and their parents in an integrated suburban school district. Am J Epidemiol 1980;111:156-165.

121. Guinn B, Crofts A. Blood pressure of low income, Mexican-American children. J School Health 1986;56:286-288.

122. Munoz S, Munoz H, Zambrano F. Blood pressure in a school-age population. Mayo Clin Proc 1980;55:623-632.

123. Whincup PH, Cook DG, Shaper AG, Macfarlane DJ, Walker M. Blood pressure in British children: associations with adult blood pressure and cardiovascular mortality. Lancet 198;2:890-893.

124. Burke GL, Webber LS, Shear CL, et al. Sources of error in measurement of children's blood pressure in a large epidemiologic study: Bogalusa Heart Study. J Chron Dis 1987;40:83–89.

125. Park MK, Menard SM. Accuracy of blood pressure measurement by the Dinamap monitor in infants and children. Pediatrics 1987;79:907–914.

126. Voors AW, Webber LS, Frerichs RR, et al. Body height and mass as determinants of basal blood pressure in children—the Bogalusa Heart Study. Am J Epidemiol 1977;106:101–108.

127. Smoak CG, Burke GL, Webber LS, Harsha DW, Srinivasan SR, Berenson GS. Relation of obesity to clustering of cardiovascular disease risk factors in children and young adults. The Bogalusa Heart Study. Am J Epidemiol 1987;125:364–372.

128. Clarke WR, Woolson RF, Lauer RM. Changes in ponderosity and blood pressure in childhood: the Muscatine Study. Am J Epidemiol 1986;124:195–206.

129. Rames LK, Clarke WR, Connor WE, Reiter MA, Lauer RM. Normal blood pressures and the evaluation of sustained blood pressure elevation in childhood: the Muscatine Study. Pediatrics 1978;61:245–251.

130. Hofman A, Hazelbroek A, Valkenburg HA. A randomized trial of sodium intake and blood pressure in newborn infants. JAMA 1983;250:370–374.

131. Hofman A, Valkenburg HA, Vaandrager GJ. Increased blood pressure in schoolchildren related to high sodium levels in drinking water. J Epidemiol Comm Health 1980;34:179–181.

132. Cooper R, Soltero I, Liu K, Berkson D, Levinson S, Stamler J. The association between urinary sodium excretion and blood pressure in children. Circulation 1980;62:97–101.

133. Frank GC, Webber LS, Nicklas TA, Berenson GS. Sodium, potassium, calcium, magnesium, and phosphorus intakes of infants and children: Bogalusa Heart Study. J Am Diet Assoc 1988;88:801–807.

134. Butcher AH, Frank GC, Harsha DW, et al. Heart Smart: a school heath program meeting the 1990 objectives for the nation. Health Educ Q 1988;5:17–34.

135. Connor SL, Connor WE, Henry H, Sexton G, Keenan EJ. The effects of familial relationships, age, body weight, and diet on blood pressure and the 24 hour urinary excretion of sodium, potassium, and creatinine in men, women and children of randomly selected families. Circulation 1984;70:76–85.

136. Jenner DA, English DR, Vandongen R, et al. Diet and blood pressure in 9-year-old Australian children. Am J Clin Nutr 1988;47:1052–1059.

137. Burns TL, Lauer RM. Blood pressure in children. In: Pierpont ME, Moller JH (eds): The genetics of cardiovascular disease. Boston: Martinus Nijhoff, 1986:305–307.

138. Zinner SH, Rosner B, Oh W, Kass EH. Significance of blood pressure in infancy. Familial aggregation and predictive effect on later blood pressure. Hypertension 1985;7:411–416.

139. Clarke WR, Schrott HG, Burns TL, Sing CF, Lauer RM. Aggregation of blood pressure in the families of children with labile high systolic blood pressure. Am J Epidemiol 1986;123:67–80.

140. Shear CL, Burke GL, Freedman GS, Berenson GS. Value of childhood blood pressure measurements and family history in predicting future blood pressure status: results from 8 years of followup in the Bogalusa Heart Study. Pediatrics 1986;77:862–869.

141. Patterson TL, Kaplan RM, Sallis JF, Nader PR. Aggregation of blood pressure in Anglo-American and Mexican-American families. Prev Med 1987;16:616–625.

142. Parker FC, Croft JB, Cresanta JL, et al. The association between cardiovascular response tasks and future blood pressure levels in children: Bogalusa Heart Study. Am Heart J 1987;113:1174–1179.

143. Siegel JM, Leitch CJ. Behavioral factors and blood pressure in adolescence: the Tacoma Study. Am J Epidemiol 1981;113:171–181.

144. Ewart CK, Harris WL, Iwata MM, Coates TJ, Bullock R, Simon B. Feasibility and effectiveness of school-based relaxation in lowering blood pressure. Health Psychol 1987;6:399–416.

145. Fraser GE, Phillips RL, Harris R. Physical fitness and blood pressure in school children. Circulation 1983;67:405–412.

146. Sallis JF, Patterson TL, McKenzie TL, Buono MJ, Atkins CJ, Nader PR. Stability of systolic blood pressure reactivity to exercise in young children. J Dev Behav Pediatr 1989;10:38–43.

147. Hagberg JM, Goldring D, Ehsani AA, et al. Effect of exercise training on the blood pressure and hemodynamic features of hypertensive adolescents. Am J Cardiol 1983;52:763–768.

148. Gifford RW Jr, Kirkendall W, O'Connor DT, Weidman W. Office evaluation of hypertension. Circulation 1989;79:721–731.

149. Frank GC, Farris RP, Ditmarsen P, Voors AW, Berenson GS. An approach to primary preventive treatment for children with high blood pressure in a total community. J Am Coll Nutr 1982;1:357–374.

150. Riopel DA, Bolerth RC, Coates TJ, Miller WW, Weidman WH, Hennekens CH. Coronary risk factor modification in children: smoking. Circulation 1986;74:1192A–1194A.

151. Baugh JG, Hunter SM, Webber LS, Berenson GS. Developmental trends of first cigarette smoking experience of children: the Bogalusa Heart Study. Am J Public Health 1982;72:1161–1164.

152. Hunter SM, Baugh JG, Webber LS, Sklov MC, Berenson GS. Social learning effects on trial and adoption of cigarette smoking in children: the Bogalusa Heart Study. Prev Med 1982;11:29–42.

153. Krohn MD, Naughton MJ, Skinner MF, Becker SL, Lauer RM. Social disaffection, friendship patterns and adolescent cigarette use: the Muscatine Study. J School Health 1986;56:146–150.

154. Byckling T, Sauri T. Atherosclerosis precursors in Finnish children and adolescents. XII. Smoking behaviour and its determinants in 12–18-year-old subjects. Acta Paediatr Scand Suppl 1985;318:195–203.

155. Freedman DS, Srinivisan SR, Shear CL, et al. Cigarette smoking initiation and longitudinal changes in serum lipids and lipoproteins in early adulthood: the Bogalusa Heart Study. Am J Epidemiol 1986;124:207–219.

156. Hunter SM, Croft JB, Burke GL, Parker FC, Webber LS, Berenson GS. Longitudinal patterns of cigarette smoking and smokeless tobacco use in youth: the Bogalusa Heart Study. Am J Public Health 1986;76:193–195.

157. Parcel GS, Bruhn JG, Murray JL. Effects of a health education curriculum on the smoking intentions of preschool children. Health Educ Q 1984;11:49–56.

158. Tell GS, Vellar OD. Noncommunicable disease risk factor intervention in Norwegian adolescents: the Oslo Youth Study. In: Hetzel B, Berenson GS (eds): Cardiovascular risk factors in childhood: epidemiology and prevention. New York: Elsevier, 1987:203–217.

159. Vartiainen E, Pallonen U, McAlister A, Koskela K, Puska P. Four year follow-up results of the smoking prevention program in the North Karelia Project. Prev Med 1986;15:692–698.

160. Flay BR, Keopke D, Thomson SJ, Santi S, Best JA, Brown KS. Six-year followup of the First Waterloo School Smoking Prevention Trial. Am J Public Health 1989;79:1371–1376.

161. Telama R, Viikari J, Valimaki I, et al. Atherosclerosis precursors in Finnish children and adolescents. X. Leisure-time physical activity. Acta Paediatr Scand Suppl 1985;318:169–180.

162. Saris WH. The assessment and evaluation of daily physical activity in children. A review. Acta Paediatr Scand Suppl 1985;318:37–48.

163. Riopel DA, Boerth RC, Coates TJ, Hennekens CH, Miller WW, Weidman WH. Coronary risk factor modification in children: exercise. Circulation 1986;74:1189A–1191A.

164. Sallis JF, Patterson TL, Buono MJ, Nader PR. Relation of cardiovascular fitness and physical activity to cardiovascular disease risk factors in children and adults. Am J Epidemiol 1988;127:933–941.

165. Strazzullo P, Cappuccio FP, Trevisan M, et al. Leisure time physical activity and blood pressure in schoolchildren. Am J Epidemiol 1988;127:726–733.

166. Burns TL, Moll PP, Lauer RM. The relation between ponderosity and coronary risk factors in children and their relatives. The Muscatine Ponderosity Family Study. Am J Epidemiol 1989;129:973–987.

167. Shear CL, Freedman DS, Burke GL, Harsha DW, Webber LS, Berenson GS. Secular

trends in obesity in early life: the Bogalusa Heart Study. Am J Public Health 1988;78:75–77.

168. Price JH, Desmond SM, Ruppert ES, Stelzer CM. Pediatricians' perceptions and practices regarding childhood obesity. Am J Prev Med 1989;2:95–103.

169. Epstein LH, Wing RR. Behavioral treatment of childhood obesity. Psychol Bull 1987;101:331–342.

170. Brownell KD, Kelman JH, Stunkard AJ. Treatment of obese children with and without their mothers: changes in weight and blood pressure. Pediatrics 1983;71:515–523.

14

management of risk in early and mid-adulthood

The major risk indicators for coronary artery disease (CAD) have been discussed in detail in earlier chapters. In chapter 13, the appearance of differentials in risk during childhood and adolescence was described. Because many young adults have no symptoms, they frequently do not have an ongoing relationship with a physician and the health care system, and do not receive continuing evaluation of their CAD risk. Further, young adults often have the responsibility for establishing health habits for their children, making it doubly important that health promotion efforts reach these two populations.

As individuals enter the middle third of their lives, some will seek evaluation even in the absence of symptoms. In many developed countries, guidelines for screening have been established for the major diseases, based on the current understanding of risk, feasibility, and cost of detection at different stages of the disease, and the efficacy and cost of treatment (1–4). Given these parameters, it is not surprising that unanimity does not exist in screening policies for many chronic diseases.

In this chapter, current policies for detection and management of CAD risk during early and mid-adulthood are re-viewed. Consideration of these topics in elderly individuals is addressed in Chapter 15.

AGE, GENDER, AND DIABETES

As described in earlier chapters, CAD risk rises in both women and men with increasing age. At any given age in early and mid-adulthood, men have at least twice the risk for CAD events as women. As indicated in Chapter 7, there have been no studies to date demonstrating significant reductions in CAD risk among diabetics who receive more vigorous management of their blood glucose levels.

Persons at higher risk because of these three factors should receive even more attention to modification of risk from modifiable factors, such as lipids/lipoprotein disorders, high blood pressure, smoking, physical inactivity, obesity, and sociobehavioral, environmental, and hematologic parameters.

LIPIDS AND LIPOPROTEINS

DETECTION OF DISORDERS

In 1987, the European Atherosclerosis Society published recommendations for

200

detection of lipid and lipoprotein disorders in adults. Based on input from scientists in 19 nations, they suggested a combination of population and individual intervention efforts. Screening of all adults is advised, with consideration of dietary modification for all persons having a blood total cholesterol in excess of 200 mg/dl (5).

In the USA, the National Cholesterol Education Program (NCEP) Expert Panel reported in 1988 their recommendations for the detection, evaluation, and treatment of dyslipidemias in adults (6). They recommended screening for blood total cholesterol in all persons age 20 or older. In those with values below 200 mg/dl, a repeat determination should occur again within five years. For those with initial values of 240 mg/dl and above, a lipoprotein analysis should be done. In measuring HDL-cholesterol and triglycerides, LDL-cholesterol can be calculated and used as a basis for further action. For individuals with values between 200 and 239 mg/dl, the presence of CAD or two or more other CAD risk indicators (one of which is male gender, see Table 3.5) indicates the need for lipoprotein analysis.

TREATMENT

When adults have calculated LDL-cholesterol levels of 130 mg/dl or more, dietary modification should be employed as the initial treatment modality. As indicated in Table 3.6, NCEP guidelines recommend that total dietary fat represent less than 30% of caloric intake, with saturated fat intake being less than 10% of all calories. Reductions in these constituents can be balanced by increases in complex carbohydrate intake. Consumption of dietary cholesterol should not exceed 300 mg/day; total calories should be adjusted to achieve and maintain desirable weight. If therapeutic goals are not met within three months, referral to a registered dietitian is indicated to facilitate adoption of step 2, which features a reduction in saturated fat to less than 7% of total calories and intake of less than 200 mg/day of dietary cholesterol.

Particular attention to limitations in specific food subgroups is important. While turkey, chicken, and fish contain cholesterol, their saturated fat content is dramatically lower than that of beef, pork, processed and organ meats. Milk and dairy products are advertised as having a given percentage of fat by weight (e.g., 2% milk, dairy dessert 97% fat free). However, the percentage of calories from fat in these products is considerably higher. For example, one cup of "low-fat" (2% by weight) milk contains 120 calories, 35% of which come from fat. A cup of whole milk has 150 calories, 50% of which are fat. In contrast, skim (nonfat) milk (80 calories per cup) can be recommended as an excellent source of protein and calcium. The latter nutrient is particularly important in women during their childbearing and later years. Similarly, one cup of ice cream (350 calories) has 60% fat; ice milk has only half the calories, of which only 23% come from fat. Cheese often contains large amounts of saturated fat; for example, in cheddar, half of all calories come from saturated fat, and another 25% arise from unsaturated fats. Low-fat cottage cheese has fewer calories, 7% of which are from saturated fat, and an equal amount are from unsaturated fats (7).

Baking, broiling, and steaming are preferable to deep-fat frying. Butter fat, lard, and beef fat should be avoided, as should "tropical oils" (coconut, palm, palm kernel) which are very high in saturated fat. Food labeling indicating hydrogenation of vegetable oils is a reliable indicator of high amounts of saturated fat. Less-solid preparations of margarine are preferable to the stick form. While egg yolk consumption should be minimized, egg whites can be used freely.

Fruits and vegetables are low in calories and high in fiber, vitamins, and minerals. Dried beans and peas provide protein and fiber; breads, cereals, and rice are generally low in fat and can be high in complex carbohydrates. Most nuts are high in fat (and therefore high in calories), but the fat in many nuts is mainly unsaturated. Minimization of other snacks and desserts will facilitate weight optimization.

The step 1 diet (30% fat) should be maintained indefinitely; diet education should be reinforced at least every three months during the first year and semiannually thereafter. If an elevated LDL-cholesterol is the only abnormality, the cost of surveillance can be minimized by using only total cholesterol determinations along with periodic assessment of hepatic and renal function. If the concerted efforts of physician, clinic staff, and consultant dietitian are insufficient to optimize lipid levels, drug treatment can be considered (Chapter 3).

HIGH BLOOD PRESSURE

DETECTION

Although most adults in the USA and Canada know their blood pressure (BP) or have had it measured, it is nevertheless recommended that blood pressure be measured at each encounter with health care professionals, since the prevalence of hypertension increases linearly with age. Chapter 4 outlines proper measurement equipment and technique; classification on the basis of two or more readings on two or more occasions is listed in Table 4.1. Follow-up frequency for adults, based on initial BP, as recommended by the USA National High Blood Pressure Program Joint National Committee is shown below (Table 14.1) (8).

TREATMENT

The goal of treatment is to achieve and maintain BP below 140/90 mm Hg.

Table 14.1. Frequency of Repeat BP Determination in Adults

Initial BP (mm Hg)	Recommended Follow-up Frequency
Diastolic BP	
< 85	Within 2 years
85–89	Within 1 year
90–104	Confirm within 2 months
105–114	Evaluate within 2 weeks
>114	Evaluate/treat immediately
Systolic (when DBP < 90)	
< 140	Within 2 years
140–199	Confirm within 2 months
> 199	Evaluate within 2 weeks

Hygienic therapy should be instituted in all cases of hypertension (5). Even if it is inadequate when used alone, it should be retained after pharmacologic treatment (outlined in Chapter 4) is begun.

A program including dietary modification and vigorous physical activity will facilitate body weight optimization, which in turn leads to significant BP reduction. Restriction of sodium, when coupled with weight loss, acts independently to lower BP in approximately half of all persons. In addition, reduction of fat and alcohol consumption will facilitate BP normalization. Dietary calcium supplementation may lower BP in young people with mildly elevated BP, particularly in those with high plasma parathyroid hormone or low serum total calcium (9).

SMOKING

The graded association of cigarette smoking with CAD risk is indisputable, as indicated in Chapter 5. Efforts at smoking cessation should begin as early in adulthood as possible, but women and men in this age group seem much less interested in quittng. A review and evaluation of smoking cessation methods used in Can-

Table 14.2. Smoking Cessation Methods

Clinical programs
   Physician counseling
   Hypnosis
   Nicotine chewing gum
Behavioral methods
   Aversive procedures (rapid smoking, shock
   therapy)
   Self-management (stimulus control, books)
Worksite policies
   Educational campaigns
   Incentives for quitting
   Restriction/elimination of smoking areas

ada and the USA was recently published (10). In the report of the Study Group of the European Atherosclerosis Society, recommendations were made for government intervention, education of health professionals and the general public, and control of smoking in public and workplaces. The report also noted that social pressures for smoking adoption by young persons should be vigorously opposed (5). A list of some of these methods appears in Table 14.2.

PHYSICAL ACTIVITY

In addition to its effects on lipid and lipoprotein parameters, enhanced BP control, and facilitation of weight control, regular aerobic physical activity makes an independent contribution to the reduction of CAD risk (see Chapter 8).

An exercise prescription can be calculated from exercise test parameters, or (in the absence of testing) from age-predicted maximal heart rates. To optimize adherence, the individual should perceive a moderate level of exertion during physical activity. Adherence to an exercise program involves many factors during early and mid-adulthood. These include enjoyment of the chosen activity, weather conditions, time and location convenience, support from family and friends, and

smoking status. The European Atherosclerosis Society has encouraged governments to provide cycle paths in urban areas, reserve thoroughfares as pedestrian precincts, and develop forest pathways and other rural exercise facilities to promote the adoption of healthy exercise habits (5).

OBESITY

As described in chapter 9, the body weight parameter most closely associated with the incidence of CAD events is weight gain from the early to middle adult years (11), making the avoidance of obesity an important factor in CAD prevention. Toward that end, development and continuation of aerobic exercise and prudent eating habits are paramount.

As part of the National Health and Nutrition Examination Survey, participants aged 25 to 74 were weighed ten years after their initial examination. The incidence of major weight gain was highest among persons aged 25 to 34, was twice as high in women as in men, and was greatest in those already obese at the initial examination (12).

SOCIOBEHAVIORAL AND ENVIRONMENTAL FACTORS

Chapter 10 describes in detail the many sociobehavioral and environmental factors that are associated with the incidence of CAD events. It appears that a strong sense of self, an ability to cope with major life events and daily hassles, and the availability of satisfying interpersonal relationships with persons supportive of good health habits are associated with lower rates of CAD. Minimizing exposure to environmental stressors, such as occupational toxins, air pollution, and cigarette smoke from others also enhances one's ability to avoid or postpone symptomatic CAD.

HORMONAL FACTORS

Women who take oral contraceptives and smoke cigarettes have a dramatically increased relative risk for myocardial infarction. At the time of menopause, various indicators of CAD risk worsen, including all lipid and lipoprotein parameters and blood pressure. Replacement estrogen therapy can counteract these adverse tendencies, while concurrent progestogen treatment weakens the favorable effects of estrogen. Estrogen therapy has the added advantage of minimizing the risk of osteoporosis, but the ultimate decision on postmenopausal hormonal treatment should be mindful of any genetic history of cancer and CAD, as well as the level of CAD risk posed by other factors, such as smoking, diabetes, hypertension, and dyslipidemias. Chapter 11 discusses these factors in more detail.

HEMATOLOGIC FACTORS

In the absence of definite CAD, the use of aspirin or other platelet-active agents in the young adult is questionable. In the USA Physicians Health Study, there were 44% fewer myocardial infarctions in the group randomized to 325 mg aspirin every other day, but this advantage accrued only to men age 50 and older. In the presence of diabetic retinopathy, poorly controlled hypertension, or a family history of hemorrhagic stroke, aspirin therapy may be contraindicated. Chapter 12 further explores the mechanisms involved in hematologic modification of CAD risk.

REFERENCES

1. Canadian Task Force on the Periodic Health Examination. The periodic health examination. Can Med Assoc J 1979;121:1193–1254.

2. American College of Physicians Medical Practice Committee. Periodic health examination: guide for designing individualized preventive health care in the asymptomatic patient. Ann Intern Med 1981;95:729–732.

3. Canadian Task Force on the Periodic Health Examination. Update: the periodic health examination. Can Med Assoc J 1984; 130:1276–1292.

4. Frame PS. A critical review of adult health maintenance. Part I: Prevention of atherosclerotic diseases. J Fam Pract 1986;22:341–346.

5. European Atherosclerosis Society Study Group. Strategies for the prevention of coronary heart disease: a policy statement of the European Atherosclerosis Society. Eur Heart J 1987;8:77–88.

6. The Expert Panel. Report of the National Cholesterol Education Program Expert Panel on detection, evaluation and treatment of high blood cholesterol in adults. Arch Intern Med 1988;148:36–69.

7. Kwiterovich PO Jr. Beyond cholesterol. Baltimore: Johns Hopkins University Press, 1989.

8. Joint National Committee. The 1988 report of the Joint National Committee on detection, evaluation, and treatment of high blood pressure. Arch Intern Med 1988;148:1023–1038.

9. Grobbee DE, Hofman A. Effect of calcium supplementation on diastolic blood pressure in young people with mild hypertension. Lancet 1986;2:703–707.

10. Schwartz JL. Review and evaluation of smoking cessation methods: the United States and Canada, 1978–1985. Washington, DC: Department of Health and Human Services, 1987. NIH Publication no. 87–2940.

11. Hubert HB, Feinleib M, McNamara PM, Castelli WP. Obesity as an independent risk factor for cardiovascular disease: A 26-year followup of participants in the Framingham Heart Study. Circulation 1983;67:968–977.

12. Williamson DF, Kahn HS, Remington PL, Anda RF. The 10-year incidence of overweight and major weight gain in US adults. Arch Intern Med 1990;150:665–672.

15

CAD risk considerations in late adulthood

In many developed countries, the most rapidly growing segment of the population consists of women and men in the latter third of their lives. Although malignant neoplasms, stroke, and infectious diseases are important contributors to mortality in this age group, coronary artery disease (CAD) remains the leading cause of death in persons 65 years and older in the USA (1). In persons 85 years of age and older, CAD deaths are three times more common than cancer deaths, and mortality from stroke exceeds that from cancer (2).

In 1985, the average life expectancy for a person aged 65 living in the USA was 19.5 years for women and 15.1 years for men. Throughout their remaining years, many older persons will continue to live independently and take great interest in promotion of their health. The cost of reparative care for cardiovascular diseases in this age group is high (more than $7 billion in the USA in 1980 (2) and more than 40% of the health care budget in Japan in 1981) (3). Efforts to educate and motivate older men and women to adopt and maintain favorable health habits appears to be highly desirable (4). Before health care resources are allocated to such a task, however, data

should demonstrate that modification of CAD risk indicators leads to reduced CAD morbidity and mortality in older persons.

In this chapter, the association of risk indicators with CAD events is explored. Where evidence is persuasive, recommendations for cardiovascular health promotion in the elderly are offered.

PATHOPHYSIOLOGY

With aging, arterial walls stiffen as a result of thickening of the intima, lipid and calcium accumulation in the media, and decreased elastin content in the adventitia (5, 6). This leads to less regulatory vasodilation in coronary arteries as well as decreased compliance in peripheral arteries and increasing blood pressure. Left ventricular myocardial compliance decreases, reducing diastolic filling (7, 8). Maximal heart rate decreases one beat per minute with each advancing year (9, 10).

CLINICAL ASSESSMENT

The physiological changes that accompany aging may mask the appearance of CAD pathology. Despite lower maximal work capacity, smaller increases in heart rate, and greater rises in systolic blood pressure, exercise testing is useful in detection of CAD in older persons (11). Rest and exercise electrocardiographic evidence of ischemia may be masked by left ventricular hypertrophy, bundle branch block, or other S-T segment and T wave disorders, as well as the use of digitalis, quinidine, and other drugs. Radionuclide ventriculography and thallium myocardial perfusion imaging will improve the predictive value of exercise testing for CAD in the elderly (12, 13).

Because of impaired pain sensation, memory, or depression (14), symptoms may be underreported, leading to a failure to diagnose angina pectoris or myocardial infarction (MI). In a Welsh study of 777 elderly MI patients, the spectrum of presentation changed significantly with increasing age. Syncope, stroke, and acute confusion were often the sole presenting symptom. In persons 85 years and older, an atypical presentation became the rule (15, 16). As noted in Chapter 17, more than one-third of all elderly subjects of the Framingham Study with MI had no symptoms or did not come to medical attention during their event. In such individuals, prognosis was no better than in those with symptomatic MI (17). Similarly, the sedentary life of many older persons may mask or mimic manifestations of heart failure (18).

EPIDEMIOLOGY

Using the World Health Organization mortality data base, Uemura has compared CAD death rates in more than 30 countries during 10-year periods from the mid-1970s to the mid-1980s. Particularly notable was the observation that CAD rates varied dramatically between countries; the ratio between countries with highest and lowest rates was 6.5 in men

and 5.8 in women. At the higher end were Ireland, Northern Ireland, Scotland, and Finland, while Japan, France, and southern European countries had the lowest rates. During the 10-year periods studied, many countries had a marked decrease in CAD rates, as shown in Table 15.1 (3).

It may be noted that CAD rate changes were more favorable in women in each country, and that this differential was particularly prominent in Scandinavian and other northern European nations. Table 15.2 indicates the median percentage changes by age during the same periods in the 32 countries analyzed.

While percentage improvement declined somewhat with age, it is clear that persons 65 years and older can make substantial improvement in preventing car-

Table 15.1.   Percentage Changes in Age-Standardized Death Rates in Selected Countries[a]

Country/Area	Period[b]	Men	Women
United States	2	− 33.9	− 37.0
Austria	3	− 27.9	− 28.5
Canada	3	− 26.2	− 27.3
Belgium	3	− 21.0	− 22.6
Japan	4	− 20.7	− 23.2
New Zealand	3	− 15.7	− 16.1
Denmark	3	− 12.2	− 20.3
Sweden	3	− 11.4	− 24.2
Scotland	4	− 10.2	− 12.2
Norway	3	− 8.6	− 18.4
Finland	3	− 6.8	− 10.0
Northern Ireland	4	− 6.7	− 10.9
Federal Republic of Germany	4	− 4.1	− 12.0
Czechoslovakia	3	− 1.5	− 7.9
Yugoslavia	1	− 0.7	− 15.2
Ireland	2	+ 1.7	− 10.2
Iceland	3	+ 2.4	− 7.1
Poland	3	+ 9.9	+ 0.3

[a]Adopted from Uemura K. International trends in cardiovascular diseases in the elderly. Eur Heart J 1988;9(Suppl D):1–8.
[b]Comparison periods: 1 = 1971–1981; 2 = 1972–1982; 3 = 1973–1983; 4 = 1974–1984.

Table 15.2. Median Percentage Change in Cardiovascular Disease Mortality by Selected Ages[a]

Age (years)	Men	Women
40–44	− 22.4	− 34.5
45–49	− 17.8	− 30.6
50–54	− 16.8	− 27.1
55–59	− 10.0	− 23.9
60–64	− 12.0	− 22.2
65–69	− 14.8	− 22.6
70–74	− 15.8	− 21.9
75–79	− 10.2	− 22.0
80–84	− 10.8	− 17.6
85 and older	− 9.1	− 10.3

[a]Adopted from Uemura K. International trends in cardiovascular diseases in the elderly. Eur Heart J 1988;9(Suppl D):1–8.

diovascular deaths, although this study did not evaluate risk indicator changes in the various countries.

SPECIFIC CAD RISK INDICATORS

While a majority of studies have focused on persons in the first seven decades (19, 20), several studies have examined the association of CAD risk indicators with cardiovascular morbidity and mortality in older individuals. Surveillance for 17 years of participants in the Alameda County (California) who were 60–94 years of age at baseline, revealed that smoking, change in body weight, and a sedentary life were associated with all-cause mortality independent of age, race, and other CAD risk indicators (21).

Aronow and colleagues performed baseline evaluation on 192 men and 516 women between the ages of 63 and 97 (mean age = 82). After 24 to 44 months of surveillance, approximately 30% of women and men had experienced MI, ventricular fibrillation, or sudden cardiac death. In persons without prior evidence of CAD, multivariate analysis revealed that age, smoking, hypertension, diabetes, serum total cholesterol, HDL-cholesterol, and triglycerides independently predicted events. In persons with preexisting CAD, age, smoking, diabetes, serum total cholesterol, HDL-C, and triglycerides were independent predictors of the cardiac outcomes listed above (22).

In the following section, available evidence on the major indicators of CAD risk in the elderly are reviewed.

LIPIDS AND LIPOPROTEINS

Although Framingham investigators originally claimed little or no association between blood total cholesterol and CAD events in older persons, further analysis of the data showed that LDL-cholesterol and HDL-cholesterol were indeed significant independent predictors of CAD in the elderly in their prospective study spanning several decades (23). In the Rancho Bernardo (CA) Study, investigators found that total cholesterol levels were significant CAD predictors in both men and women 65 years of age and older. During a 10-year surveillance of women, aged 65 to 79, those who had an initial total cholesterol level of 260 mg/dl or more had a relative risk of 2.5, compared with women with lower values (24).

Trials of fat-modified diets in the elderly have been few in number. In the Los Angeles Veterans Administration Domiciliary Facility Study, men (mean age 65) participated in a randomized controlled trial of institutional feeding of a diet low in saturated fat and cholesterol. Although efficacy was more marked in younger men, those above the age of 65 consuming the healthier diet also had fewer atherosclerotic events during an 8.5-year surveillance (25). Other large-scale trials of dietary intervention have been concentrated in younger subjects (26). The European Atherosclerosis Society has suggested that "when risk factors are detected for the first time in older persons, less-intensive treatment may be appropriate" (27).

However, the guidelines issued by the USA National Cholesterol Education Program Expert Panel made no distinction by age in recommending cholesterol screening, dietary treatment, and pharmacologic intervention in adults. They acknowledge the aforementioned association of LDL-cholesterol and CAD events and cite clinical-trial evidence that improving the lipid and lipoprotein profile in persons with advanced CAD results in decreased CAD mortality. Finally, they emphasize that "the fact that age is associated with a high risk of CHD in the later decades of life means that the absolute magnitude of the potential benefits of intervention remains substantial in the elderly" (28).

HYPERTENSION

Applegate has discussed the large differences in hypertension prevalence among persons more than 65 years of age, attributing the disparities in part to threshold value selection and to the frequency and accuracy of measurements (29). Guidelines for measurement (30) are discussed in Chapter 4.

In general, diastolic blood pressure rises during the first six decades, after which it tends to decline (31) or remain constant (32), while systolic blood pressure continues to increase with age.

The influence of posture and postprandial effects have also been documented. In the Normative Aging Study of 1359 men, the difference between sitting and standing systolic and diastolic blood pressure (BP) values was a significant predictor of MI during a follow-up of more than eight years (33). Systolic BP drops of 10 to 20 mm Hg may be seen in elderly persons during the first hour after eating (34, 35); these changes may not be accompa-

nied by symptoms in robust older individuals (36).

When diastolic BP is below 95 mm Hg, but systolic BP is elevated, persons are nonetheless at increased risk for CAD morbidity and mortality. In the Framingham Study, relative risk was at least three in women and men aged 65 to 74 with a systolic BP of 190 mm Hg or more (37). After 30 years of follow-up, those with treated hypertension continued to display risks of that magnitude compared with normotensive subjects (38). Framingham investigators have confirmed the predictive value of left ventricular hypertrophy (LVH) for CAD events in persons aged 60 to 90, even after controlling for BP levels (39). In persons 90 years of age and older, electrocardiographic sensitivity for LVH is low, necessitating the use of echocardiography for its detection (40).

In the Hypertension Detection and Followup Program (HDFP) trial, persons with diastolic BP below 90 mm Hg at baseline, but with systolic BP above 160 mm Hg, had an 8-year death rate approximately twice that of individuals with the same diastolic BP but lower systolic values (41). The Systolic Hypertension in the Elderly Program (SHEP) multicenter trial pilot project followed more than 500 women and men 60 years of age and older (42). Completion of the full-scale trial should allow definitive recommendations to be made for older persons with isolated systolic hypertension.

In a study of 561 persons (82% female) aged 85 years or more in Tampere, Finland, investigators found that 5-year mortality was least in persons with systolic BP above 160 mm Hg and diastolic BP greater than 90 mm Hg. In this trial, even frail elderly persons were included, so that baseline BPs may have been a consequence of concurrent illness, although results did not differ by place of residence (home vs. institutional care) (43).

Treatment of hypertension in the elderly also begins with weight reduction and modification of diet to lower the intake of sodium and fat and to ensure adequate calcium intake; sodium restriction is probably more effective in older patients (44). Physical activity can be encouraged when not contraindicated by other chronic diseases.

When pharmacologic therapy is contemplated, other considerations arise. It is possible that regulation of cerebral blood flow may be critically dependent on a certain BP level. However, several large-scale trials have demonstrated the relative safety and clinical efficacy of treatment with drugs. These investigations include the Veterans Administration Study, the HDFP, the Australian Mild Hypertension Trial, and the European Working Party on Hypertension in the Elderly (EWPHE) trial. Overall results of these trials are shown in Figure 4.4 and are discussed in the accompanying paragraphs. In their recent review of these trials, Birkenhager and de Leeuw advocate thiazides in low doses and a mindful eye on potassium levels as initial therapy for most elderly hypertensives. They acknowledge the potential benefits of β-adrenergic blockers, calcium-channel blockers, and converting-enzyme inhibitors for this category of patients (45).

Diuretics offer documented efficacy (HDFP, EWPHE, SHEP feasibility trials) and relatively low cost, but they may worsen the lipid and lipoprotein profiles, and they can make the individual particularly susceptible to hypokalemia. β-blockers offer a concurrent antianginal effect and protection from MI and sudden cardiac death (46), but they may worsen the lipid and lipoprotein levels, increase peripheral vascular resistance, and worsen glucose control. Calcium-channel blockers are also useful in persons with angina, but their vasodilatory effects make postural

hypotension a concern in the elderly. Verapamil can cause or exacerbate conduction disorders and further impair cardiac contractility. Converting-enzyme inhibitors appear to be well tolerated in older patients, given their low probability of central nervous system side effects, but experience in the elderly is limited at present. Applegate has provided a useful table indicating the effects of these agents on peripheral resistance, cardiac output, lipids, glucose homeostasis, and left ventricular hypertrophy (29). Relative costs for these agents are found in Table 4.5 of this volume.

SMOKING

Although older smokers are less interested in quitting, evidence suggests that an excess risk of CAD mortality is associated with persistent smoking. (47) Subjects in the Chicago Stroke Study were urban poor men and women, initially aged 65 to 74 years, who were not institutionalized. During the 5-year study, the relative risk of CAD death was 1.5 times greater in smokers (48). A similar relative risk was present in Framingham men, aged 65 to 94 years, who smoked more than 40 cigarettes per day (38). In the SHEP pilot project, men and women (mean age 72 years) who were current smokers were two to three times more likely to have a first CAD event, MI, or sudden cardiac death (42).

Recent advances in the understanding and implementation of smoking cessation are discussed in Chapter 5.

DIABETES

The prevalence of diabetes mellitus increases with age; 10% of USA residents aged 60 have diabetes; prevalence increases to 16 to 20% by age 80. An additional 20% have age-related hyperglycemia (49).

The independent contribution of diabetes to CAD risk was particularly pronounced in older women subjects in the Framingham Study (50). In addition to the risk of CAD events, older women with insulin-dependent diabetes mellitus were at significantly higher risk for development of congestive heart failure (51). After 30 years of follow-up, blood glucose level was highly correlated with CAD incidence in women and men aged 65 to 94 years (23). Glucose metabolism becomes progressively impaired with aging. Elderly men and women who were more than 40% overweight were twice as likely to be diabetic (52). Unfortunately, there is little evidence currently that closer control of hyperglycemia reduces the individual's risk of CAD (38). This fact adds additional impetus for normalization of lipids, lipoproteins, blood pressure, and weight in the elderly (53).

PHYSICAL ACTIVITY

As indicated in Chapter 8, the majority of studies linking physical activity levels with CAD have been done in young and middle-aged men (54). However, Paffenbarger and colleagues included men up to age 74 in their studies of San Francisco longshoremen and of Harvard alumni. In the former study population, men aged 65 to 74 years, who had expended 8500 kcal/week at work, had only two-thirds the CAD mortality rate of those with less-energetic duties (55). Among 16,936 Harvard alumni aged 65 to 74 years, those with habitual and leisure exercise expenditure of 2000 kcal/week or more had a relative risk of 0.51 of CAD events during 12 to 16 years of surveillance compared to less-active men (56).

In the Honolulu Heart Program, men age 65 and older who were most active had a relative risk less than half of those with more sedentary lives (57). In the Framingham Heart Study, less-active men, aged 55 to 64 years, had a relative risk of CAD incidence 1.3 times higher than more active

subjects. An identical relative risk was seen in men aged 45 to 54 years (58); no data have been provided for men 65 years and older (38).

Physical activity was also associated with a reduced risk of cardiac arrest in a case-control study of Seattle, Washington residents. Compared with those with the highest intensity of physical activity, those women and men, aged 60 years and older, who were most sedentary were at more than double the risk for primary cardiac arrest (59).

The exercise prescription is calculated as it is for younger persons (Chapter 8). A longer warm-up period preceding exercise is recommended. Davidson and Maloney found that light calisthenics are both safe and useful in elderly persons, even in those recovering from MI (60). Davidson and Murphy found that women and men, aged 65 years and older, can improve their level of fitness and cardiac risk indicators substantially by participation in an exercise-based cardiac rehabilitation program after MI or coronary artery bypass surgery (61).

OBESITY

As indicated in Chapter 9, obesity adversely affects other CAD risk indicators. Further, recent evidence from the Framingham Study confirms that obesity makes a strong, independent contribution to CAD development. In women, aged 65 to 94 years, relative risk is increased when relative weight exceeds 120% of desirable levels. In men of the same ages, this effect is noted at the same level; when relative weight exceeds 135%, risk doubles (38).

SOCIOBEHAVIORAL FACTORS

Gentry and colleagues recently reviewed a variety of behavioral, cognitive, and emotional considerations in the development and treatment of CAD in the elderly (62). In one study, cognitive function improved after successful treatment of hypertension (63). Social support appears to have a beneficial effect in reduction of all-cause and cardiovascular mortality (64, 65), but the "coronary-prone (type A)" behavior pattern is not associated with increased risk in elderly persons (66).

HEMATOLOGIC FACTORS

Chapter 12 discusses the use of antiplatelet therapy for the prevention of CAD and its recurrence, but few primary prevention studies have included older subjects (67).

In the USA Physicians' Health Study, only men aged 50 years and older had significant reduction in risk from alternate-day aspirin (325 mg) therapy (68).

DRUG TREATMENT CONSIDERATIONS

Because conduction system disorders and syncope are more common in the elderly, care must be taken in determining dosages for a number of cardiovascular medications, including calcium-channel blockers, β-blockers, digoxin, and antihypertensive agents (69). In addition, the metabolism of most drugs used for treating rhythm disorders is altered with aging (70).

REFERENCES

1. Fried LP, Bush TL. Morbidity as a focus of preventive health care in the elderly. Epidemiol Rev 1986;10:48–64.

2. Feinleib M, Gillum RF. Coronary heart disease in the elderly: the magnitude of the problem in the United States. In: Wenger NK, Furberg CD, Pitt E (eds): Coronary heart disease in the elderly. New York: Elsevier, 1986:29–56.

3. Uemura K. International trends in cardiovascular diseases in the elderly. Eur Heart J 1988;9(Suppl D):1–8.

4. Wenger NK, Marcus FI, O'Rourke RA. Cardiovascular disease in the elderly. J Am Coll Cardiol 1987;10:80A–87A.

5. Berman ND. Geriatric cardiology. Toronto: Collamore Press, 1982.

6. Roberts WC. The very elderly heart. In: Wenger NK, Furberg CD, Pitt E (eds): Coronary heart disease in the elderly. New York: Elsevier, 1986:233–248.

7. Gardin JM, Davidson DM, Rohan MK, et al. Relationship between age, body size, gender, and blood pressure and Doppler flow measurements in the aorta and pulmonary artery. Am Heart J 1987;113:101–109.

8. Gardin JM, Rohan MK, Davidson DM, et al. Doppler transmitral flow velocity parameters: relationship between age, body surface area, blood pressure and gender in normal subjects. Am J Noninvasive Cardiol 1987;1:3–10.

9. Fleg JL. The aging heart: anatomic and physiologic alterations. In: Wenger NK, Furberg CD, Pitt E (eds): Coronary heart disease in the elderly. New York: Elsevier, 1986:253–273.

10. Lakatta EG, Mitchell JH, Pomerance A, Rowe GG. Human aging: changes in structure and function. J Am Coll Cardiol 1987; 10:42A–47A.

11. Gaul G. Stress testing in persons above the age of 65 years: applicability and diagnostic value of a standardized maximal symptom-limited testing protocol. Eur Heart J 1984;5(suppl E):51–53.

12. Cobb FR, Higginbotham M, Mark D. Diagnosis of coronary disease in the elderly. In: Wenger NK, Furberg CD, Pitt E (eds): Coronary heart disease in the elderly. New York: Elsevier, 1986:303–319.

13. Lam JY, Chaitman BR, Glaenzer M, et al. Safety and diagnostic accuracy of dipyridamole thallium imaging in the elderly. J Am Coll Cardiol 1988;11:585–589.

14. Tresch DD, Folstein MF, Rabins PV, Hazzard WR. Prevalence and significance of cardiovascular disease and hypertension in elderly patients with dementia and depression. J Am Geriatr Soc 1985;33:530–537.

15. Bayer AJ, Chadha JS, Farag RR, Pathy MS J. Changing presentation of myocardial infarction with increasing old age. J Am Geriatr Soc 1986;34:263–266.

16. Gersh BJ. Clinical manifestations of coronary heart disease in the elderly. In: Wenger NK, Furberg CD, Pitt E (eds): Coronary heart disease in the elderly. New York: Elsevier, 1986:276–297.

17. Kannel WB, Abbott RD. Incidence and prognosis of unrecognized myocardial infarction: an update on the Framingham Study. N Engl J Med 1984;311:1144–1147.

18. Wenger NK, Franciosa JA, Weber KT. Heart failure. J Am Coll Cardiol 1987;10:73A–76A.

19. Chesney MA, Hunt JC, Applegate WB, Aronson MK, Davidson DM, Farrand M, et al. Primary and secondary prevention of coronary heart disease in the elderly. In: Wenger NK, Furberg CD, Pitt E (eds): Coronary heart disease in the elderly. New York: Elsevier, 1986:211–230.

20. Satler LF, Green CE, Wallace RB, Rackley CE. Coronary artery disease in the elderly. Am J Cardiol 1989;63:245–248.

21. Kaplan GA, Seeman TE, Cohen RD, Knudsen LP, Guralnik J. Mortality among the elderly in the Alameda County Study: behavioral and demographic risk factors. Am J Public Health 1987;77:307–312.

22. Aronow WS, Herzig AH, Etienne F, D'Alba P, Ronquillo J. 41-month follow-up of risk factors correlated with new coronary events in 708 elderly patients. J Am Geriatr Soc 1989;37:501–506.

23. Kannel WB, Doyle JT, Shephard RJ, Stamler J, Vokonas PS. Prevention of cardiovascular disease in the elderly. J Am Coll Cardiol 1987;10:25A–28A.

24. Barrett-Connor E, Suarez L, Khaw KT, Criqui MH, Wingard DL. Ischemic heart disease risk factors after age 50. J Chronic Dis 1984;37:903–908.

25. Dayton S, Pearce ML, Hashimoto S, Dixon WJ, Tomiyasu U. A controlled clinical trial of a diet high in unsaturated fat in preventing complications of atherosclerosis. Circulation 1969;39/40(suppl II):1–63.

26. Hjermann I. Dietary trials for the prevention of coronary heart disease. Eur Heart J 1987;8(Suppl E):39–44.

27. European Atheroscelerosis Society Study Group. Strategies for the prevention of coronary heart disease: a policy statement of the European Atherosclerosis Society. Eur Heart J 1987;8:77–88.

28. The Expert Panel. Report of the National Cholesterol Education Program Expert Panel on Detection, Evaluation, and Treatment of High Blood Cholesterol in Adults. Arch Intern Med 1988;148:36–69.

29. Applegate WB. Hypertension in elderly patients. Ann Intern Med 1989;110:901–915.

30. Frolich ED, Grim C, Labarthe DR, Maxwell MH, Perloff D, Weidman WH. Recommendations for human blood pressure determination by sphygmomanometers. Circulation 1988;77:502A–514A.

31. Frohlich ED, Gifford RW, Hall WD. Hypertensive cardiovascular disease. J Am Coll Cardiol 1987;10:57A–59A.

32. Hypertension Detection and Follow-up Program Cooperative Group. Blood pressure studies in 14 communities. A two-stage screen for hypertension. JAMA 1977;237:2385–2391.

33. Sparrow D, Tifft CP, Rosner B, Weiss ST. Postural changes in diastolic blood pressure and the risk of myocardial infarction: the Normative Aging Study. Circulation 1984;70:533–537.

34. Lipsitz LA, Nyquist RP, Wei JY, Rowe JW. Postprandial reductions in blood pressure in the elderly. N Engl J Med 1983;309:81–83.

35. Liptsitz LA, Fullerton KJ. Postprandial blood pressure reduction in healthy elderly. J Am Geriatr Soc 1986;34:267–270.

36. Peitzman SJ, Berger SR. Postprandial blood pressure decrease in well elderly persons. Arch Intern Med 1989;149:286–288.

37. Schoenberger JA. Epidemiology of systolic and diastolic systemic blood pressure elevation in the elderly. Am J Cardiol 1986;57:45C–51C.

38. Kannel WB, Vokonas PS. Primary risk factors for coronary heart disease in the elderly: the Framingham Study. In: Wenger NK, Furberg CD, Pitt E (eds): Coronary heart disease in the elderly. New York: Elsevier, 1986:60–92.

39. Levy D, Garrison RJ, Savage DD, Kannel WB, Castelli WP. Left ventricular mass

and incidence of coronary heart disease in an elderly cohort. The Framingham Heart Study. Ann Intern Med 1989;110:101–107.

40. Tuzcu EM, Golz SJ, Lever HM, Salcedo EE. Left ventricular hypertrophy in persons age 90 years and older. Am J Cardiol 1989;63:237–240.

41. Borhani NO. Prevalence and prognostic significance of hypertension in the elderly. J Am Geriatr Soc 1986;34:112–114.

42. Siegel D, Kuller L, Lazarus NB, et al. Predictors of cardiovascular events and mortality in the Systolic Hypertension in the Elderly Program pilot project. Am J Epidemiol 1987;126:385–399.

43. Mattila K, Haavisto M, Rajala S, Heikinheimo R. Blood pressure and five year survival in the very old. Br Med J 1988;296:887–889.

44. Grobbee DE, Hofman A. Does sodium restriction lower blood pressure? Br Med J 1986;293:27–29.

45. Birkenhager WH, de Leeuw PW. Treatment of the elderly hypertensive: a clinical perspective. Eur Heart J 1988;9:63–67.

46. Wikstrand J, Westergren G, Berglund G, et al. Antihypertensive treatment with metoprolol or hydrocholorothiazide in patients aged 60 to 75 years. JAMA 1986;255:1304–1310.

47. Luepker RV. Feasibility of risk factor reduction in the elderly. In: Wenger NK, Furberg CD, Pitt E (eds): Coronary heart disease in the elderly. New York: Elsevier, 1986:134–152.

48. Jajich CL, Ostfeld AM, Freeman DH Jr. Smoking and coronary heart disease mortality in the elderly. JAMA 1984;252:2831–2834.

49. Lipson LG. Diabetes in the elderly: diagnosis, pathogenesis, and therapy. Am J Med 1986;80(Suppl 5A):10–21.

50. Kannel WB, McGee DL. Diabetes and cardiovascular disease. The Framingham Study. JAMA 1979;241:2035–2038.

51. Kannel WB, Hjortland M, Castelli WP. Role of diabetes in congestive heart failure: the Framingham Study. Am J Cardiol 1974;34:29–34.

52. Wilson PW, Anderson KM, Kannel WB. Epidemiology of diabetes mellitus in the elderly. Am J Med 1986;80(Suppl 5A):3–9.

53. Kannel WB, Garrison RJ, Wilson PW. Obesity and nutrition in elderly diabetic patients. Am J Med 1986;80(suppl 5A):22–30.

54. Powell KE, Thompson PD, Caspersen CJ, Kendrick JS. Physical activity and the incidence of coronary heart disease. Annu Rev Public Health 1987;8:253–287.

55. Paffenbarger RS Jr, Hale WE. Work activity and coronary heart mortality. N Engl J Med 1975;292:545–550.

56. Paffenbarger RS Jr, Hyde RT, Wing AL, Hsieh CC. Physical activity, all-cause mortality, and longevity of college alumni. N Engl J Med 1986;314:605–613.

57. Donahue RP, Abbott RD, Reed DM, Yano K. Physical activity and coronary heart disease in middle-aged and elderly men: the Honolulu Heart Program. Am J Public Health 1988;78:683–685.

58. Kannel WB, Sorlie P. Some health benefits of physical activity. The Framingham Study. Arch Intern Med 1979;139:857–861.

59. Siscovick DS, Weiss NS, Fletcher RH, Schoenbach VJ, Wagner EH. Habitual vigorous exercise and primary cardiac arrest: effect of other risk factors on the relationship. J Chron Dis 1984;37:625–631.

60. Davidson DM, Maloney CA. Energy costs of calisthenic exercises in post myocardial infarction patients. Circulation 1985;72(suppl III):III68.

61. Davidson DM, Murphy CR. Exercise training in elderly persons: do women benefit as much as men? In: McPherson BD (ed): Sport and aging. Champaign, IL: Human Kinetics Press, 1985:273–278.

62. Gentry WD, Aronson MK, Blumenthal J, Costa PT Jr, DiGiacomo JN. Behavioral, cognitive and emotional considerations. J Am Coll Cardiol 1987;10:38A–41A.

63. Miller RE, Shapiro AP, King HE, Ginchereau EH, Hosutt JA. Effect of antihypertensive treatment on the behavioral consequences of elevated blood pressure. Hypertension 1984;6:202–208.

64. Blazer DG. Social support and mortality in an elderly community population. Am J Epidemiol 1982;115:684–694.

65. Davidson DM, Shumaker SA. Social support and cardiovascular disease. Arteriosclerosis 1987;7:101–104.

66. Sparacino J. The type A (coronary-prone) behavior pattern, aging, and mortality. J Am Geriatr Soc 1979;27:251–257.

67. Miller KP, Frishman WH. Platelets and antiplatelet therapy in ischemic heart disease. Med Clin North Am 1988;72:117–184.

68. The Steering Committee of the Physicians' Health Study and Research Group. Final report on the aspirin component of the ongoing Physicians' Health Study. N Engl J Med 1989;321:129–135.

69. Montamat SC, Cusack BJ, Vestal RE. Management of drug therapy in the elderly. N Engl J Med 1989;321:303–309.

70. Marcus FI, Ruskin JN, Surawicz B. Arrhythmias. J Am Coll Cardiol 1987;10:66A–72A.

Section IV

Prevention of CAD Events after Detection of Risk

16

management of ischemia before MI or bypass surgery

Myocardial ischemia results from a disparity between myocardial oxygen supply and myocardial oxygen demand. Supply can be limited by reductions in coronary artery blood flow from fixed atherosclerotic obstructions, dynamic constriction (spasm), or thrombotic or embolic occlusion of the coronary arteries, as well as from reduced cardiac ouput or decreased oxygen content in the blood. Myocardial oxygen demand is directly related to heart rate, mean blood pressure ("afterload"), cardiac contractility, and left ventricular size ("preload"). During exercise, demand is increased due to increases in the first three factors, while coronary dilatation results from neural and hormonal signals to the richly innervated muscular layers of the arterial walls.

If there is insufficient supply to meet myocardial oxygen demands, contractility decreases and cardiac output is reduced. In some individuals, angina pectoris develops, warning the individual to stop or slow current activities. As the heart rate and blood pressure subside, the supply/demand balance is restored.

Prior to myocardial infarction (MI) or coronary artery bypass surgery (CABS),

myocardial ischemia is usually first detected (a) through reports of angina pectoris at rest or exercise or (b) by notation of S-T segment changes during exercise testing or ambulatory electrocardiography. Radionuclide testing during exercise can confirm initial observations.

Angina pectoris that is consistent in frequency, intensity, and response to medication is termed stable, while acute disruption in these patterns is designated unstable angina and is treated with hospitalization (1).

When ischemia occurs in the absence of angina, it is termed "silent," but the prognosis is no better than for symptomatic ischemia. Asymptomatic ischemia can occur during exercise, cold weather, or mental stress (2, 3). This may result from constriction of diseased arterial segments, while normal arteries may dilate under similar conditions (4). Myocardial ischemia is traditionally treated pharmacologically, along with improvement of other indicators of CAD risk through weight reduction, aerobic exercise, and optimization of blood pressure and blood lipids. If these measures prove insufficient, but CABS is not immediately indicated, coronary an-

nary angioplasty is appropriate. These topics form the basis for this chapter.

MANAGEMENT AND PROGNOSIS OF STABLE ANGINA

In the two centuries following Heberden's classic description of angina pectoris, many types of therapy have been tried and abandoned. As with many medical innovations, enthusiasm waxes, then wanes; some have suggested that the placebo effect accounts for some relief of angina (5). Rose and colleagues at the London School of Hygiene developed a questionnaire on chest pain, later revised for self-administration. If the respondent indicates "any pain or discomfort in your chest," subsequent questions inquire about its presence during walking on the level or uphill and the location and duration of the pain, as well as its disappearance after stopping, slowing down, or standing still (6). Associations between "Rose questionnaire angina" and objective evidence of CAD are greater in older persons and in younger men than in women (7), but, within age and gender groups, are equal among blacks, whites, and Mexican-Americans in the United States (8).

In 1972, the Canadian Cardiovascular Society proposed a grading of angina pectoris which has been widely adopted (9). Its four categories are shown in Table 16.1.

Because attribution of chest pain to CAD remains problematic in the absence of objective evidence of ischemia, some have advocated not using angina pectoris as an end-point in large-scale cardiovascular studies, particularly in women. However, it appears that indicators of risk for developing angina are similar to those for other CAD manifestations. In a study of 9764 Israeli men, anxiety and severe psychosocial problems (especially family-related) accompanied blood cholesterol level,

Table 16.1. Canadian Cardiovascular Society Angina Categories[a]

I. Angina with strenuous, rapid, or prolonged exertion at work or recreation.
II. Angina while walking or climbing stairs rapidly, walking uphill, on exertion slowly after waking, while under emotional stress, after meals, or in cold weather.
III. Angina when walking 1–2 blocks on the level or climbing one flight of stairs at a normal pace under ordinary conditions.
IV. Inability to carry on any physical activity without discomfort, or angina at rest.

[a]Adapted from Campeau L. Grading of angina pectoris. Circulation 1976;54:522–523.

blood pressure, and diabetes in predicting new cases of angina over a five-year period (10). In a group of apparently healthy men in the United States, exercise electrocardiographic abnormalities were predictive of subsequent development of angina (11). In the Göteborg (Sweden) Primary Prevention Trial, angina accompanying MI was predicted by blood cholesterol level, hypertension, and smoking at baseline, while angina alone was predicted by stress, diabetes mellitus, and increased relative body weight (12).

Prognosis

The natural history of angina pectoris (when only nitrates were available and CABS was not yet widespread) was described in the Framingham population after a 14-year follow-up (ascertainment in 1963–1966). Angina was the presenting symptom of CAD in 65% of women and 37% of men. One in four men had an MI within five years after the onset of angina; incidence was only half that rate in women. One-fourth of the MIs were not recognized clinically until the next biennial examination. Approximately 30% of new angina patients died within the subsequent eight years, nearly half of these suddenly (13). Longer follow-up of Framingham participants with new angina showed smoking persistence was accompanied by a 2- to 4-fold risk of new CAD events (14). Other investigators have documented a significant interference of smoking with the efficacy of nifedipine and propranolol treatment; the therapeutic effect of atenolol is much less impaired in smokers (15). While the prevalence of angina is relatively stable, mortality from CAD has decreased in recent years (16).

In the Göteborg population, men with angina at baseline had a relative risk of fatal and nonfatal MI three times higher than that of asymptomatic men, over 11 years of follow-up. Similar risk was incurred by men developing new angina during the first four years and followed seven more years. Indicators of CAD event risk were elevated serum cholesterol, hypertension, and smoking, suggesting preventing efforts are equally as important in persons with new angina as they are in asymptomatic individuals and survivors of MI and CABS (17).

In the Leiden Intervention Trial, investigators prescribed a vegetarian diet for 39 patients with stable angina pectoris. In those persons with significant drops in their total/HDL cholesterol ratios and in those with low values throughout the study, no progression of lesions was noted (18). If dietary intervention, weight reduction, and aerobic exercise training do not significantly reduce anginal attacks, medication is indicated.

Drug Treatment

To decrease myocardial oxygen demand and/or improve coronary artery blood supply, nitrates, β-adrenergic blockers, and calcium-channel blockers are commonly employed, alone or in combination. The choice of agents will depend upon concomitant disorders and medications as described below (19).

NITRATES

Direct effects on coronary artery supply include dilation of large coronary arteries, small intramural coronary arteries, and conduit vessels that provide collateral flow distal to obstructions, as well as dilation of coronary artery stenoses themselves. Peripherally, venous dilation results in lowered left ventricular pressure and volume. Systemic arterial dilation also reduces the systemic blood pressure, reducing the left ventricular afterload and the myocardial oxygen demand. Numerous studies have documented the improvement in exercise tolerance in angina patients after nitrate administration.

However, tolerance to frequent or continuous dosing occurs commonly, particularly with transdermal preparations. Intermittent dosing, with nitrate levels dropping substantially between doses, may retard development of tolerance (20). Although nitrates are useful as afterload reducers in congestive heart failure, hemodynamic resistance can develop rapidly (21).

β-ADRENERGIC BLOCKERS

β-Blockers lower the myocardial oxygen demand through reductions in heart rate, blood pressure, and contractility. At least eight β-blockers are available in the United States, with considerably more in use in European countries (22). Table 16.2 lists characteristics of various agents and their average wholesale prices in the United States in 1989 (23).

Several pharmacologic features will affect suitability for individual patients. Acebutolol, atenolol, and metoprolol selectively block β_1-receptors in the heart at concentrations below those that block β_2-receptors in the bronchi and peripheral arteries. These agents, used in lower doses, are most suitable for patients with coexisting pulmonary or peripheral artery disease. Nonselective β-blockers may also potenti-

Table 16.2.   Properties of β-Adrenergic Blocking Agents[a]

Drug	Activity	Half-life (Hours)	Daily Dose[b] (mg)	Daily Cost ($)
Acebutolol	B1S,PAA	3–6	400	$0.80
Atenolol	B1S	6–9	50	$0.63
Labetalol	A1S,NOS	3–8	400	$0.80
Metoprolol	B1S	3–6	100	$0.60
Nadolol	NOS	12–24	40	$0.64
Pindolol	PAA	3–4	10	$0.63
Propranolol	NOS			
Inderal		3–6	160	$1.48
Generic		3–6	160	$0.30
Inderal-LA		8–10	160	$1.30
Timolol	NOS	3–5	20	$0.76

[a]Data from Annual Pharmacists' Reference. Orodell, NJ: Medical Economics Inc.; 1990.
[b]Abbreviations: Daily dose = lowest typical maintenance dosage; A1S = α_1-selective; B1S = β_1-selective; NOS = nonselective β-blockade; PAA = partial sympathetic agonist activity.

ate coronary vasoconstriction, probably due to unopposed α-adrenergic stimulation (24).

Atenolol, nadolol, and the active metabolite of acebutolol are more water-soluble and less lipid-soluble than other agents. Lipophylic drugs are absorbed more rapidly and completely in the gut and eliminated rapidly, necessitating more frequent dosages. Hydrophylic agents tend to be eliminated unchanged by the kidney and have longer half-lives in plasma. Several investigators have suggested that the hydrophilic drugs cross the blood-brain barrier less readily. In several trials, atenolol has caused fewer sleep disturbances than other β-blockers.

Acebutolol and pindolol exhibit partial agonist activity (intrinsic sympathomimetic activity) while occupying receptor sites. The main advantage of this feature in persons at risk for CAD is that partial agonist β-blockers have less negative effect on blood lipids and lipoproteins. They may also produce less peripheral vasoconstriction and thereby improve skin blood flow (25). When sympathetic tone is high, the β-blocking effect predominates. However, with low basal sympathetic tone, the ago-

nist effect may increase heart rate and may worsen rest angina (19).

Calcium-Channel Blockers

Diltiazem, nicardipine, nifedipine, and verapamil are all effective in reducing exertional and rest angina, but they have different molecular structures and effects on the heart. Nicardipine and nifedipine have the greatest vasodilating effect, including improved coronary blood flow, but they can cause edema, flushing, headache, and reflex tachycardia. Daily therapeutic doses for angina range from 60 to 120 mg for nicardipine and 30 to 120 mg for nifedipine (26).

Verapamil decreases atrioventricular conduction, making it useful for treatment of supraventricular dysrhythmias, but unsuitable in angina patients with existing conduction disorders. It can also decrease myocardial contractility. Effective dosages range from 240 to 360 mg per day. Its most common side effect is constipation.

Of the three, diltiazem has the fewest side effects in its effective daily doses of 120 to 360 mg. It may have a slowing effect on AV node conduction (19).

Combination Therapy

Nitrates and β-blockers act in a complementary fashion, producing vasodilation as well as reduced heart rate and blood pressure. The tendency of nitrates to cause a reflex increase in contractility can balance the opposite effect of β-blockers. Likewise, the direct coronary artery effects of nitrates can counter the potential for vasoconstriction by the adrenergic blockers.

β-Blockers and calcium-channel blockers also offer the advantage of two different antianginal mechanisms, with the therapeutic choice largely determined by the particular calcium-channel blocker. Nicardipine and nifedipine have sufficient vasodilating effect to lower blood pressure significantly. This effect can cause reflex tachycardia, which can be balanced by β-blocker administration. Verapamil and β-blockers are seldom used concomitantly because of the risk for extreme bradycardia or hypotension from cardiodepressant effects. These concerns are true to a much smaller extent for diltiazem, nicardipine, and nifedipine.

Nitrates and calcium-channel blockers have been used less often in combination, probably due to their additive effects on peripheral vasodilation and the potential for resultant hypotension. These effects might be desirable, however, in a younger person with congestive heart failure and CAD. Because of the potential for reflex tachycardia with nicardipine and nifedipine, diltiazem or verapamil may be better choices for combination therapy with nitrates when treating angina.

Rarely, treatment with drugs from all three categories is instituted, but a number of studies show little additive benefit beyond optimal doses of two-drug treatment (27). Table 16.3 lists recommendations for specific antianginal medications for persons with other medical conditions.

MANAGEMENT AND PROGNOSIS OF SILENT ISCHEMIA

In recent years, myocardial ischemia in the absence of angina or other symptoms has been recognized as a frequent occurrence, as detected by exercise testing

Table 16.3.   Selection of Antianginal Agents in Patients with Other Conditions

Condition	Advantageous	Disadvantageous
Congestive heart failure (CHF)	NIT,[a] NIC, NIF	BBL
Diabetes mellitus, insulin dependent		BBL (esp nonsel)
Dysrhythmias/conduction disorders		
Sinus bradycardia; sinus or AV nodal dysfunction	NIC, NIF	BBL, VER
Sinus tachycardia (no CHF)	BBL	NIC, NIF
Supraventricular tachycardia/atrial fibrillation	VER, BBL	NIC, NIF
Ventricular dysrhythmias	BBL	
Hypertension	All	
Myocardial infarction, recent and without CHF	BBL	
Peripheral vascular disease	NIC, NIF	BBL (esp nonsel)
Pulmonary disease (COPD, asthma)	NIT, CCB	BBL (esp nonsel)
Smoking, no COPD	ATN	
Valvular disease		
Aortic or mitral regurgitation	NIT, NIC, NIF	BBL

[a]Abbreviations: ATN = atenolol; BBL = β-blockers; CCB = calcium-channel blockers; COPD = chronic obstructive pulmonary disease; DIL = diltiazem; NIC = nicardipine; NIF = nifedipine; NIT = nitrates; Nonsel = nonselective β-blocker; VER = verapamil.

and ambulatory electrocardiography (28). It is now clear that episodes of "silent" ischemia occur in patients who also have angina on other occasions; the frequency of both types of ischemic episode appears to be poorly correlated with disease severity (29).

Several theories have been proposed to explain painless ischemia, including those of increased pain threshold and increased β-endorphin levels (30–32). Silent ischemia appears to be more common in diabetics (33) and the elderly (34). It often occurs at relatively low heart rates, and with a circadian rhythm that parallels changes in the release of catecholamines. The latter feature has led several investigative teams to document the effects of personally relevant mental stress on silent ischemia (35). Freeman and colleagues measured urinary secretion of noradrenaline as an indicator of stress during discussions of coronary angiography and the need for CABS, comparing these values to later determinations. Persons with high noradrenalin secretion on the first occasion have significantly more silent ischemia (36).

Cohn suggests that assessment of the clinical significance is facilitated by considering three groups of patients with silent ischemia: (a) asymptomatic patients with no other evidence of CAD, (b) persons asymptomatic after MI, and (c) individuals exhibiting both angina and silent ischemia (29).

When silent ischemia on routine exercise testing is the only indication of CAD, β-blocker therapy may be useful in limiting heart rate and blood pressure excursions into the ischemic range, as well as minimizing the probability of sudden cardiac death (37). If S-T segment depression is marked (0.2 mV or more), thallium myocardial perfusion imaging with exercise can be undertaken. If exercise-induced reversible perfusion defects are noted, coro-

nary angiography to rule out left main coronary artery disease may be considered. Modifications of CAD risk indicators should also be undertaken.

In persons asymptomatic after MI, prognostic exercise testing (38) and ambulatory electrocardiography may disclose silent ischemia (39). Prognosis for patients in this group is similar to that for those displaying angina after MI (40). Similarly, subjects from the Coronary Artery Surgery Study Registry with only silent ischemia on exercise testing had nearly identical risk of MI or sudden cardiac death as those who displayed angina and ischemic S-T depression during exercise. In those with three-vessel disease, the likelihood of cardiac events was higher in those with silent ischemia alone (41). Treatment for persons with both symptomatic and silent ischemic episodes is similar to that described above for angina pectoris.

When medical management is insufficient to control symptoms, coronary angioplasty may be considered.

CORONARY ANGIOPLASTY

During the 1980s, transluminal coronary angioplasty (PTCA) became a popular intervention for the treatment of coronary artery disease patients with a suboptimal response to pharmacologic management in whom CABS was not immediately indicated. By 1987, more than 175,000 PTCA procedures were undertaken in the United States alone (42). Similar growth patterns were noted in other countries as well.

In 1979, the National Heart, Lung, and Blood Institute (NHLBI) in the United States established a registry to facilitate evaluation of this new technique (43). In 1986, the investigators reported a mean follow-up of 4.3 years for 1390 patients from 16 centers. In this early group of patients, 75% of subjects had single-vessel angioplasty. PTCA was initially successful in 64%; 17% underwent a second angioplasty within the first year and 11% had coronary artery bypass surgery (CABS) during that same period. Those surviving the initial hospitalization had a cumulative mortality of 4.2% (1% per year), and 8% had nonfatal myocardial infarction (MI) (44). In 1985, the NHLBI reopened the registry; during the next several years, it became apparent that a majority of patients being enrolled had multivessel disease. Less than one-third of all patients had "complete revascularization" (no residual proximal lesions narrowed greater than 50% diameter); this included 16% of patients with triple-vessel disease, 30% of those with two-vessel involvement, and 78% of persons with single-vessel disease (45). In single-vessel patients enrolled during 1985 and 1986, the incidence of perioperative death, nonfatal MI, and emergency CABS was 0.2, 3.5, and 2.9%, respectively (46); 84% were successfully dilated without mortality, MI, or emergency CABS. Initial dilation was successful in 86 to 88% of persons with two- or three-vessel disease. The incidence of an event (death, MI, or emergency CABS) was 8 and 10% in double- and triple-vessel disease (47). Women have a much greater incidence of coronary dissection and in-hospital mortality associated with PTCA, but long-term results are similar to those in men (48).

In comparing PTCA with CABS, the lack of complete revascularization becomes important. In a Mayo Clinic study of patients with multivessel disease, those with incomplete revascularization had more than twice the rate of development of angina and necessity for CABS than those with complete revascularization (49).

In recent years, angioplasty has been done in saphenous vein grafts at the site of total coronary occlusions, and soon after acute myocardial infarction. Management

and assessment of prognosis after PTCA may be categorized in three periods: during hospitalization, in the interval after hospital discharge, and from 8 months onward (50).

Hospitalization Period

During the first 24 hours, from 2 to 10% of dilated vessels will abruptly reocclude. Half of these acute closures occur within the catheterization laboratory; approximately 84% occur within the first six hours after the procedure. Lesion length, lesion location at a bifurcation, dissection, spasm at distal or dilation site, and the presence of coronary thrombus have been correlated with acute closure rate (50, 51). Electrocardiographic detection of ischemia should result in immediate treatment with nitroglycerin; if ischemia episodes are repetitive or unresponsive to nitroglycerin, repeat angiography is indicated. Prompt redilation is successful in approximately 50% of cases; in others, emergency CABS should be quickly undertaken where appropriate (52).

Pretreatment with aspirin has reduced acute vessel closure from approximately 10 to 2%. In patients with preexisting thrombus or unstable angina, continuous heparin infusion is indicated for several days before the procedure (50).

Success rates in single-vessel disease angioplasty done for unstable angina are similar to those in stable angina patients, but they are often less satisfactory in unstable angina patients with multivessel disease (53). Elderly patients can safely undergo PTCA for unstable angina with low rates of morbidity, mortality, and restenosis (54).

Immediately after acute MI, angioplasty is usually done only in the infarct-related artery; success rates may reach 90%. Other lesions can be dilated electively at a later time (53). Angioplasty may follow ineffective thrombolytic therapy; success rates of 70 to 80% have been reported; however, in-hospital mortality is still higher than in cases of successful lytic reperfusion; bleeding and the need for emergency CABS are also recognized complications (55).

In a Mayo Clinic study, PTCA of saphenous vein grafts was successful in more than 80% of cases; more than 70% were asymptomatic after 20 months (56).

Several studies have examined the prognostic utility of predischarge testing using exercise myocardial perfusion imaging (thallium-201) or radionuclide ventriculography. Some have found that patients with early abnormalities are more likely to develop subsequent restenoses, while others have failed to find prognostic significance (50, 57).

Pharmacologic prophylaxis may also be considered prior to discharge. Studies of anticoagulants, antiplatelet agents, and calcium-channel blockers showed no improvement in reducing restenosis rates, although many clinicians continue to prescribe aspirin for at least six months after PTCA (50). Omega-3 fatty acid administration through fish oil capsules has reduced early restenosis when given in daily dosages of 3.2 g eicosapentanoic (with or without 1.3 g docasahexanoic acid) for six months (58, 59).

Longer Follow-up after PTCA

During the eight months following hospital discharge, from 20 to 50% of patients will have restenosis of the dilated segment(s), a process that appears to be progressive, despite daily aspirin and other agents (60). Restenosis and disease progression is 50% higher in subjects who continue to smoke; recurrence of angina is also greater in those who do not quit smoking (61). Repeat PTCA can be undertaken for restenosis; even a third PTCA has proven safe and effective therapy (62).

Six months after PTCA, patients display better return to work, sexual activities, and family satisfaction than CABS patients. In one study, however, only the improvement in work performance was significantly different between the two groups of patients after 15 months (63).

Despite the high rates of reocclusion and repeat angioplasty, PTCA still represents a less expensive treatment of symptomatic CAD (64). Within the United States medical care system, forces of competition and regulation will have a large impact on the further proliferation of PTCA (65). Recipients of PTCA are currently eligible for reimbursement for cardiac rehabilitation outpatient training programs.

REFERENCES

1. Bashour TT, Myler RK, Andrae GE, Stertzer SH, Clark DA, Ryan CJ. Current concepts in unstable myocardial ischemia. Am Heart J 1988;115:850–861.

2. Shea MJ, Deanfield JE, deLandsheere CM, Wilson RA, Kensett M, Selwyn AP. Asymptomatic myocardial ischemia following cold provocation. Am Heart J 1987;114:469–476.

3. Barry J, Selwyn AP, Nabel EG, et al. Frequency of ST-segment depression produced by mental stress in stable angina pectoris from coronary artery disease. Am J Cardiol 1988;61:989–993.

4. Selwyn AP, Ganz P. Myocardial ischemia in coronary disease. N Engl J Med 1988;318:1058–1060.

5. Benson H, McCallie DP Jr. Angina pectoris and the placebo effect. N Engl J Med 1979;300:1420–1429.

6. Rose G, McCartney P, Reid DD. Self-administration of a questionnaire on chest pain and intermittent claudication. Br J Prev Soc Med 1977;31:42–48.

7. Wilcosky T, Harris R, Weissfeld L. The prevalence and correlates of Rose questionnaire

angina among women and men and the Lipid Research Clinics Program Prevalence Study population. Am J Epidemiol 1987;125:400–409.

8. LaCroix AZ, Haynes SG, Savage DD, Havlik RJ. Rose questionnaire angina among United States black, white and Mexican-American women and men. Am J Epidemiol 1989;129:669–686.

9. Campeau L. Grading of angina pectoris. Circulation 1976;54:522–523.

10. Medalie JH, Goldbourt U. Angina pectoris among 10,000 men. II. Psychosocial and other risk factors as evidenced by a multivariate analysis of a five-year incidence study. Am J Med 1976;60:910–921.

11. McHenry PL, O'Donnell J, Morris SN, Jordan JJ. The abnormal exercise electrocardiogram in apparently healthy men: a predictor of angina pectoris as an initial coronary event during long-term follow-up. Circulation 1984;70:547–551.

12. Hagman M, Wilhelmsen L, Wedel H, Pennert K. Risk factors for angina pectoris in a population study of Swedish men. J Chron Dis 1987;40:265–275.

13. Kannel WB, Feinleib M. Natural history of angina pectoris in the Framingham Study. Prognosis and survival. Am J Cardiol 1972;29:154–163.

14. Hubert HB, Holford TR, Kannel WB. Clinical characteristics and cigarette smoking in relation to prognosis of angina pectoris in Framingham. Am J Epidemiol 1982;115:231–242.

15. Deanfield J, Wright C, Krikler S, Ribeiro P, Fox K. Cigarette smoking and the treatment of angina with propranolol, atenolol and nifedipine. N Engl J Med 1984;310:951–954.

16. Pryor DB, Harrell FE Jr, Lee KL, Califf RM, Rosati RA. An improving prognosis over time in medically treated patients with coronary artery disease. Am J Cardiol 1983;52:444–448.

17. Hagman M, Wilhelmson L, Pennert K, Wedel H. Factors of importance for prognosis in men with angina pectoris derived from a random population sample. The Multicenter Primary Prevention Trial, Gothenburg, Sweden. Am J Cardiol 1988;61:530–535.

18. Arntzenius AC, Kromhout D, Barth JD, et al. Diet, lipoproteins, and the progression of coronary atherosclerosis. The Leiden Intervention Trial. N Engl J Med 1985;312:805–811.

19. Shub C, Vlietstra RE, McGoon MD. Selection of optimal drug therapy for the patient with angina pectoris. Mayo Clin Proc 1985;60:539–548.

20. Abrams J. A reappraisal of nitrate therapy. JAMA 1988;259:396–401.

21. Kulick D, Roth A, McIntosh N, Rahimtoola SH, Elkayam U. Resistance to isosorbide dinitrate in patients with severe chronic heart failure: incidence and attempt at hemodynamic prediction. J Am Coll Cardiol 1988; 12:1023–1028.

22. Vedin A, Wilhelmson C. Medical treatment of ischaemic heart disease—β blockers. Eur Heart J 1985;6(suppl A):13–27.

23. Annual Pharmacists' Reference. Orodell, NJ: Medical Economics Inc., 1990.

24. Kern MJ, Ganz P, Horowitz JD, et al. Potentiation of coronary vasoconstriction by β-adrenergic blockade in patients with coronary artery disease. Circulation 1983;67:1178–1185.

25. Breckenridge A. Which beta blocker? Br Med J 1983;286:1085–1088.

26. Julian DG. Nicardipine—A vasoselective calcium antagonist. Am J Cardiol 1987; 59:37J.

27. Julian DG. Comparisons and combinations in anti-anginal therapy. Eur Heart J 1985;6(suppl A):37–45.

28. Rozanski A, Berman DS. Silent myocardial ischemia. Am Heart J 1987;114:615–638.

29. Quyyumi AA, Wright CM, Mockus LJ, Fox KM. How important is a history of chest pain in determining the degree of ischaemia in patients with angina pectoris? Br Heart J 1985;54:22–26.

30. Cohn PF. Silent myocardial ischemia. Ann Intern Med 1988;109:312–317.

31. Falcone C, Specchia G, Rondanelli R, et al. Correlation between beta-endorphin plasma levels and anginal symptoms in patients with coronary artery disease. J Am Coll Cardiol 1988;11:719–723.

32. Falcone C, Sconocchia R, Guasti L, Codega S, Montemartini C, Specchia G. Dental

pain threshold and angina pectoris in patients with coronary artery disease. J Am Coll Cardiol 1988;12:348–352.

33. Murray DP, O'Brien T, O'Sullivan DJ. Silent myocardial ischaemia in diabetes mellitus. J Am Coll Cardiol 1988;11:23A.

34. Kurita A, Takase B, Horiuchi K, et al. Painless myocardial ischemia in elderly patients with coronary heart disease compared with middle-aged patients and its relation to treadmill testing and coronary hemodynamics. J Am Coll Cardiol 1988;11:50A.

35. Rozanski A, Bairey CN, Krantz DS, et al. Mental stress and the induction of silent myocardial ischemia in patients with coronary artery disease. N Engl J Med 1988;318:1005–1012.

36. Freeman LJ, Nixon PG, Sallabank P, Reaveley D. Psychological stress and silent myocardial ischemia. Am Heart J 1987;114:477–482.

37. Sharma B, Asinger R, Francis GS, Hodges M, Wyeth RP. Demonstration of exercise-induced painless myocardial ischemia in survivors of out-of-hospital ventricular fibrillation. Am J Cardiol 1987;59:740–745.

38. Davidson DM, DeBusk RF. Prognostic value of a single exercise test 3 weeks after uncomplicated myocardial infarction. Circulation 1980;61:236–242.

39. Cohn PF, Sodums MT, Lawson WE, Vlay SC, Brown EJ Jr. Frequent episodes of silent myocardial ischemia after apparently uncomplicated myocardial infarction. J Am Coll Cardiol 1986;8:982–985.

40. Weiner DA, Ryan TJ, McCabe CH, et al. Significance of silent myocardial ischemia during exercise testing in patients with coronary artery disease. Am J Cardiol 1987;59:725–729.

41. Weiner DA, Ryan TJ, McCabe CH, et al. Risk of developing an acute myocardial infarction or sudden coronary death in patients with exercise-induced silent myocardial ischemia. A report from the Coronary Artery Surgery Study (CASS) Registry. Am J Cardiol 1988;62:1155–1158.

42. Bourassa MG, Alderman EL, Bertrand M, et al. Report of the Joint ISFC/WHO Task Force on Coronary Angioplasty. Circulation 1988;78:780–789.

43. ACC/AHA Task Force. Guidelines for percutaneous transluminal angioplasty. J Am Coll Cardiol 1988;12:529–545.

44. Kent KM, Cowley MJ, Kelsey CF, Costigan TM, Detre KM. Long-term follow-up of the NHLBI-PTCA Registry. Circulation 1986;74(suppl II):II-280.

45. Bourassa MG, David PR, Costigan T, et al. Completeness of revascularization early after coronary angioplasty (PTCA) in the NHLBI PTCA Registry. J Am Coll Cardiol 1987;9:19A.

46. Holmes DR Jr, Holubkov R, Vlietstra RE, et al. Comparison of complications during percutaneous transluminal coronary angioplasty (PTCA) in the NHLBI PTCA Registry. J Am Coll Cardiol 1988;12:1149–1155.

47. Detre K, Holubkov R, Kelsey S, et al. Percutaneous transluminal coronary angioplasty in 1985–1986 and 1977–1981: The NHLBI Registry. N Engl J Med 1988;318:265–270.

48. Cowley MJ, Mullin SM, Kelsey SF, et al. Sex differences in early- and long-term results of coronary angioplasty in the NHLBI PTCA Registry. Circulation 1985;71:90–97.

49. Mabin TA, Holmes DR, Smith HC, et al. Follow-up clinical results in patients undergoing percutaneous transluminal coronary angioplasty. Circulation 1985;71:754–760.

50. Popma JJ, Dehmer GJ. Care of the patient after coronary angioplasty. Ann Intern Med 1989;110:547–559.

51. Ellis SG, Roubin GS, King SB III, et al. Angiographic and clinical predictors of acute closure after native vessel coronary angioplasty. Circulation 1988;77:372–379.

52. Sinclair IN, McCabe CH, Sipperly ME, Baim DS. Predictors, therapeutic options and long-term outcome of abrupt reclosure. Am J Cardiol 1988;61G–66G.

53. Holmes DR Jr, Vlietstra RE. Balloon angiography in acute and chronic coronary artery disease. JAMA 1989;261:2109–2115.

54. Holt GW, Sugrue DD, Bresnahan JF, et al. Results of percutaneous transluminal coronary angioplasty for unstable angina pectoris in patients 70 years of age and older. Am J Cardiol 1988;61:994–997.

55. Califf RM, Topol EJ, George BS, et al. Characteristics and outcome of patients in

whom reperfusion with intravenous tissue-type plasminogen activator fails: results of the Thrombolysis and Angioplasty in Myocardial Infarction (TAMI) Trial. Circulation 1988; 77:1090–1099.

56. Reeder GS, Bresnahan JF, Holmes DR Jr, et al. Angioplasty for aortocoronary bypass graft stenosis. Mayo Clin Proc 1986;61:14–19.

57. Vlay SC, Chernillas J, Lawson WE, Dervan JP. Restenosis after angioplasty: don't rely on the exercise test. Am Heart J 1989;117:980–986.

58. Dehmer GJ, Popma JJ, Van den Berg EK, et al. Reduction in the rate of early restenosis after coronary angioplasty by a diet supplemented by n-3 fatty acids. N Engl J Med 1988;319:733–740.

59. Milner R, Gallino RA, Leffingwell A, et al. Usefulness of fish oil supplements in preventing clinical evidence of restenosis after percutaneous transluminal coronary angioplasty. Circulation 1980;64:294–299.

60. Serruys PW, Luitjen HE, Beatt KJ, et al. Incidence of restenosis after successful coronary angioplasty: A time-related phenomenon. A quantitative angiographic study in 342 consecutive patients at 1, 2, 3 and 4 months.

61. Galan KM, Deligonul U, Kern MJ, Chaitman BR, Vandormael MG. Increased frequency of restenosis in patients continuing to smoke cigarettes after percutaneous transluminal coronary angioplasty. Am J Cardiol 1988;61:260–263.

62. Joly P, Bonan R, Palisaitis D, et al. Treatment of recurrent restenosis with repeat percutaneous transluminal coronary angioplasty. Am J Cardiol 1988;61:905–908.

63. Raft D, McKee DC, Popio KA, Haggerty JJ Jr. Life adaptation after percutaneous transluminal angioplasty and coronary bypass grafting. Am J Cardiol 1985;56:395–398.

64. Reeder GS, Krishan I, Nobrega FT, et al. Is percutaneous transluminal angioplasty less expensive than bypass surgery? N Engl J Med 1984;311:1157–1162.

65. Robinson JC, Garnick DW, McPhee SJ. Market and regulatory influences on the availability of coronary angioplasty and bypass surgery in U.S. hospitals. N Engl J Med 1987;317:85–90.

Section V

Prevention of CAD Event Recurrence

17

prognosis and management after myocardial infarction

Approximately one million persons experience myocardial infarction (MI) in Canada and the United States each year. Of those who survive the event and hospitalization, some 10 to 15% will die within the following year. A majority of these deaths will occur in the first few months after the MI (1). From years one to five, another 10 to 15% will have a cardiovascular-related death (2–3).

There are several prognostic indicators that guide the clinician's testing and intervention decisions. As Table 17.1 indicates, these reflect (a) myocardial cumulative damage and residual function, (b) recurrent myocardial ischemia, (c) dysrhythmias and conduction disorders, (d) prophylactic medications, (e) noninvasive and invasive testing, (f) standard coronary artery disease (CAD) risk indicators, including age, gender, race, and other demographic factors, (g) psychosocial and behavioral considerations, and (h) the provision of cardiac rehabilitation services.

This chapter discusses these topics and outlines a four-phase program of cardiac rehabilitation services that is designed to optimize the recovery of the MI survivor.

MYOCARDIAL CUMULATIVE DAMAGE AND RESIDUAL FUNCTION

Previous MI or Angina

A history of prior MI, when added to the damage incurred from the current infarction, correlated well with the risk of subsequent cardiovascular death in several studies with follow-up ranging from one month to 15 years (4–10). Lie and coworkers noted a worse prognosis in those with two or more previous MIs, in those with MI less than three months previously, and in those with a previous anterior wall infarction (4). In the Coronary Drug Project, which enrolled men at least three months after their most recent MI, the number of previous MIs was related to mortality over a five-year follow-up period (7).

Other studies suggest that a diagnosis of angina pectoris before the MI indicates a poorer prognosis, whether noted alone (11–13) or in the presence of previous infarction (14–19). Pierard and colleagues studied 732 consecutive patients admitted for a first MI; 27% had angina for one month or more preinfarction, 24% had

Table 17.1. Prognostic Indicators after Myocardial Infarction

- Myocardial cumulative damage and residual function
- Recurrent myocardial ischemia
- Dysrhythmias and conduction disorders
- Prophylactic medications
- Noninvasive and invasive test results
- CAD risk indicators
  Smoking
  Lipids and lipoproteins
  Hypertension
  Diabetes
  Obesity
  Age and gender
  Race and ethnicity
  Psychosocial and behavioral risks

developed new-onset angina within the preceding month, and the remaining 39% had no angina prior to the infarction. Patients in the two groups with angina were older, were more likely to be women, and had a higher frequency of anterior MI and early postinfarction angina. While angina and nonangina patients had a similar in-hospital mortality (10 and 8%), the angina patients discharged alive had a 16% three-year mortality compared to 7% in those without angina before their MI (13). Extension of the MI, which occurs in approximately 10% of patients during their hospitalization, also worsens the prognosis (20–21). Extension is more likely to occur in patients with a history of previous MI, S-T segment depression on the admission electrocardiogram (ECG), and recurrent ischemic pain on the second hospital day (21).

Extension, Location, and Type of Current MI

The extent and damage during MI can be quantitated from the appearance of myocardial enzymes in the serum. Several studies, ranging in mean follow-up duration from two weeks to six years, have doc-

umented the prognostic value of such enzyme rises (11, 12, 17, 22).

Conventional clinical wisdom holds that anterior MIs are associated with a worse prognosis than inferior infarctions. Norris and co-workers found this to be true, and included that measure in their coronary prognostic index (15). Among the possible explanations for this association is one based on the increased likelihood that an anterior MI reflects left ventricular damage with consequent greater hemodynamic impairment, while enzyme elevations from an inferior MI may result from damage to both right and left ventricles. As with other factors described in this chapter, the prognosis may vary considerably depending on the composition of the study population.

For example, Robinson and colleagues followed 28-day survivors of MI for periods up to 15 years. Mortality and nonfatal MI recurrences were equal in anteroseptal and inferior wall infarction patients, as was the reappearance of angina (23). One could postulate that anterior MIs, with their more serious impairment of left ventricular function, do most of their damage within the hospitalization period or the first month thereafter.

The type of infarction also has prognostic implications. In the past, the terms transmural and nontransmural were used to classify infarcts. However, autopsy studies indicated that the electrocardiographic findings do not reliably predict the presence of transmural necrosis, so current classification is based on the presence of Q waves on the surface electrocardiogram (24). Because long-term mortality and MI recurrence after non–Q wave infarcts is similar to that of Q wave MIs (and higher in older patients without previous infarction), further studies exploring the underlying mechanisms have been undertaken (8, 13, 16, 19, 25, 26).

DeWood et al. note reports that suggest incomplete coronary artery occlusion in non-Q wave infarctions early in its course, with subsequent progression of luminal obstruction. In their own series of patients undergoing coronary angiography soon after non–Q wave MI, they found total occlusion of the infarct-related vessel in 26, 37, and 42% of subjects studied less than 24 hours, 1 to 3 days, and 3 to 7 days after MI, respectively (25). Given this propensity for closure, immediate therapy might be directed at thrombolysis, inhibition of platelet aggregation, and prevention of coronary artery spasm. It is clear that non–Q wave infarctions are frequently followed by infarct extension and recurrence of angina pectoris or MI (8).

Nicod and his colleagues also noted the prognostic equality of Q wave and non–Q wave infarction patients under the age of 70. In older patients with a first MI, a higher mortality after hospital discharge was noted in patients with a non–Q wave MI (26).

Hemodynamic Impairment

Several methods for classifying patients with acute MI have been utilized in recent years. Killip and Kimball proposed four categories (27):

I. No congestive heart failure (CHF)
II. Mild-to-moderate CHF (S3, rales)
III. Pulmonary edema
IV. Cardiogenic shock

These criteria have proved useful in estimating prognosis from clinical examination. In their 1968 report, the authors noted in-hospital rates for the four categories of 6 to 8%, 7 to 30%, 33 to 44%, and 80 to 100%, respectively (28).

To further characterize the relation between clinical and hemodynamic variables, Forrester, Diamond, and Swan studied 200 consecutive MI patients. They de-

Table 17.2. Classification of Clinical and Hemodynamic Function after MI[a]

Clinical subsets
I.   No pulmonary congestion or peripheral hypoperfusion
II. Isolated pulmonary congestion
III. Isolated peripheral hypoperfusion
IV. Both pulmonary congestion and peripheral hypoperfusion

Hemodynamic subsets
I.   Normal cardiac index and pulmonary capillary pressure
II. Elevated pulmonary capillary pressure only
III. Depressed cardiac index only
IV. Both depressed cardiac index and elevated pulmonary capillary pressure

[a]Adapted from Forrester JS, Diamond GA, Swan HJ. Correlative classification of clinical and hemodynamic function after myocardial infarction. Am J Cardiol 1988;39:137–145.

veloped parallel clinical and hemodynamic subsets as shown in Table 17.2.

The diagnosis of pulmonary congestion required the presence of both auscultatory and radiographic findings. Peripheral hypoperfusion was defined as the presence of decreased skin temperature, confusion, or oliguria in patients with either arterial hypotension or sinus tachycardia. A cardiac index of 2.2 liter min/m^2 or less was defined as depressed; pulmonary capillary pressures of 18 mm Hg or greater were considered elevated. The clinical and hemodynamic subsets were equally predictive of in-hospital mortality; I = 2.2%, II = 10.1%, III = 22.4%, and IV 55.5% (29).

Assessment of Residual Myocardial Function

Thallium-201 myocardial perfusion imaging has proved useful prognostically. One study, done with MI patients within 15 hours of admission, showed if less than 40% of the left ventricle was visualized at rest, in-hospital and six-month mortality rates were 46% and 62%, respectively. In contrast, those with a lower defect score (representing less infarction and/or ischemia) had rates of 3 and 7% for the same periods (30).

While thallium-201 imaging offers information on the adequacy of regional myocardial perfusion, the technique of radionuclide ventriculography, using technetium 99–labeled red blood cells, offers quantitative information regarding left and right ventricular function. This technique, when used at rest during the first week after MI, adds significantly to the prognostic power of clinical and radiologic findings. This is particularly true in Killip class II patients, who display a broad range of mild-to-moderate congestive heart failure (31, 32).

RECURRENT MYOCARDIAL ISCHEMIA

Persons with persistent or recurrent angina or silent ischemia soon after MI have an increased risk of recurrence or death. In one study, 12% of patients had angina within 48 hours after the infarction. By 3 and 12 months thereafter, 25 and 37% of these patients with early angina recurrence had died (33). Kassis and colleagues performed autopsies on 57 victims of myocardial rupture following MI; 33% had occurred within the first 24 hours after MI, 52% by 4 days and 81% by one week. In 26 of 39 patients who were observed to suddenly lose consciousness, pulse, and respiration as a consequence of the rupture, angina preceded the fatal episode (34). Singer et al. found that 13% of 536 consecutive MI patients were readmitted to the coronary care unit an average of 2.7 days after initial transfer from the unit; 32% of these had recurrent chest pain after the first 24 hours in hospital. In contrast, only 7% of those not readmitted has such symptoms (35). In a Stanford University study of 195 patients who had experienced a clin-

ically uncomplicated MI three weeks previously, angina developed on exercise testing in 30 (15.4%). Along with exercise-induced S-T segment depression of 0.2 mV or more, angina was predictive of medical and surgical events during the ensuing year. All persons who died suddenly had manifested one of the two indicators of ischemia on the treadmill test three weeks after MI (36).

Recurrent ischemia may reflect subtotal arterial occlusion either in the zone of the infarction (which is often nontransmural) or distant from that area. Schuster and colleagues noted transient S-T segment or T wave changes in 18% of MI survivors within 10 days; 6-month mortality of these patients was 57%. Among their patients who had left ventricular ejection fraction measured at catheterization or with radionuclide ventriculography within a week after the MI, individuals who survived the 6 months had a greater mean ejection fraction than those who died (60 versus 45%) (37).

In a Stanford University study of 665 men, 70 years of age and younger, previous MI and recurrence of angina in the coronary care unit were the best predictors of the clinical course during the subsequent six months. Ten percent of that study population had one or both characteristics, but they accounted for 25% of medical events and 33% of medical or surgical events (18). The nine-center Multicenter Postinfarction Research Group study had a nearly identical population; 51 of their 866 men experienced recurrent MI. Of these, 54% had experienced angina before hospital discharge (38).

The incidence of recurrent angina over the first and subsequent years following MI has varied in the past five decades. Studies done from 1937 to 1954 show rates of 45 to 71%; Framingham participants experiencing MI before 1972 had a 49% recurrence rate. A Montreal study reported in 1979 showed a one-year incidence of recurrent angina of 61%; of those with preinfarction angina or a positive post-MI exercise test, 96% developed angina, compared with 26% of those having neither characteristic (39).

The relatively poor prognosis associated with recurrent ischemia noted in these earlier studies has stimulated intervention with thrombolytic agents, coronary angioplasty, and bypass surgery, favorably altering the course of many MI patients (40–42).

Lange and co-workers reviewed coronary arteriograms from 45 subjects, studied within 60 days of MI, who had significant narrowing of only the infarct-related artery, but with residual antegrade flow in that vessel. Of the 45, 26 had experienced postinfarction angina. In those 26, stenoses were more than twice as long. An eccentric plaque with irregular borders, a condition often associated with a ruptured, ulcerated plaque and unstable angina, was present in 46% of those with recurrent angina but only in 32% of those without such symptoms. However, percentage diameter narrowing, absolute stenosis diameter, and absolute stenosis were similar in the two groups. Multivariate stepwise discriminant analysis revealed stenosis length to be the most significant predictor of postinfarction angina; logistic progression analysis revealed that stenosis length had a sensitivity and specificity of 80% in such prediction. The authors caution that their findings might not be applicable in persons with multivessel disease or those with totally occluded single vessel disease following myocardial infarction (43).

Silent ischemia in the early post-MI period also has an ominous prognosis (44). In two similar studies of exercise testing soon after MI, painless S-T depression was seen in 18 to 20% of subjects (36, 45). Gottlieb and colleagues studied 103 high-risk postinfarction patients with ambulatory electrocardiography; 30 displayed ischemic S-T segments, of whom only one-third had in-hospital angina. Mortality at one year was 30% in this group, compared to only 8 of 73 (11%) in those without ischemic changes (46).

DYSRHYTHMIAS AND CONDUCTION DISORDERS

Complex dysrhythmias and conduction disorders also adversely affect prognosis in the post-MI patient. In the Aspirin Myocardial Infarction Study, 194 of 235 witnessed deaths during the first 24 hours after admission were attributed to cardiac dysrhythmias (47). In-hospital deaths are twice as likely when primary ventricular fibrillation accompanies acute MI (48). Approximately 20% of patients with acute MIs experience cardiac arrest in-hospital; one-third of these occur on the first day. Case-fatality rate is 78% for such patients, compared with 4% for those who do not have cardiac arrest (49). Invasive electrophysiologic studies should be undertaken in all survivors of cardiac arrest; inducible ventricular tachycardia is the best predictor of such poor prognosis in patients experiencing cardiac arrest following MI (50).

Other dysrhythmias early in the hospital course are much less prognostic during long-term follow-up. Ambulatory ECG monitoring later in the hospitalization is more predictive, with prognostic yield depending upon the length of the monitoring period (51). In examining ventricular premature complex (VPC) repetitiveness on predischarge ambulatory ECG recordings, Bigger found a one-year mortality rate three times higher in those with 3 or more successive VPCs (defined as ventricular tachycardia) than in those without that feature (52). In the Multicenter Postinfarction Research Group study, the two-year incidence of sudden cardiac death was

17% in patients with repetitive VPCs compared with 3% in those without (53). A Swedish collaborative study found that ventricular tachycardia noted in the coronary care unit was significantly predictive in identifying women and men at high risk for sudden coronary death (54). In the Multicenter Investigation of the Limitation in Infarct Size, VPCs (10 or more per hour) and a radionuclide left ventricular ejection fraction of 0.40 or less were independent risk factors for such cardiac death over the two years following hospital discharge (55). Using a six-hour predischarge ambulatory ECG recording, Moss et al. found that complex ventricular dysrhythmias, defined as bigeminal, multiform, repetitive, or early cycle (R on T) patterns, indicated increased risk of cardiac mortality during a mean follow-up period of 3 years (56). VPC frequency can also be a useful prognostic indicator. Single VPCs occurring 10 or more times per hour was an independent predictor of mortality (9). Sturzenhofecker and colleagues had similar findings in their study of postinfarction patients under the age of 40 (57).

Cardiac dysrhythmias retain their predictive power when measured after hospital discharge. Bigger et al. noted a relative risk of 2.7 of death in the subsequent six months in patients with ventricular tachycardia occurring within two weeks of MI (58). Marchilinski found that, of patients with ventricular tachycardia documented during the first two months after MI, half were dead (75% sudden) during a mean 20 month follow-up period (59). After a three-year follow-up, participants in the Coronary Drug Project with VPCs on a resting ECG had a significantly higher risk of death than those without the dysrhythmia; subjects were recruited into the study at least 3 months after their MI (60). Ruberman et al. also recruited men some months after their MI; five-year mortality in subjects with complex ventricular dysrhythmias was higher, both for sudden and nonsudden death (61).

In the presence of dysrhythmias and myocardial dysfunction, digitalis can increase cardiac mortality (62), causing clinicians to abandon routine use of this agent after MI. Heavy or binge drinking of ethanol can also substantially worsen prognosis in persons with underlying cardiac dysrhythmias, especially in those with borderline or frank congestive heart failure (63).

Although trials of phenytoin, tocainide, mexiletine, and aprinidine were compelted in postinfarction patients, none showed significant improvement in mortality in the treatment groups. In the Cardiac Arrhythmia Suppression Trial, subjects in the encainide and flecainide groups had higher mortality rates than those in the placebo group (64). In contrast, trials have shown β-adrenergic blocking agents to be efficacious in reducing mortality (65).

Several studies have demonstrated an adverse prognosis in patients with acute MI that is associated with a new diagnosis of complete heart block (11), right bundle branch block (11), block in two or more fascicles (51), and left bundle branch block (66). Repolarization abnormalities, as reflected in a prolonged Q-T interval, are significantly correlated with subsequent sudden death in myocardial infarction survivors (67).

PROPHYLACTIC MEDICATIONS

Aspirin and Other Platelet-Active Medications

As noted in Chapter 12 ("Hematologic Considerations"), aspirin and sulfinpyrazone each significantly reduced mortality in patients recovering from acute MI, and aspirin cut in half the rate of reinfarction during the first 15 months of follow-up in the ISIS-2 study (68). Table 12.2

lists studies of long-term treatment of MI survivors with platelet-active agents. Metaanalysis by British scientists led them to conclude that such drugs reduce vascular mortality by 15% and nonfatal vascular events, such as MI and stroke, by 30% (69).

β-Adrenergic Blocking Drugs

In 1985, Yusef et al. published their extensive review of more than 60 trials of β-blockade during and after myocardial infarction. They divided trials into three categories: (a) those beginning β-blockade within a few hours of symptoms, while the MI is still evolving; (b) those starting medication within the subsequent few days, and (c) those initiating therapy some weeks or months after the MI (70).

When administration of β-blockers begins within the first few hours of MI, infarct size, as judged by peak myocardial enzyme release, is reduced some 14 to 30% (71–73). Long-term survival is significantly better in those patients receiving intravenous β-blockers early, followed by oral maintenance medication. In the International Study of Infarct Survival, MI patients who received atenolol had a 15% lower mortality than those in the placebo group (74). Subjects in the MIAMI (Metoprolol in Acute Myocardial Infarction) study assigned to intravenous/oral metoprolol therapy had a 13% mortality reduction 15 days post-MI (75).

When β-blockers are begun beyond the first 24 hours after MI, mortality reductions approximating 25% have been noted for periods up to six years (70, 76–78). While all β-blockers show appreciable benefit, those with significant intrinsic sympathomimetic activity may be less effective (70).

β-Blockers may exert their long-term protective action through an antidysrhythmic effect or through an increase in the ventricular fibrillation threshold (79). While the wisdom of suppressing asymptomatic or mildly symptomatic ventricular ectopic activity after MI is still debated, the benefit of starting long-term β-blockade before hospital discharge (in the absence of congestive heart failure) has been clearly established (80).

Calcium-Channel Blocking Medications

Although postinfarction trials of verapamil and nifedipine have not demonstrated reduced morbidity or mortality, diltiazem appears to confer benefit on certain groups of MI survivors. In a 14-day study of diltiazem (320 mg/day), early reinfarction and the frequency of refractory postinfarction angina were significantly reduced after non–Q wave infarctions (81). During the Multicenter Diltiazem Postinfarction Trial, 2466 MI survivors were randomized to diltiazem (240 mg/day) or placebo groups. Although no overall effect on morbidity or mortality was noted, those in the diltiazem group who had normal left ventricular function did have significantly fewer cardiac events. The authors caution that the differences noted in the responses of the normal and abnormal myocardial function groups should be confirmed in a propsective study, since such differences were not part of their orginal hypothesis (82).

NONINVASIVE AND INVASIVE TESTING AFTER MI

Of all persons dying within the first year after MI, 50% do so within the first three weeks and another 25% die within the next ten weeks. Fortunately, several testing procedures allow further prognostic discrimination and evaluation of functional capacity in MI survivors beyond that available from the hospital course.

These tests become especially useful in persons with a silent MI; such individuals comprise as many as a third of all MI survivors, and they have a similar prognosis as those with a symptomatic course (83). Useful procedures include exercise and radionuclide testing, coronary angiography and electrophysiologic evaluation. Stepwise evaluation, such as that recommended by DeBusk, allows identification of patients at high risk due to irreversible left ventricular dysfunction, those at moderate risk due to myocardial ischemia, and those at low risk who are free of myocardial dysfunction and ischemia (32).

Exercise and Radionuclide Testing

Exercise testing in the late hospitalization or early home periods can be accomplished in a majority of MI survivors with little risk and reasonable cost-effectiveness. Functional capacity is usually quantitated in METs (multiples of resting oxygen consumption); the ability to complete 5 METs or more without electrocardiographic abnormalities, angina, exertional hypotension (10 mm Hg drop from earlier peak blood pressure), or complex ventricular dysrhythmias places the individual in the lowest risk category (32, 36). The presence of any of the aforementioned conditions places the individual at the least at twice the risk for reinfarction or cardiac death (32).

Radionuclide ventriculography offers further prognostic discrimination in the MI survivor. If the ejection fraction rises with exercise, the risk of subsequent events is low. In contrast, an exercise-induced fall in the ejection fraction usually reflects a reversible myocardial ischemia, and correlates well with thallium myocardial perfusion imaging defects noted during exercise. These findings are associated with significantly increased risk of rein-farction, death, or the need for coronary artery bypass surgery (84, 85).

Ross et al. have recommended that persons who do not have an exercise test, but have a resting radionuclide ejection fraction between 0.20 and 0.44, should go directly to angiography. Persons who displayed ischemia on exercise testing or stop at a low-peak workload (11% one-year mortality) should receive angiography as well (86).

Coronary Angiography

Using their database of 1848 patients surviving beyond day 5 of hospitalization, Ross et al. examined published decision schemes for coronary angiography after acute MI. Their findings led them to recommend the following patients (under age 75) for angiography without further testing: (a) those with severe resting ischemia anytime beyond the first 24 hours (18% mortality between day 6 and one year); and (b) hospital survivors with clinical and radiographic signs of left ventricular failure and a history of previous MI (25% mortality from discharge to one year). They recommend that angiography decisions for persons 75 and older be made on an individual basis (86).

Electrophysiologic Testing

While the benefits of programmed electrical stimulation to induce ventricular dysrhythmias during electrophysiologic testing have been established for predicting sudden death (87), they are not clearly useful prognostically after a myocardial infarction uncomplicated by cardiac arrest.

STANDARD CAD RISK INDICATORS

Smoking

In most studies of MI survivors, the risk of recurrence can be cut in half by smoking cessation. This is true in young as well as in elderly patients, in both women and men, and in cigar and pipe smokers as well as cigarette users. The relative risk of smoking continuance is attenuated somewhat after the initial postinfarction years (88–91). Recurrence of angina after MI occurs twice as often in continuing smokers as in those who quit after the infarction (92), and the risk of recurrent cardiac arrest is significantly lowered by smoking cessation (93). Salonen has estimated that 28% of the deaths in Finnish postinfarction patients are attributable to smoking continuance (94). Approximately half of MI patients stop smoking after their infarction, but as many as 40 to 75% of smokers resume their habit after hospital discharge (95).

Smoking cessation success after MI correlates with higher socioeconomic status and more severe MI. Individual and community programs can significantly aid MI survivors in modifying their risk in this regard (96). Women apparently find it more difficult to give up smoking after cardiac events. In one study of 129 cardiac rehabilitation patients who were smoking at the time of their event, 14% of the men were smoking six months later compared with 59% of the women (97). Facilitation of initiation and adherence to smoking cessation is discussed more fully in Chapter 5 ("Smoking").

Dyslipidemias and Nutrition

Studies of the prognostic value of serum total cholesterol measurements after MI have been limited by several factors. Because of the relative unreliability of lipid measurements made late in a hospitalization for MI, most studies recorded their baseline cholesterol levels months to years after the MI (98), during which time, many patients may make considerable dietary changes. However, recent evidence

indicates that measurements made within 24 hours of acute symptoms are reasonably accurate indicators of pre-MI lipid levels (99).

Nevertheless, a majority of investigations show an increased relative risk of an elevated total cholesterol level in the post-MI period. The Framingham Study, which did have preinfarction lipid and lipoprotein levels, estimated an excess of risk of 30% for every 50 mg/dl increment in total cholesterol (100).

The Coronary Drug Project had a niacin-treated group among their subjects who had survived MI some years earlier. Active treatment ended after six years of study; however, nine years later, persons originally treated with niacin were still at significantly less risk for both total mortality and coronary heart disease mortality (101). Niacin, in pharmacologic doses, lowered triglycerides and raised HDL-cholesterol in two major investigations. In the Stockholm Ischaemic Heart Disease Secondary Prevention study, lowered triglyceride levels were associated with reduced mortality (102). In the Coronary Drug Project, five-year mortality was twice as high in men with HDL-cholesterol levels below 35 mg/dl as in subjects with higher values (103).

Physical exercise can raise HDL-cholesterol levels (104), and, through reduction of obesity, lower triglyceride levels. Gemfibrozil treatment can do likewise in MI survivors (105). Management of lipid disorders is discussed more comprehensively in Chapter 3 ("Lipids").

Blood Pressure

In the Framingham Study, Kannel and co-workers confirmed that MI often results in decreased blood pressure, secondary to myocardial damage. This effect is noted even after controlling for age and pharmacologic treatment. Such individuals were at twice the risk of recurrence; the larger the post-MI drop, the greater the mortality. When persons with more than a 10 mm Hg blood pressure drop were excluded from subsequent analyses, persons with hypertension after MI had five times the mortality of persons who remained normotensive post-infarct (100, 106). In the Coronary Drug Project, patients with a post-MI blood pressure drop had a worse prognosis. They also noted that persistence of combined systolic and diastolic hypertension as well as isolated systolic hypertension were adverse prognostic factors (107). These blood pressure effects may partly explain the relatively poorer prognosis post-MI in black patients (108).

Treatment of hypertension in MI survivors appears beneficial; those assigned to the treatment group in the Hypertension Detection and Follow-up Program had a 20% reduction in total mortality compared with those assigned to the control group (109). Current hypertension treatment guidelines are found in the 1988 Joint National Committee Report (110) and in Chapter 4 ("Hypertension").

Diabetes Mellitus

Diabetic MI survivors have morbidity and mortality rates at least double that of nondiabetic patients (100, 111–113). The risk of recurrent MI in diabetic women is twice that of diabetic men. Diabetic women are also twice as likely as nondiabetic women to have recurrent MI, and were four times as likely to develop congestive heart failure (114). Diabetologists agree that proper management of type II (non–insulin dependent) diabetes requires close attention to the accompanying lipid disorders, but such awareness is often lacking in patient and clinician, particularly in lower socioeconcomic groups (115).

Obesity

Karvetti and Knuts noted a significant weight reduction in their cardiac rehabilitation patients (116). Similarly, Boston investigators have observed concurrent decreases in weight and lipids in their patients, along with a reduction in frequency of angina and S-T segment depression (117). Holt and colleagues reviewed the course of overweight patients after MI. Obesity strongly influenced early mortality in older patients, but had no significant influence on one-year outcome or on early prognosis in patients younger than 65 years (118). Management of obesity in cardiac patients is discussed more fully in Chapter 9 ("Obesity").

Age and Gender

As might be expected, almost every major study of post-MI prognosis shows age to be a major determinant of survival, even after controlling for the presence or level of the major physiologic risk indicators mentioned above (10).

Several studies have indicated a poorer prognosis for women after MI, particularly with regard to early morbidity and mortality (8, 11, 119). Many factors have been hypothesized to account for this observed difference, including increased severity of disease and an increased prevalence of comorbid conditions such as diabetes, hypertension, dyslipidemias, or obesity before and after the MI. Adjustments for these factors reduces the observed differences in long-term prognosis between men and women to insignificant levels, since women MI survivors are older, more likely to be diabetic, and have higher blood cholesterol and blood pressure readings after the infarction than their male counterparts (7, 100).

In the Multicenter Postinfarction Research Study, the relative risk of recurrence was similar in women and men categorized by degree of ventricular dysrhythmias, but women had a worse prognosis if baseline left ventricular ejection fraction was less than 30% (120). In the Beta-Blocker Heart Attack Trial, which enrolled patients during hospitalization, prognosis in the propranolol group was equal in women and men during a mean 25-month follow-up period, although women in the placebo group did have higher event rates than men so assigned (121). The Aspirin Myocardial Infarction Study, which accepted women and men with an MI anytime in the previous five years, mortality rates for women were half those of men among those assigned placebo, despite higher levels of cardiovascular risk indicators in women at baseline. In the aspirin group, women had lower rates of subsequent angina, cerebral transient ischemic attacks, stroke, and nonfatal recurrent MI, but did have a higher overall mortality (121).

Race and Ethnicity

Until recently, postinfarction prognosis studies have focused almost exclusively on whites. Information is now available on blacks in the United States, but little is known about post-MI survival in any other racial or ethnic groups.

Data from the National Hospital Discharge Survey in the United States indicates that, during the years 1973 to 1984, in-hospital case fatality rates after MI were 10 to 70% higher in blacks than in whites for all 10-year age groups through age 70, after which a crossover occurred (122). One possible explanation may be increased delay times from symptom onset to arrival at the emergecy room; in a Chicago study, the delay was two to three times as long for blacks as for whites (123). In a North Carolina study, significantly

more blacks than whites did not see a physician after experiencing chest pain (124).

Long-term prognosis is similarly worse in blacks, particularly in black women. In the Beta-Blocker Heart Attack Trial, whites and blacks randomized to propranolol had a relative risk of death of 0.74 compared to the placebo group. However, deaths among blacks in both groups were 72% higher than among whites. Adjustment for social class reduces the black-white survival differential substantially, as does lack of access to health care facilities and higher levels of baseline cardiovascular risk in poorer persons (125).

Psychosocial and Behavioral Factors

ANXIETY AND DEPRESSION

Almost all MI patients display significant anxiety while hospitalized. This reaction is particularly seen during a first infarction, but the intensity of the anxiety seems to be independent of the severity of the MI. If anxiety has not disappeared by four months after hospital discharge, there is little improvement expected without treatment during the remainder of the first year after infarction. In such cases, readjustment to family and work life is much poorer. Engaging the patient and family in education and cardiac rehabilitation programs is helpful in this regard for most; if severe depression persists, referral to a mental health professional is indicated.

Likewise, depression is seen in most MI patients during the early phases of recovery, but it is present least often in patients from higher socioeconomic and educational strata (126). Goble and colleagues suggest that such depression is similar to that seen in bereavement; in this case, the grief is for loss of self and one's sense of immortality. Mood changes reflecting this depression are fatigue, irritability, early waking, and reduced libido. Anxiety may accompany the depression; both may resolve if the patient and family recognize the transient nature of this response to the MI. Education and exercise programs add to the pace of emotional recovery (127).

CORONARY-PRONE (TYPE A) BEHAVIOR

Several studies have investigated outcome in post-MI patients classified by their coronary-prone (Type A) behavior. As noted in Chapter 10, comparability of these studies is made difficult by their use of a variety of instruments to categorize such behavior. In the Recurrent Coronary Prevention Project, type A behavior was significantly related to sudden, but not nonsudden, cardiac death (128). However, in the absence of intervention, many studies show no additional risk incurred by exhibiting type A behavior at baseline (129). Given type A behavior, does it help to change? Friedman et al. randomized post-MI patients into type A behavior counseling and cardiac counseling groups, and compared their outcomes with postinfarction patients from another area who received no counseling. After 4.5 years, a reduction in type A behavior was documented in 35% and 10% of the behavior counseling and cardiac counseling groups, respectively. During that period, cardiac recurrence rate was 12.9% and 21.2% in the two groups, and was 28.2% in the no-counseling group (130). One year after the cessation of counseling, these distinctions between groups had persisted (131). Powell and Thoresen found that this apparent protective of behavior modification was most evident in those with a mild prior MI. In those with more severe earlier infarctions, residual left ventricular dysfunction was much more important prognostically (132).

At present, it is somewhat difficult to reconcile the conflicting findings of the studies. One interpretation involves recognizing that persons with type A behavior may actively change other risk indicators after their MI, counterbalancing the risk of persistence of their time-urgent behavior. If such patients can concurrently lower their risk through dietary modification, adoption of a vigorous exercise program, and modification of their other behaviors, an improved prognosis might be expected.

EDUCATION

In a follow-up study of men who had survived an MI some years before and had complex premature ventricular beats (VPB) at baseline, participants with less than nine years of formal education had three times the rate of sudden death as those with more education. This differential was not seen in the absence of VPBs, and there was no relation between education and recurrent MI (133).

CARDIAC REHABILITATION SERVICES

Recovery from MI may be divided into four phases: hospitalization, early home period, outpatient active training period, and maintenance. In addition to physical recuperation, emotional, social, and economic recovery is facilitated by an integrated, interdisciplinary program such as that described below (134).

Hospitalization

In the past three decades, the length of hospital stay after an uncomplicated MI has decreased from eight weeks to less than one week; in one study, patients were safely discharged three days after coronary reperfusion therapy (135). Early ambulation and discharge minimizes the rapid deconditioning of peripheral and cardiac muscle noted in earlier decades and does not seem to impair health behavior changes such as diet modification or smoking cessation (136).

Patients frequently display anxiety, denial, depression, and anger before accepting the reality of their infarction. Initial anxiety may be manifested in an inability to concentrate, understand, or retain information. Subsequent denial is usually transient, and may be helpful in the early recovery period (137). Depression, which reflects a loss of self-esteem, may follow. Anger may be directed at staff members, who should be psychologically prepared for such outbursts (138).

Most hospitals have a stepped-care program for the MI patient, which includes supervised ambulation and exercise, educational sessions, and counseling by dietitians as well as physical and occupational therapists. Appropriate goals for discharge include adoption of stretching, light calisthenics, and walking activities, as well as a thorough understanding of educational materials and presentations. If exercise testing is done for prognostic reasons prior to discharge, an exercise prescription can be written to guide the patient and family during the early days at home (134).

The social support provided by a family can exert an immediate effect after MI (138, 139); in a Baltimore study, in-hospital case fatality rates were 40 to 50% higher in unmarried women and men compared to those who were married (140). Investigators in the Beta-Blocker Heart Attack Trial identified two psychosocial factors associated with poorer prognosis. Persons who were both socially isolated and reported a high degree of life stress had mortality rates four times higher than those with neither characteristics (141). In a Swedish study, being unmarried was significantly related to an increased risk of cardiovascular events and death over a two-to-five-year period after MI (142).

Even the presence of animal companions can significantly improve survival during the year following MI (143).

Early Home Period

The patient's return to the home environment requires a readjustment of roles for each of the family members. Men are often faced with household management problems that escaped their attention prior to the infarction. Patients of both genders often complain at this time of overprotective spouses. In a Canadian study, 75% of wives reported that their husbands took less responsibility after their MI (144). During a five-year study of 400 German cardiac patients and their wives, interpersonal problems led to a decreased sense of the patient's personal competence. In contrast, positive health perceptions and a strong sense of marital intimacy predicted a positive sense of well-being at later examination (145).

Optimally, contact with the rehabilitation team continues during the early weeks after discharge. Both patients and spouses report that they would benefit from more frequent contact with the physician during the early home period. Patients and their family members can be invited to return to the hospital for educational and support group sessions, which should smooth the process of reintegration into their former activities (134).

UCLA researchers hypothesized that family fears and overprotectiveness might be mitigated by offering a class on cardiopulmonary resuscitation (CPR). Unexpectedly, anxiety and depression scores in the CPR-trained family members were higher at six months than at baseline. The authors suggested that the training may have vividly reminded the family members of their primary responsibility, making denial harder. They also reported that some patients felt increased anxiety when away from their CPR-trained family members (146). Alonzo found that family members, especially a spouse, might provide sufficient reassurance that the cardiac patient may delay in seeking medical help during a life-threatening episode (147).

Stanford University investigators have studied self-efficacy in male patients in relation to exercise testing three weeks after an uncomplicated MI. They first demonstrated significant improvement in self-efficacy for walking, running, lifting, and sexual activity when measured (a) before and after a symptom-limited treadmill test, and (b) before and after counseling that followed the treadmill test. In a subsequent study, the researchers involved subjects' wives by randomizing couples to one of three groups: (a) wife present only at counseling; (b) wife present at husband's treadmill test and at counseling; (c) wife present at test and counseling plus she walked three minutes on the treadmill at the same speed and grade as her husband. Progressively better long-term outcomes were noted with increasing involvement of the wife on the day of the treadmill test (148, 149).

Additionally, family participation in support groups has been helpful. Probably the greatest benefits are the opportunity to know other families who are several weeks farther along in their recovery process and to learn that issues such as fear and overprotectiveness are not unique to their family (138).

Outpatient Active Training Period

The typical outpatient cardiac rehabilitation program in the United States is largely exercise-based. If an exercise test has not been done before hospital discharge, one should be done before beginning the training period. Symptom-limited testing is safe at this time (36), but care

must be taken with type A patients, who tend to suppress reports of fatigue and other symptoms (150).

Patients participating in training programs can recieve: (a) careful monitoring for dysrhythmias and symptoms of congestive heart failure; (b) safe progression of physical activity based on the hospital discharge (or program entry) exercise test, (c) social support from program staff and other participants, and (d) dietary counseling and monitoring to improve diet quality and facilitate weight reduction (134).

To examine the possibility that low-risk post-MI patients might achieve the same exercise benefits by undergoing training at home, Stanford University investigators randomized 198 men to no training, home training, or outpatient-supervised training groups. Home training and group training were equally effective in improving exercise tolerance; both had better results at six months than the no-training group (151). The same team examined the efficacy of high-intensity and low-intensity home training. Peak oxygen consumption rose 17% in the high-intensity group, 8% in those training at low intensity, and did not change in the control group (152).

Although exercise improvement occurs, patients training at home do not have the opportunity to learn from other cardiac patients, as do those training in groups, who have been noted to have lower anxiety and depression scores six months after the MI (153). Social support can be offered by telephone from the cardiac rehabilitation staff for those who train at home. When appropriate, this contact can be augmented by transtelephonic electrocardiographic monitoring and by the availability of a lidocaine injector for home use (154).

Active training, regardless of location, confers physiological conditioning benefits, such as improved exercise tolerance, reduction of heart rate and blood pressure at a given total body workload, improvement of lipid and lipoprotein profiles, weight loss, reduction in platelet aggregation and enhancement of fibrinolysis, and increased likelihood of abstention from smoking (134). Women may achieve smaller benefits than men in such programs, for reasons not currently clear (139). Sessions limited to women only may appeal to older women unaccustomed to exercising vigorously in the presence of men. Older men progress comparably to their younger counterparts (155). The safety of exercise in the immediate post-MI period has been well-established (156).

Several individual trials of outpatient exercise training have noted lower morbidity and mortality in the training group, but study size has been inadequate for these differences to achieve statistical significance. However, Oldridge and colleagues did a metaanalysis on such trials, noting a significant improvement in mortality from such participation (157).

In a Finnish study, post-MI women and men were randomized to treatment and control groups. Two weeks after hospital discharge, the former group began a program that included monthly examinations by an internist and contact with a physical therapist, a psychologist, a nutritionist, and a social worker. The subjects participated in a supervised exercise program that was most intense during the first three months after MI. At the end of three years, sudden death in the treatment group was less than that of the controls, and total mortality was only 18.6% compared with 29.4% in those not receiving the intervention (158).

Maintenance Phase

After the first few months post-MI, patients face an even greater challenge: lifelong maintenance of their newly developed health habits.

Oldridge and colleagues found that certain categories of patients adhere less well to a maintenance exercise plan. These include those with (a) two or more previous MIs; (b) a coronary-prone behavior pattern; (c) a cigarette smoking habit; (d) blue-collar occupation; and (e) leisure-time inactivity (159). Those who adhere to treatment regimens may be different from nonadherers in other ways presently unmeasurable. In the Coronary Drug Project, good adherers to placebo had lower mortality rates than poor adherers to the study medication (160).

Return to work after MI is often used as a measure of the entire rehabilitation program. However, individuals rarely return to work above a culturally determined age (60 in the United States, 55 in Scandinavian countries, 50 in Spain and Ireland) (161). Patients who remain symptomatic after MI rarely return to work; those who are asymptomatic show little correlation between residual cardiac dysfunction and work reentry. Persons discharged early appear to return to work earlier than others (40). Individuals who remain depressed return to work slowly, if at all. In contrast, type A persons often return quickly (161).

Equally important are the patient's attributions and expectations. Those who attribute their MI to job stress have a much slower rate of return to work (162). Patients who attribute their MI to external, uncontrollable causes had a poorer outcome six months later than those who cited a more complex causal pattern (163). The best indicator of return to work is the patient's prediction at the time of hospital discharge. Some individuals use the time after MI to rethink and reorder their life's priorities, so such delays may favorably improve long-term prognosis (161). In many individuals, however, encouragement by the physician to return to work early can have important psychological and financial benefits for the patient and the health care system (164).

Return to sexual activity is another important indicator of MI recovery. Most MI patients previously active have resumed their preinfarction levels within six months, although many accomplish this much sooner. As with return to work, patients can accurately predict the time at which they will resume sexual activity. Reasons advanced for not reengaging in sexual activity are anxiety, depression, fear of relapse or death, fatigue, decreased desire, angina pectoris, impotence, and a dissatisfaction with the prior activity (138).

For a typical middle-aged couple, heart rate and blood pressure responses during intercourse do not exceed those already performed by the patient on exercise testing; this fact should be used during the counseling that follows the exercise test to reassure the couple about the safety of sexual activity. β-Adrenergic blockade can complement exercise training in lowering heart rate and blood pressure responses to exercise (138).

REFERENCES

1. Epstein SE, Palmeri ST, Patterson RE. Evaluation of patients after acute myocardial infarction. Indications for cardiac catheterization and surgical intervention. N Engl J Med 1982;307:1487–1492.

2. Weinblatt E, Goldberg JD, Ruberman W, Frank CW, Monk MA, Chaudhary BS. Mortality after first myocardial infarction. Search for a secular trend. JAMA 1982;247:1576–1581.

3. Ulvenstam G, Aberg A, Bergstrand R, et al. Recurrent myocardial infarction. 1. Natural history of fatal and non-fatal events. Eur Heart J 1985;6:294–302.

4. Lie KI, Tans AC, Louridtz WJ, Durrer D, Wellens HJ. Immediate prognosis in recurrent myocardial infarction. Lancet 1975;1:647–648.

5. Helmers C, Lundman T. Early and late deaths after myocardial infarction. A report from the Swedish CCU Study. Acta Med Scand 1979;205:3–9.

6. Taylor GJ, Humphries JO, Mellits ED, et al. Predictors of clinical course, coronary anatomy and left ventricular function after recovery from acute myocardial infarction. Circulation 1980;62:960–970.

7. Schlant RC, Forman S, Stamler J, Canner PL. The natural history of coronary heart disease: Prognostic factors after recovery from myocardial infarction in 2789 men. The five-year findings of the Coronary Drug Project. Circulation 1982;66:401–414.

8. Marmor A, Geltman EM, Schechtman K, Sobel BE, Roberts R. Recurrent myocardial infarction: clinical predictors and prognostic implications. Circulation 1982;66:415–421.

9. The Multicenter Postinfarction Research Group. Risk stratification and survival after myocardial infarction. N Engl J Med 1983;309:331–336.

10. Merrilees MA, Scott PJ, Norris RM. Prognosis after myocardial infarction: Results of 15-year follow-up. Br Med J 1984;288:356–359.

11. Beaune J, Touboul P, Boissel JP, Delahaye JP. Quantitative assessment of myocardial infarction prognosis to 1 and 6 mth—from clinical data. Eur J Cardiol 1978;8:629–647.

12. Ulvenstam G, Aberg A, Pennert K, et al. Recurrent myocardial infarction. 2. Possibilities of prediction. Eur Heart J 1985;6:303–311.

13. Pierard LA, Dubois C, Smeets JP, Boland J, Carlier J, Kulbertus HE. Prognostic significance of angina pectoris before first acute myocardial infarction. Am J Cardiol 1988;61:984–987.

14. Peel AA, Semple T, Wang I, Lancaster WH, Dall JL. A coronary prognostic index for grading the severity of infarction. Br Heart J 1962;24:745–760.

15. Norris RM, Brandt PW, Caughey DE, Lee AJ, Scott PJ. A new coronary prognostic index. Am Heart J 1970;79:428–431.

16. Fabricius-Bjerre N, Munkvad M, Knudsen JB. Subendocardial and transmural myocardial infarction. A five-year survival study. Am J Med 1979;66:986–990.

17. Chapelle JP, Albert A, Smeets JP, et al. Early assessment of risk in patients with acute myocardial infarction. Eur Heart J 1981;2:187–196.

18. DeBusk RF, Kraemer HC, Nash E. Stepwise risk stratification soon after acute myocardial infarction. Am J Cardiol 1983;52:1161–1166.

19. Hsu L, Senaratne MP, De Silva S, Rossall RE, Kappagoda T. Prediction of coronary events following myocardial infarction using a discriminant function analysis. J Chron Dis 1986;39:543–552.

20. Baker JT, Bramlet DA, Lester RM, Harrison DG, Roe CR, Cobb FR. Myocardial infarct extension: incidence and relationship to survival. Circulation 1982;65:918–923.

21. Muller JE, Rude RE, Brawnwald E, et al. Myocardial infarct extension: occurrence, outcome and risk factors in the Multicenter Investigation of Limitation of Infarct Size. Ann Intern Med 1988;108:1–6.

22. Grande P, Nielsen A, Wagner GS, Christiansen C. Quantitative influence of serum creatinine kinase isoenzyme MB estimated infarct size and other prognostic variables on one year mortality after acute myocardial infarction. Br Heart J 1985;53:9–15.

23. Robinson K, Conroy R, Mulcahy R. Fifteen-year comparative follow-up in patients with anterior and inferior myocardial infarction. J Am Coll Cardiol 1988;11:222A.

24. Kennedy JW. Non–Q wave myocardial infarction. N Engl J Med 1986;315:451–453.

25. DeWood MA, Stiffler WF, Simpson CS, et al. Coronary arteriographic findings soon after non–Q wave myocardial infarction. N Engl J Med 1986;315:417–423.

26. Nicod P, Gilpin E, Dittrich H, et al. Short- and long-term clinical outcome after Q-wave and non–Q wave myocardial infarction in a large patient population. Circulation 1989;79:528–536.

27. Killip T III, Kimball JT. Treatment of myocardial infarction in a coronary care unit. A two-year experience with 250 patients. Am J Cardiol 1967;20:457–464.

28. Killip T, Kimball JT. A survey of the coronary care unit: Concept and results. Prog Cardiovasc Dis 1968;11:45–51.

29. Forrester JS, Diamond GA, Swan HJ. Correlative classification of clinical and hemodynamic function after acute myocardial infarction. Am J Cardiol 1977;39:137–145.

30. Silverman KJ, Becker LC, Bulkley BH, et al. Value of early thallium-201 scintigraphy for predicting mortality in patients with acute myocardial infarction. Circulation 1980;61:996–1003.

31. Sanford CF, Corbett J, Nicod P, et al. Value of radionuclide ventriculography in the initial characterization of patients with acute myocardial infarction. Am J Cardiol 1982;49:637–643.

32. DeBusk RF. Specialized testing after recent acute myocardial infarction. Ann Intern Med 1989;110:470–481.

33. Chaturvedi NC, Walsh MJ, Evans A, Munro P, Boyle DM, Barber JM. Selection of patients for early discharge after myocardial infarction. Br Heart J 1974;36:533–535.

34. Kassis E, Vogelsang M, Lyngborg K. Cardiac rupture complicating myocardial infarction. A study concerning early diagnosis and possible management. Dan Med Bull 1981;28:164–167.

35. Singer DE, Mulley AG, Thibault GE, Barnett GO. Unexpected readmissions to the coronary-care unit during recovery from acute myocardial infarction. N Engl J Med 1981;304:625–629.

36. Davidson DM, DeBusk RF. Prognostic value of a single exercise test 3 weeks after uncomplicated myocardial infarction. Circulation 1980;61:236–242.

37. Schuster EH, Bulkley BH. Early postinfarction angina. Ischemia at a distance and ischemia in the infarct zone. N Engl J Med 1981;305:1101–1105.

38. Dwyer EM, McMaster P, Greenberg H. Nonfatal cardiac events and recurrent infarction in the year after acute myocardial infarction. J Am Coll Cardiol 1984;4:695–702.

39. Waters DD, Theroux P, Halphen C, Mizgala HF. Clinical predictors of angina following myocardial infarction. Am J Med 1979;66:991–996.

40. Topol EJ. Coronary angioplasty for acute myocardial infarction. Ann Intern Med 1988;109:970–980.

41. White HD, Rivers JT, Maslowski AH, et al. Effect of intravenous streptokinase as compared with that of tissue plasminogen activator on left ventricular function after first myocardial infarction. N Engl J Med 1989;320:817–821.

42. Kennedy JW, Ivey TD, Misbach G, et al. Coronary artery bypass graft surgery early after acute myocardial infarction. Circulation 1989;79(suppl I):I73–I78.

43. Lange RA, Cigarroa RG, Hillis LD. Angiographic characteristics of the infarct-related coronary artery in patients with angina pectoris after myocardial infarction. Am J Cardiol 1989;64:257–260.

44. Epstein SE, Quyyumi AA, Bonow RO. Myocardial ischemia—silent or symptomatic. N Engl J Med 1988;318:1038–1043.

45. Theroux P, Waters DD, Halphen C, Debaisieux JC, Mizgala HF. Prognostic value of exercise testing soon after myocardial infarction. N Engl J Med 1979;301:341–345.

46. Gottlieb SO, Gottlieb SH, Achuff SC, et al. Silent ischemia on Holter monitoring predicts mortality in high-risk post-infarction patients. JAMA 1988;259:1030–1035.

47. Goldstein S, Friedman L, Hutchinson R, et al. Timing, mechanism and clinical setting of witnessed deaths in postmyocardial infarction patients. J Am Coll Cardiol 1984;3:1111–1117.

48. Volpi A, Maggioni A, Franzosi MG, Pampillona S, Mauri F, Tognoni G. In-hospital prognosis of patients with acute myocardial infarction complicated by primary ventricular fibrillation. N Engl J Med 1987;317:257–261.

49. Goldberg RJ, Gore JM, Haffajee CI, Alpert JS, Dalen JE. Outcome after cardiac arrest during acute myocardial infarction. Am J Cardiol 1987;59:251–255.

50. Richards D, Ross D, Cooper M, Skinner M, Uther J. What is the best predictor of sudden death following myocardial infarction? J Am Coll Cardiol 1988;11:26A.

51. Rosenthal ME, Oseran DS, Gang E, Peter T. Sudden cardiac death following acute myocardial infarction. Am Heart J 1985; 109:865–876.

52. Bigger JT, Weld FM, Rolnitzky LM. Prevalence, characteristics, and significance of ventricular tachycardia (3 or more complexes) detected with ambulatory electrocardiographic recording in the late hospital phase of acute myocardial infarction. Am J Cardiol 1981; 48:815–823.

53. Bigger JT, Fleiss JL, Kleiger R, Miller VP, Rolnitzky LM. The relationships among ventricular arrhythmias, left ventricular dysfunction, and mortality in the 2 years after myocardial infarction. Circulation 1984;69:250–258.

54. Helmers C, Lundman T. Sudden coronary death after acute myocardial infarction. Adv Cardiol 1978;25:176–182.

55. Mukarji J, Rude RE, Poole K, et al. Risk factors for sudden death after acute myocardial infarction: two-year follow-up. Am J Cardiol 1984;54:31–36.

56. Moss AJ, Davis HT, DeCamilla J, Bayer LW. Ventricular ectopic beats and their relation to sudden and nonsudden cardiac death after myocardial infarction. Circulation 1979;60:998–1003.

57. Sturzenhofecker P, Samek L, Droste C, Gohlke H, Peterson J, Roskamm H. Prognosis of coronary heart disease and progression of coronary arteriosclerosis in postinfarction patients under the age of 40. In: Roskamm H (ed): Myocardial infarction at a young age. New York: Springer-Verlag, 1981.

58. Bigger JT Jr, Heller CA, Wenger TL, Weld FM. Risk stratification after myocardial infarction. Am J Cardiol 1978;42:202–210.

59. Marchilinski FE, Waxman HL, Buxton AE, Josephson ME. Sustained ventricular tachycardia during the early post-infarction period: electrophysiologic findings and prognosis for survival. J Am Coll Cardiol 1983;2:240–250.

60. The Coronary Drug Project Research Group. The prognostic importance of the electrocardiogram after myocardial infarction. Experience in the Coronary Drug Project. Ann Intern Med 1972;77:677–689.

61. Ruberman W, Weinblatt E, Goldberg J, Frank CW, Chaudhary BS, Shapiro S. Ventricular premature complexes and sudden death after myocardial infarction. Circulation 1981;64:297–305.

62. Moss AJ, Davis HT, Conard DL, DeCamilla JJ, Odoroff CL. Digitalis-associated cardiac mortality after myocardial infarction. Circulation 1981;64:1150–1156.

63. Davidson DM. Cardiovascular effects of alcohol. West J Med 1989;151:430–439.

64. The Cardiac Arrhythmia Suppression Trial (CAST) Investigators. Preliminary report: effect of encainide and flecainide on mortality in a randomized trial of arrhythmia suppres-

sion after myocardial infarction. N Engl J Med 1989;321:406–412.

65. May GS, Eberlein KA, Furberg CD, Passamani ER, DeMets DL. Secondary prevention after myocardial infarction: a review of long-term trials. Prog Cardiovasc Dis 1982;24:331–352.

66. Brush JE Jr, Brand DA, Acampora D, Chalmer B, Wackers FJ. Use of the initial electrocardiogram to predict in-hospital complications of acute myocardial infarction. N Engl J Med 1985;312:1137–1141.

67. Schwartz PJ, Wolf S. QT interval prolongation as a predictor of sudden death in patients with myocardial infarction. Circulation 1978;57:1074–1077.

68. ISIS-2 (Second International Study of Infarct Survival) Collaborative Group. Randomized trial of intravenous streptokinase, oral aspirin, both, or neither among 17,187 cases of suspected acute myocardial infarction: ISIS-2. Lancet 1988;2:349–360.

69. Antiplatelet Trialists' Collaboration. Secondary prevention of vascular disease by prolonged antiplatelet treatment. Br Med J 1988;296:320–331.

70. Yusuf S, Peto R, Collins R, Sleight P. Beta blockade during and after myocardial infarction: an overview of the randomized trials. Prog Cardiovasc Dis 1985;27:335–371.

71. Boyle DM, Barber JM, McIlmoyle EL, et al. Effect of very early intervention with metoprolol on myocardial infarct size. Br Heart J 1983;49:229–233.

72. Herlitz J, Elmfeldt D, Hjalmarson A, et al. Effect of metoprolol on indirect signs of the size and severity of acute myocardial infarction. Am J Cardiol 1983;51:1282–1288.

73. The International Collaborative Study Group. Reduction of infarct size with the early use of timolol in acute myocardial infarction. N Engl J Med 1984;310:9–15.

74. ISIS-1 (First Collaborative Study of Infarct Survival) Collaborative Group. Randomized trial of intravenous atenolol among 16,027 cases of suspected acute myocardial infarction: ISIS-1. Lancet 1986;2:57–66.

75. The MIAMI Trial Research Group. Metoprolol in acute myocardial infarction (MIAMI). A randomized placebo-controlled international trial. Eur Heart J 1985;6:199–226.

76. Baber NS, Lewis JA. Confidence in results of beta-blocker postinfarction trials. Br Med J 1982;284:1749–1750.

77. Herlitz J, Hjalmarson A, Swedberg K, Ryden L, Waagstein F. Effects on mortality during five years after early intervention with metoprolol in suspected acute myocardial infarction. Acta Med Scand 1988;223:227–231.

78. Pedersen TR for the Norwegian Multicenter Study Group. Six-year follow-up of the Norwegian Multicenter Study on Timolol after acute myocardial infarction. N Engl J Med 1985;313:1055–1058.

79. Luketich J, Friehling TD, O'Connor KM, Kowey PR. The effect of beta adrenergic blockade on vulnerability to ventricular fibrillation and inducibility of ventricular arrhythmia in short- and long-term feline infarction models. Am Heart J 1989;118:265–271.

80. Ruskin JN. The Cardiac Arrhythmia Suppression Trial (CAST). N Engl J Med 1989;321:386–388.

81. Gibson RS, Boden WE, Theroux P, et al. Diltiazem and reinfarction in patients with non–Q wave myocardial infarction. N Engl J Med 1986;315:423–429.

82. The Multicenter Diltiazem Postinfarction Trial Research Group. The effect of diltiazem on mortality and reinfarction after myocardial infarction. N Engl J Med 1988;319:385–392.

83. Kannel WB, Abbott RD. Incidence and prognosis of unrecognized myocardial infarction: an update on the Framingham Study. N Engl J Med 1984;311:1144–1147.

84. Hung J, Goris ML, Nash E, Kraemer HC, DeBusk RF. Comparative value of maximal treadmill testing, exercise thallium myocardial perfusion scintigraphy and exercise radionuclide ventriculography for distinguishing high- and low-risk patients soon after myocardial infarction. Am J Cardiol 1984;53:1221–1227.

85. Gibson RS, Watson DD, Craddock GB, et al. Prediction of cardiac events after uncomplicated myocardial infarction: a prospective study comparing predischarge exercise thallium-201 scintigraphy and coronary angiography. Circulation 1983;68:321–336.

86. Ross J Jr, Gilpin EA, Madsen EB, et al. A decision scheme for coronary angiography

after acute myocardial infarction. Circulation 1989;79:292–303.

87. Denniss AR, Baaljens H, Cody DV, et al. Value of programmed stimulation and exercise testing in predicting one-year mortality after acute myocardial infarction. Am J Cardiol 1985;56:213–220.

88. Wilhelmsen L. Cessation of smoking after myocardial infarction: effects on mortality after ten years. Br Heart J 1983;49:416–422.

89. Mulcahy R. Influence of cigarette smoking on morbidity and mortality after myocardial infarction. Br Heart J 1983;49:410–415.

90. Hickey N, Mulcahy R, Daly L, Graham I, O'Donoghue S, Kennedy S. Cigar and pipe smoking related to four-year survival of coronary patients. Br Heart J 1983;49:423–426.

91. Hermanson B, Omenn GS, Kronmal RA, Gersh BJ and participants in the Coronary Artery Surgery Study. Beneficial six-year outcome of smoking cessation in older men and women with coronary artery disease. Results from the CASS Registry. N Engl J Med 1988;319:1365–1369.

92. Daly LE, Graham IM, Hickey N, Mulcahy R. Does stopping smoking delay onset of angina after infarction? Br Med J 1985;291:935–937.

93. Hallstrom AP, Cobb LA, Ray R. Smoking as a risk factor for recurrence of sudden cardiac arrest. N Engl J Med 1986;314:271–275.

94. Salonen JT. Stopping smoking and long-term mortality after acute myocardial infarction. Br Heart J 1980;43:463–469.

95. Blumenthal JA, Levenson RM. Behavioral approaches to secondary prevention of coronary heart disease. Circulation 1987;76:(suppl I):I130–I137.

96. Salonen JT, Hamynen H, Heinonen OP. Impact of a health education program and other factors on stopping smoking after heart attack. Scand J Soc Med 1985;13:103–108.

97. Higgins C, Schweiger MJ. Smoking termination patterns in a cardiac rehabilitation program. J Cardiac Rehabil 1983;3:55–59.

98. Phillips AN, Shaper AG, Pocock SJ, Walker M, MacFarlane PW. The role of risk factors in heart attacks occurring in men with pre-existing ischaemic heart disease. Br Heart J 1988;60:404–410.

99. Gore JM, Goldberg RJ, Matsumoto AS, Castelli WP, McNamara PM, Dalen JE. Validity of serum total cholesterol level obtained within 24 hours of acute myocardial infarction. Am J Cardiol 1984;54:722–725.

100. Wong ND, Cupples LA, Ostfeld AM, Levy D, Kannel WB. Risk factors for long-term coronary prognosis after initial myocardial infarction: the Framingham Study. Am J Epidemiol 1989;130:469–480.

101. Canner PI, Berge KG, Wenger NK, et al. Fifteen-year mortality in Coronary Drug Project patients: long-term benefit with niacin. J Am Coll Cardiol 1986:8:1245–1255.

102. Carlson LA, Rosenhamer G. Reduction of mortality in the Stockholm Ischaemic Heart Disease Secondary Prevention Study by combined treatment with clofibrate and nicotinic acid. Acta Med Scand 1988;223:405–418.

103. Berge KG, Canner PL, Hainline A. High-density lipoprotein cholesterol and prognosis after myocardial infarction. Circulation 1982;66:1176–1178.

104. Ballantyne FC, Clark RS, Simpson HS, Ballantyne D. The effect of moderate physical exercise on the plasma lipoprotein subfractions of male survivors of myocardial infarction. Circulation 1982;65:913–918.

105. Kaukola S, Manninen V, Malkonen M, Ehnholm C. Gemfibrozil in the treatment of dyslipidaemias in middle-aged male survivors of myocardial infarction. Acta Med Scand 1981;209:69–73.

106. Kannel WB, Sorlie P, Castelli WP, McGee D. Blood pressure and survival after myocardial infarction: the Framingham study. Am J Cardiol 1980;45:326–330.

107. The Coronary Drug Project Research Group. Blood pressure in survivors of myocardial infarction. J Am Coll Cardiol 1984;4:1135–1147.

108. Castaner A, Simmons BE, Mar M, Cooper R. Myocardial infarction among black patients: poor prognosis after hospital discharge. Ann Intern Med 1988;109:33–35.

109. Langford HG, Stamler J, Wassertheil-Smoller S, Prineas RJ. All-cause mortality in the Hypertension Detection and Follow-up Program: findings for the whole cohort and for persons with less severe hypertension, with and without other traits related to the risk of mor-

tality. Prog Cardiovasc Dis 1986;29(3 suppl 1):29–54.

110. The 1988 Joint National Committee. The 1988 report of the Joint National Committee on Detection, Evaluation, and Treatment of High Blood Pressure. Arch Intern Med 1988;148:1023–1038.

111. Heliovaraa M, Karvonen MJ, Punsar S, et al. Importance of coronary risk factors in the presence or absence of myocardial ischemia. Am J Cardiol 1982;50:1248–1252.

112. Smith JW, Marcus FI, Serokman R. Prognosis of patients with diabetes mellitus after myocardial infarction. Am J Cardiol 1984;54:718–721.

113. Ulvenstam G, Aberg A, Bergstrand R, et al. Long-term prognosis after myocardial infarction in men with diabetes. Diabetes 1985;34:787–792.

114. Abbott RD, Donahue RP, Kannel WB, Wilson PW. The impact of diabetes on survival following myocardial infarction in men vs. women. JAMA 1988;260:3456–3460.

115. Stern MP, Patterson JK, Haffner SM, Hazuda HP, Mitchell BD. Lack of awareness and treatment of hyperlipidemia in type II diabetes in a community survey. JAMA 1989;262:360–364.

116. Karvetti RL, Knuts LR. Effects of comprehensive rehabilitation on weight reduction in myocardial infarction patients. Scand J Rehab Med 1983;15:11–16.

117. Ribiero JH, Hartley LH, Sherwood J, Herd A. The effectiveness of a low lipid diet and exercise in the management of coronary disease. Am Heart J 1984;108:1183–1189.

118. Hoit BD, Gilpin EA, Maisel AA, Henning H, Carlisle J, Ross J Jr. Influence of obesity on morbidity and mortality after acute myocardial infarction. Am Heart J 1987; 114:1334–1341.

119. Fiebach NH, Viscoli CM, Horwitz RI. Differences between women and men in survival after myocardial infarction. Biology or methodology? JAMA 1990;263:1092–1096.

120. Moss AJ, Carleen E, and the Multicenter Postinfarction Research Group. Gender differences in the mortality risk associated with ventricular arrhythmias after myocardial infarction. In: Eaker ED, Packard B, Wenger NK, Clarkson TB, Tyroler HA (eds): Coronary heart

disease in women. Proceedings of an NIH workshop. New York: Haymarket Doyma, Inc., 1987:204–207.

121. Furberg CD, Friedman LM, MacMahon SW. Women as participants in trials of the primary and secondary prevention of cardiovascular disease: part II. Secondary prevention: The Beta-Blocker Heart Attack Trial and the Aspirin Myocardial Infarction Study. In: Eaker ED, Packard B, Wenger NK, Clarkson TB, Tyroler HA (eds): Coronary heart disease in women. Proceedings of an NIH workshop. New York: Haymarket Doyma, Inc., 1987:241–246.

122. Roig E, Castaner A, Simmons B, Patel R, Ford E, Cooper R. In-hospital mortality rates from acute myocardial infarction by race in U.S. hospitals: findings from the National Hospital Discharge Survey. Circulation 1987;76:280–288.

123. Cooper RS, Simmons B, Castaner A, Prasad R, Franklin C, Ferlinz J. Survival rates and prehospital delay during myocardial infarction among black persons. Am J Cardiol 1986;57:208–211.

124. Strogatz DS. Use of medical care for chest pain: differences between blacks and whites. Am J Public Health 1990;80:290–294.

125. Haywood LJ. Coronary heart disease mortality/morbidity and risk in blacks. I.: Clinical manifestations and diagnostic criteria: the experience with the Beta-Blocker Heart Attack Trial. Am Heart J 1984;108:787–793.

126. Guiry E, Conroy RM, Hickey N, Mulcahy R. Psychological response to an acute coronary event and its effect on subsequent rehabilitation and lifestyle change. Clin Cardiol 1987;10:256–260.

127. Goble AJ, Biddle N, Worcester MC. Depression after acute cardiac illness. Qual Life Cardiovasc Care 1989;5:60–65.

128. Brackett CD, Powell LH. Psychosocial and physiological predictors of sudden cardiac death after healing acute myocardial infarction. Am J Cardiol 1988;61:979–983.

129. Ragland DR. Type A behavior and the outcome of coronary disease. N Engl J Med 1989;321:394.

130. Friedman M, Thoresen CE, Gill JJ, et al. Alteration of type A behavior and its effect on cardiac recurrences in post-myocardial in-

farction patients: summary results of the recurrent coronary prevention project. Am Heart J 1986;112:653-665.

131. Friedman M, Powell LH, Thoresen CE, et al. Effect of discontinuance of type A behavioral counseling on type A behavior and cardiac recurrence rate of post-myocardial infarction patients. Am Heart J 1987;114:483-490.

132. Powell LH, Thoresen CE. Effects of type A behavioral counseling and severity of prior acute myocardial infarction on survival. Am J Cardiol 1988;62:1159-1163.

133. Weinblatt E, Ruberman W, Goldberg JD, Frank CW, Shapiro S, Chaudhary BS. Relation of education to sudden death after myocardial infarction. N Engl J Med 1978;299:60-65.

134. Davidson DM, Maloney CA. Recovery after cardiac events. Phys Ther 1985;65:1820-1827.

135. Topol EJ, Burek K, O'Neill WW, et al. A randomized controlled trial of hospital discharge three days after myocardial infarction in the era of reperfusion. N Engl J Med 1988;318:1083-1088.

136. West RR, Evans DA. Lifestyle changes in long term survivors of acute myocardial infarction. J Epidemiol Community Health 1986;40:103-109.

137. Levine J, Warrenburg S, Kerns R. The role of denial in recovery from coronary heart disease. Psychosom Med 1987;49:109-117.

138. Davidson DM. Family and sexual adjustments after cardiac events. Qual Life Cardiovasc Care 1989;5:66-71, 77-79.

139. Davidson DM. Social support and cardiac rehabilitation: a review. J Cardiopulm Rehabil 1987;7:196-200.

140. Chandra V, Szklo M, Goldberg R, Tonascia J. The impact of marital status on survival after an acute myocardial infarction: a population-based study. Am J Epidemiol 1983;117:320-325.

141. Ruberman W, Weinblatt E, Goldberg JD, Chaudhary BS. Psychosocial influences on mortality after myocardial infarction. N Engl J Med 1984;311:552-559.

142. Wiklund I, Oden A, Sanne H, Ulvenstam G, Wilhelmsson C, Wilhelmsson L. Prognostic importance of somatic and psychosocial variables after a first myocardial infarction. Am J Epidemiol 1988;128:786-795.

143. Friedmann E, Katcher AH, Lynch JJ, Thomas SA. Animal companions and one-year survival of patients after discharge from a coronary care unit. Publ Health Rep 1980;95:307-312.

144. Kavanagh T, Shephard RJ. Sexual activity after myocardial infarction. Can Med Assoc J 1977;116:1250-1253.

145. Waltz M, Badura B. Subjective health, intimacy, and perceived self-efficacy after heart attack: predicting life quality five years afterward. Soc Indicators Res 1988;20:303-332.

146. Dracup K, Guzy PM, Taylor SE, Barry J. Cardiopulmonary resuscitation (CPR) training. Consequences for family members of high-risk cardiac patients. Arch Intern Med 1986;146:1757-1761.

147. Alonzo AA. The impact of the family and lay others on care-seeking during life-threatening episodes of coronary artery disease. Soc Sci Med 1986;22:1297-1311.

148. Ewart CK, Taylor CB, Reese LB, DeBusk RF. Effects of early postmyocardial infarction exercise testing on self-perception and subsequent physical activity. Am J Cardiol 1983;51:1076-1080.

149. Taylor CB, Bandura A, Ewart CK, Miller NH, DeBusk RF. Exercise testing to enhance wives' confidence in their husbands' cardiac capability soon after clinically uncomplicated acute myocardial infarction. Am J Cardiol 1985;55:635-638.

150. Carver CS, Coleman AE, Glass DC. The coronary-prone behavior pattern and the suppression of fatigue on a treadmill test. J Pers Soc Physiol 1976;33:460-466.

151. Miller NH, Haskell WL, Berra K, DeBusk RF. Home versus group exercise training for increasing capacity after myocardial infarction. Circulation 1984;70:645-649.

152. Gossard D, Haskell WL, Taylor CB. Effects of low- and high-intensity home-based exercise training on functional capacity in healthy middle-aged men. Am J Cardiol 1986;57:446-449.

153. Taylor CB, Houston-Miller N, Ahn DK, Haskell W, DeBusk RF. The effects of ex-

ercise training programs on psychosocial improvement in uncomplicated postmyocardial infarction patients. J Psychosom Res 1986; 30:581–587.

154. Follick MJ, Gorkin L, Smith TW, Capone RJ, Visco J, Stablein D. Quality of life post–myocardial infarction: effects of transtelephonic coronary intervention system. Health Psychology 1988;7:169–182.

155. Davidson DM, Murphy CR. Exercise training in elderly persons: do women benefit as much as men? In: McPherson BD(ed): Sport and aging. Champaign, IL: Human Kinetics Press, 1985:273–278.

156. VanCamp SP, Peterson RA. Cardiovascular complications of outpatient cardiac rehabilitation programs. JAMA 1986;256:1160–1163.

157. Oldridge N, Guyatt G. Mortality and morbidity after combining randomized trials of cardiac rehabilitation. Circulation 1986;74(suppl II):II-9.

158. Kallio V, Hamalainen H, Hakkila J, Luurila OJ. Reduction in sudden deaths by a multifactoral intervention programme after acute myocardial infarction. Lancet 1979;2:1091–1094.

159. Oldridge NB, Donner AP, Buck CW, et al. Predictors of dropout from cardiac exercise rehabilitation. Ontario Exercise-Heart Collaborative Study. Am J Cardiol 1983;51:70–74.

160. The Coronary Drug Project Group. Influence of adherence to treatment and response of cholesterol on mortality in the Coronary Drug Project. N Engl J Med 1980;303:1038–1041.

161. Davidson DM. Return to work after cardiac events: a review. J Cardiac Rehabil 1983;3:60–67.

162. Davidson DM. Work reentry after myocardial infarction. Arch Phys Med Rehabil 1983;64:526.

163. Bar-On D, Cristal N. Causal attributions of patients, their spouses and physicians, and the rehabilitation of the patients after their first myocardial infarction. J Cardiopulm Rehabil 1987;7:285–298.

164. Picard MH, Dennis C, Schwartz RG, et al. Cost-benefit analysis of early return to work after uncomplicated acute myocardial infarction. Am J Cardiol 1989;63:1308–1314.

18

prognosis and management after coronary artery bypass surgery

From 1979 to 1986, the number of coronary artery bypass surgery (CABS) procedures done annually in the United States rose from 114,000 to 228,000; the latter figure is approximately 1 per 1000 citizens of all ages. This growth occurred despite the increase of coronary angioplasty procedures from 200 to 133,000 during the same period (1), and continuing attention to the appropriateness of CABS in certain subgroups of patients (2). This chapter reviews the prognosis of post-CABS patients and discusses management to reduce the risk of another cardiac event.

PROGNOSIS AFTER CABS

In three large multicenter trials, participants were randomized to surgical or medical therapy; 2334 persons were enrolled in these trials between 1972 and 1979 (3). The Veterans Administration (VA) trial in the United States initially sought to evaluate intramyocardial implantation of an internal mammary artery in patients with stable angina, but the sa-

phenous vein bypass graft procedure became the standard procedure. Eleven-year follow-up of the 686 subjects in the VA trial is now available (4). The Coronary Artery Surgery Study (CASS) in the United States enrolled 780 persons (5), while the European Coronary Surgery Study (ECSS) included 768 participants with a left ventricular ejection fraction greater than 0.50 (6). Neither the VA nor the CASS trials showed a significant difference in long-term survival between medical and surgical groups; in the ECSS, initial differences favoring the surgical group narrowed after 10 years (3). Surgical techniques and patient survival have continued to improve in the decade since enrollment in these studies was closed (7).

Further analyses of these and other studies have identified various indicators of risk for progression of atherosclerosis, graft closure, recurrent cardiac events, and death, which are discussed in the following sections. These include residual myocardial function, indications for surgery (angina, stable or unstable; failed angioplasty), other cardiac events and disease, type of graft (internal thoracic artery vs. saphenous vein graft), the occurrence of perioperative MI, asymptomatic myocardial ischemia after surgery, dysrhythmias, prophylactic medications, noninvasive testing, and standard CAD risk indicators.

Residual Myocardial Function

Compared with medical therapy alone, CABS offers the greatest advantage in symptomatic patients with extensive disease (8). CASS investigators reviewed subjects with baseline left ventricular ejection fractions of 0.35 to 0.49; with a mean follow-up of seven years, the surgical group had 16% mortality compared with 30% in the group randomized to medical therapy alone. This difference arose mainly from subjects with three-vessel disease, in whom the mortality rates were 12% and 35%, respectively (9). Participants with an ejection fraction of 25% or less also had improved survival if randomized to surgery (10). Despite the benefits of surgery in patients at all levels of pump dysfunction, left ventricular dysfunction remains the most powerful determinant of operative mortality and long-term survival after CABS for stable angina (11).

Indications for Surgery

STABLE ANGINA

Perioperative risk for patients undergoing CABS for stable angina is largely determined by left ventricular dysfunction and age. These factors, along with the extent of associated diseases, are the most powerful predictors of event-free survival and long-term mortality (11).

UNSTABLE ANGINA

In their review of 14 studies of myocardial revascularization for unstable angina from 1978 to 1988, Kaiser and colleagues noted an average operative

mortality of 3.7% and a perioperative MI rate of 9.8%. While operative mortality is largely related to left ventricular dysfunction, age, and the presence of significant left main disease, risk indicators for perioperative infarction are less clear (12). In the VA Cooperative Study of unstable angina, the three-year mortality for participants with left ventricular dysfunction (ejection fraction less than 0.50 or left ventricular end diastolic pressure exceeding 15 mm Hg) was 6.1% in surgical patients and 17.1% in those randomized to medical treatment only (13).

Other Cardiac Events and Diseases

RECENT MYOCARDIAL INFARCTION

CABS within 30 days after myocardial infarction carries operative mortality rates of 2%, similar to those in patients undergoing CABS for stable angina. In this setting, however, elderly patients or those with left ventricular dysfunction have a significantly higher mortality rate in both women and men (14, 15). After a recurrent MI, however, bypass surgery no longer improves prognosis in the absence of disabling angina or left main disease (16).

FAILED ANGIOPLASTY

Patients enrolled in the NHLBI angioplasty registry during 1985 and 1986 had a 5.6% referral rate for CABS; slightly more than half of these required emergency surgery. Coronary artery dissection is the most common cause for such intervention, and this often occurs on the first vessel to undergo angioplasty. Nonfatal Q wave infarction may develop in one-fourth of emergency CABS patients, while in-hospital death approximates 2% (17).

REPEAT CABS

Although operative mortality is higher during a repeat CABS, persons undergoing a second or subsequent operation for recurrent angina have long-term survival chances similar to those having an initial CABS (18, 19). In one study of persons with at least two prior bypass operations, five-year survival was 76.4% for the entire series of patients and was 87.3% in hospital survivors (19).

CHRONIC CONGESTIVE HEART FAILURE AND VALVULAR DISEASE

Some 3 to 5% of persons having CABS have moderate to severe congestive heart failure. In two recent studies, predictors of subsequent mortality in such subjects included mitral regurgitation in addition to the other risks mentioned herein (20). In patients who have concurrent mitral valve repair and CABS, the operative mortality is higher than for either procedure alone. For such combined procedures, the risk is greater if valve dysfunction has resulted from CAD, if severe left ventricular dysfunction is present, or if emergency operation is required (21).

Type of Graft

Throughout most of the past two decades, the saphenous vein has been the conduit most often used for coronary artery revascularization. However, vein grafts are subject to processes leading to their obstruction. Fuster et al. describe several stages of vein graft disease. During the first postoperative month, thrombosis is largely responsible for occlusion. At the end of that period, smooth muscle cell proliferation and intimal hyperplasia can be detected histologically. The high-pressure pulsatile stress on the vein probably leads to endothelial damage and a platelet–vessel wall interaction. Occlusion occurring later in the first year appears to be related to rapid progression of intimal hyperplasia. Beyond the first year, lipid may be in-

corporated into the lesions, histologically resembling atherosclerosis (22).

Occlusion rates in vein grafts during the first year range from 10 to 20% and from 2 to 4% annually for the next 4 to 5 years. Thereafter, the occlusion rate doubles, meaning approximately 50% of saphenous vein grafts will be occluded 10 years after the initial operation (23). Angioplasty has proven useful in reopening stenosed vein grafts (24).

In recent years, use of the internal thoracic (mammary) artery (ITA) has dramatically improved the survival of patients and the patency of their conduits. Although they are more technically demanding, ITA grafts can be used for up to 70% of all distal anastomoses and in up to 95% of patients (25). In the Cleveland Clinic experience, patients who had only vein grafts during CABS had double the risk of reoperation and 1.6 times the risk of death during a 10-year follow-up when compared to patients having at least one ITA graft. Improvement was noted in patients with one-, two-, or three-vessel disease (26). In CASS participants, ITA use resulted in significantly improved survival in both women and men, in those with and without significant left ventricular dysfunction, in those above and below the age of 65, and in those with and without critical stenosis of the left main coronary artery (27).

Perioperative MI

Perioperative myocardial infarction increases the risk of subsequent MI after CABS as well as the risk for developing congestive heart failure. In the Seattle Heart Watch angiography registry, patients who developed Q-wave infarction during CABS had a 76% five-year survival compared to 90% in those without perioperative infarction (28). Perioperative MI may result from vein graft closure, emboli, reperfusion injury, or occlusive coronary artery spasm (29).

Asymptomatic Myocardial Ischemia after CABS

In one study, one-third of CABS survivors displayed asymptomatic ischemia on ambulatory ECG monitoring three months after surgery. During the remainder of the first postoperative year, 75% of cardiac events occurred in that third of the population, indicating a doubling of relative risk that accompanies asymptomatic ischemia after CABS (30).

Dysrhythmias

Reports from the long-term studies of CABS rarely indicate a prognostic value of ventricular dysrhythmias. In some cases, dysrhythmias are not routinely measured postoperatively, while in others, multivariate analyses reveal that ventricular dysrhythmias are not independently predictive of outcome (31). Postoperative atrial fibrillation is associated with an increased risk of stroke after CABS (32).

MANAGEMENT AFTER CABS

Prophylactic Medications

PLATELET-ACTIVE DRUGS

In 1984, Mayo Clinic investigators reported the beneficial effects of dipyridamole (started two days before surgery) and aspirin (started seven hours after CABS). After one month, 2% of vein-graft distal anastomoses were occluded in the treated group versus 10% in those taking placebo. Six percent of the treated group had one or more grafts occluded, compared with 22% of the placebo group (33). At one year, these effects were less striking. Of patients with all grafts patent one month after CABS, 16% developed one or more occlusions in the treated group, compared with 27% in those taking placebo (34).

Similar early and late results have been reported in the Veterans Administration Cooperative Study population. Subjects received either (a) aspirin (ASA) 325 mg/day; (b) ASA 325 mg t.i.d.; (c) ASA 325 mg t.i.d. and dipyridamole 75 mg t.i.d.; (d) sulfinpyrazone 267 mg t.i.d.; or (e) placebo t.i.d. All groups receiving aspirin had significantly less occlusion than the placebo group (35). Aspirin in doses as low as 100 mg/day can also improve graft patency (36). Long-term warfarin therapy to preserve the patency of saphenous vein grafts is not recommended (37).

NONINVASIVE TESTING

Exercise testing in the early postoperative period can document improvement in functional capacity after CABS. Serial testing during the years that follow is correlated with patency of vein grafts (38). Myocardial perfusion imaging with thallium 201 also offers objective evaluation of the results of revascularization (39).

STANDARD CAD RISK INDICATORS

Smoking

Among CASS registry subjects who had CABS, the progression of disease was slower in those who stopped smoking after surgery (40). There was no diminution of this effect with age over a six-year follow-up (41). Among CASS subjects randomized to treatment groups, only 20% of those smoking at the time of their assignment to surgery successfully quit (42).

Postoperative morbidity is also reduced with smoking cessation; pulmonary complications were significantly less in Mayo Clinic patients who had stopped smoking at least two months before CABS (43).

Dyslipidemias and Nutrition

In a study completed just before the publication of the National Cholesterol Education Panel guidelines (44), nearly half of patients admitted for CABS at Johns Hopkins Hospital had elevated total blood cholesterol levels; half of these were unaware of their risk, and few were undergoing active treatment (45).

Campeau and colleagues in Montreal measured blood total cholesterol and triglycerides in patients at the time of CABS and 10 years later; values of both parameters were higher in persons with new atherosclerotic lesions. Multivariate analysis revealed that low plasma HDL-cholesterol and high plasma LDL-apolipoprotein-B were the best predictors of disease progression (46). Cleveland Clinic investigators found that event-free survival after 10 years correlated inversely with both total blood cholesterol and triglycerides in their 4913 patients; saphenous vein graft patency after two years was also inversely correlated with the two lipid parameters (47). Neitzel and colleagues compared CABS patients who required reoperation after five years of follow-up with those who did not. The former group had higher baseline levels of blood total cholesterol and triglycerides and lower HDL-cholesterol levels than those who did not develop symptoms requiring reoperation (48).

In the Cholesterol Lowering Atherosclerosis Study (CLAS), 162 men aged 40 to 59 years with previous CABS were randomized to one of two groups: the "drug" group received colestipol and niacin therapy along with a diet limited to 22% of calories from fat (4% from saturated fat) and 125 mg dietary cholesterol daily. The "placebo" group had a target diet consisting of 26% of calories from fat (5% saturated fat) and 250 mg dietary cholesterol daily. After two years of treatment, the treatment group had 26% lower plasma total choles-

terol, 43% lower LDL-cholesterol, and 37% higher HDL-cholesterol. This was associated with a significant reduction in the average number of lesions that progressed and with the percentage of patients with new atheroma formation in native arteries. The percentage of patients with new lesions in bypass grafts was also significantly reduced. Atherosclerosis regression occurred in 16% of the colestipol-niacin treated subjects versus 2% of the placebo group (49).

High Blood Pressure

Despite its prognostic value in primary CAD prevention and in post-MI patients, hypertension has not been demonstrated to be predictive in CABS patients. Campeau et al. found a similar prevalence of hypertension in patients with and without new lesions on angiography after CABS (46).

Diabetes

Salomon and co-workers found that the extent of diffuse CAD, operative mortality, sternotomy complications, renal insufficiency, and hospital stay were all greater in diabetics; long-term survival was lower (50). Neitzel et al. noted that diabetes was more than twice as likely in their subjects undergoing repeat CABS as in those not requiring such treatment (48).

Age

Hospital morbidity and mortality rates for elderly CABS patients are somewhat higher than those for younger persons, but this can largely be attributed to the greater levels of risk in patients over the age of 70. Longer-term follow-up is similar in younger or older patients (51). Edmunds et al. operated on 100 octagenarians, 90 of whom had New York Heart Association class IV disease. Eighty-five had unstable or postinfarction angina, syncope, acute pulmonary edema, or cardiogenic shock; 69 had coronary artery disease. Twenty-nine died within 90 days after the operation, but the majority were in New York Heart Association class I or II several years later (52). It appears that an older age, in the absence of other significant risk, is not an absolute contraindication for CABS.

Gender

Several studies have documented a higher operative mortality rate for women undergoing CABS (53–55). When matched for age, severity of angina, and extent of atherosclerosis, women still had twice the operative mortality of men. However, after adjusting for body size, gender was no longer significantly associated with operative deaths. After two years, women had a lower graft patency rate, but at 10 years, mortality rates were equal for the two genders (53). Women are also more likely to have angina before and after CABS (54, 56).

A review of preoperative variables among CASS participants revealed that women were more likely to be hypertensive and diabetic, but less likely to have prior cardiac events. There was no difference between men and women in predictors of six-year mortality (55).

Race and Ethnicity

From the CASS registry, Maynard et al. analyzed clinical outcomes in 202 blacks and 13,105 whites who were not part of the randomized CASS program. Physicians recommended CABS to 47% of blacks and 59% of whites; of those with surgery recommended, 81% of blacks and 90% of whites had CABS. Overall, 38% of blacks had surgery versus 58% of whites. Higher percentages of black women and men had hypertension, were diabetic, and smoked cigarettes, but there were no significant black-white differences in serum total cholesterol (57, 58). The small number of blacks in large, randomized clinical trials leaves the issue of long-term survival by race unresolved. Data are not available on CABS for other racial and ethnic groups in the United States.

PSYCHOSOCIAL AND BEHAVIORAL FACTORS

Although their surgery is usually elective, CABS patients experience many of the same emotions as MI patients (Chapter 18); transient anxiety and depression often resolves in persons without such characteristics prior to surgery (59). In contrast, preoperative depression often persists after CABS, leading to a poor psychosocial outcome after surgery (60).

CARDIAC REHABILITATION SERVICES

CABS patients are offered similar services as MI patients during hospitalization, the early home period, and outpatient exercise training periods. Patients over 65 can benefit from these programs as well as younger individuals (61).

However, CABS patients often fail to return to sexual activity and to work as might be expected with their new asymptomatic status. Kornfeld et al. found that sexual abstinence in their CABS patients increased from 11% preoperatively to 31% nine months after surgery (62). Papadapoulos and colleagues found that discussions of sexual activity resumption are still not being initiated by the physician and other rehabilitation team members (63). The counseling that follows a postsurgical exercise test provides an ideal opportunity to relate heart rate and blood pressure changes during coitus with those just experienced on the exercise test (64).

RETURN TO WORK

Many persons do not return to work following CABS, despite having good functional capacity (65). As with myocardial infarction, few men undergoing CABS after the age of 60 return to work (66). Little is known about return to work in women after surgery (67).

In one series, fewer individuals who had CABS returned to work than those who had medical treatment only (68). Investigators in another study determined that 90% of CABS survivors were capable of returning to work, but only 50% did so (69). The patient's perception of health (regardless of its actual state) is probably more important as a predictor of return to work (70).

Alabama researchers found that relief of angina, presurgical employment, and higher educational levels were correlated with higher rates of return to work, but these factors still only accounted for 40% of the variance (71). Almeida et al. found that failure to return to work correlated with residual angina, presurgical unemployment, age, lower educational level, female gender, incomplete myocardial revascularization, left ventricular dysfunction, and previous MIs (72). Gohlke and co-workers found that an improved exercise tolerance after CABS was positively correlated with return-to-work rates (73).

When nonwork income compensation approximates that which can be achieved from working, the percentage of patients returning to work decreases, particularly in persons doing manual labor (70, 74).

REFERENCES

1. Feinleib M, Havlik RJ, Gillum RF, Pokras R, McCarthy E, Moien M. Coronary heart disease and related procedures. National Hospital Discharge Survey data. Circulation 1989;79(suppl I):I13–I18.

2. Winslow CM, Kosecoff JB, Chassin M, Kanouse DE, Brook RH. The appropriateness of performing coronary artery bypass surgery. JAMA 1988;260:505–509.

3. Killip T. Twenty years of coronary bypass surgery. N Engl J Med 1988;319:366–368.

4. The Veterans Administration Coronary Artery Bypass Surgery Cooperative Study Group. Eleven-year survival in the Veterans Administration randomized trial of coronary artery surgery for stable angina. N Engl J Med 1984;311:1333–1339.

5. CASS Principal Investigators and Associates. Coronary artery surgery study (CASS): a randomized trial of coronary artery bypass surgery: survival data. Circulation 1983;68:939–950.

6. Varnauskas E and the Europan Coronary Surgery Study Group. Twelve-year follow-up of survival in the randomized European Coronary Surgery Study. N Engl J Med 1988; 319:332–337.

7. Califf RM, Harrell FE Jr, Lee KL, et al. The evolution of medical and surgical therapy for coronary artery disease. A fifteen year perspective. JAMA 1989;261:2077–2086.

8. Frye RL, Fisher L, Schaff HV, Gersh BJ, Vliestra RE, Mock MB. Randomized trials in coronary artery bypass surgery. Prog Cardiovasc Dis 1987;30:1–22.

9. Passamani E, Davis KB, Gillespie MJ, Killip T, and the CASS Principal Investigators and Associates. A randomized trial of coronary artery bypass surgery. Survival of patients with a low ejection fraction. N Engl J Med 1985; 312:1665–1671.

10. Alderman EL, Fisher LD, Litwin P, et al. Results of coronary artery surgery in patients with poor left ventricular function. Circulation 1983;68:785–795.

11. Gersh BJ, Califf RM, Loop FD, Akins CW, Pryor DB, Takaro TC. Coronary bypass surgery in chronic stable angina. Circulation 1989;79(suppl I):I46–I59.

12. Kaiser GC, Schaff HV, Killip T. Myocardial revascularization for unstable angina pectoris. Circulation 1989;79(suppl I):I60–I67.

13. Scott SM, Luchi RJ, Deupree RH, and the Veterans Administration Unstable Angina Cooperative Study Group. Veterans Administration Cooperative Study for treatment of patients with unstable angina. Results in patients with abnormal left ventricular function. Circulation 1988;78(suppl I):I113–I121.

14. Naunheim KS, Kesler KA, Kanter KR, et al. Coronary artery bypass for recent infarction. Predictors of mortality. Circulation 1988;78(suppl I):I122–I128.

15. Kennedy JW, Ivey TD, Misbach G, et al. Coronary artery bypass graft surgery early after acute myocardial infarction. Circulation 1989;79(suppl I):I73–I78.

16. Norris RM, Agnew TM, Brandt PW, et al. Coronary surgery after recurrent myocardial infarction: progress of a trial comparing surgical with nonsurgical management for asymptomatic patients with advanced coronary disease. Circulation 1981;63:785–792.

17. Talley JD, Jones EL, Weintraub WS, King SB III. Coronary artery bypass surgery after failed elective percutaneous transluminal coronary angioplasty. A status report. Circulation 1989;79(suppl I):I126–I131.

18. Cameron A, Kemp HG Jr, Green GE. Reoperation for coronary artery disease. Ten years of clinical follow-up. Circulation 1988;78(suppl I):I158–I162.

19. Brenowitz JB, Johnson WD, Kayser KL, Saedi SF, Dorros G, Schley L. Coronary artery bypass grafting for the third time or more. Results of 150 consecutive cases. Circulation 1988;78(suppl I):I166–I170.

20. Wechsler AS, Junod FJ. Coronary bypass grafting in patients with chronic congestive heart failure. Circulation 1989;79(supp I):I92–I96.

21. Karp RB, Mills N, Edmunds LH Jr. Coronary artery bypass grafting in the presence of valvular disease. Circulation 1989;79(suppl I):I182–I184.

22. Fuster V, Adams PC, Badimon JJ, Chesebro JH. Platelet inhibitor drugs' role in coronary artery disease. Prog Cardiovasc Dis 1987;29:325–346.

23. Grondin CM, Campeau L, Thornton JC, Engle JC, Cross FS, Schreiber H. Coronary artery bypass grafting with saphenous vein. Circulation 1989;79(suppl I):I24–I29.

24. Cote G, Myler RK, Stertzer SH, et al. Percutaneous transluminal angioplasty of stenotic coronary artery bypass grafts: 5 years' experience. J Am Coll Cardiol 1987;9:8–17.

25. Green GE. Use of internal thoracic artery for coronary artery grafting. Circulation 1989;79(suppl I):I30–I33.

26. Loop FD, Lytle BW, Cosgrove DM, et al. Influence of the internal mammary artery graft on 10-year survival and other cardiac events. N Engl J Med 1986;314:1–6.

27. Cameron A, Davis KB, Green GE, Myers WO, Pettinger M. Clinical implications of the internal mammary artery bypass grafts: the Coronary Artery Surgery Study experience. Circulation 1988;77:815–819.

28. Namay DL, Hammermeister KE, Zia MS, DeRouen TA, Dodge HA, Namay K. Effect of perioperative myocardial infarction on late survival in patients undergoing coronary artery bypass surgery. Circulation 1982;65:1066–1071.

29. Fischell TA, McDonald TV, Grattan MT, Miller DC, Stadius ML. Occlusive coronary artery spasm as a cause of acute myocardial infarction after coronary-artery bypass grafting. N Engl J Med 1989;320:400–401.

30. Egstrup K. Asymptomatic myocardial ischemia as a predictor of cardiac events after coronary artery bypass grafting for stable angina pectoris. Am J Cardiol 1988;61:248–252.

31. Kirklin JW, Naftel DC, Blackstone EH, Pohost GM. Summary of consensus concerning death and ischemic events after coronary artery bypass grafting. Circulation 1989;79(suppl I):I81–I91.

32. Reed GL III, Singer DE, Picard EH, DeSanctis RW. Stroke following coronary artery bypass surgery. A case-control estimate of the risk from carotid bruits. N Engl J Med 1988;319:1246–1250.

33. Chesebro JH, Clements IP, Fuster V, et al. A platelet-inhibitor drug trial in coronary artery bypass operations. N Engl J Med 1982;307:73–78.

34. Chesebro JH, Fuster V, Elveback LR, et al. Effect of dipyridamole and aspirin on late vein-graft patency after coronary bypass operations. N Engl J Med 1984;310:209–214.

35. Goldman, S, Copeland J, Moritz T, et al. Improvement in early saphenous vein graft patency after coronary artery bypass surgery with antiplatelet therapy: results of a Veterans Administration Cooperative Study. Circulation 1988;77:1324–1332.

36. Lorenz RL, Weber M, Kotzur J, et al. Improved aortocoronary bypass patency by low-dose aspirin (100 mg daily). Lancet 1984;1:1261–1264.

37. Stein PD, Kantrowitz A. Antithrombotic therapy in mechanical and biological prosthetic heart valves and saphenous vein by-

pass grafts. Chest 1989;95(2)(suppl):107S–117S.

38. Gohlke H, Gohlke-Barwolf C, Samek L, Sturzenofecker P, Schmuziger M, Roskamm H. Serial exercise testing up to six years after coronary bypass surgery: behavior of exercise parameters in groups with different degrees of revascularization determined by postoperative angiography. Am J Cardiol 1983;51:1301–1306.

39. Robinson PS, Williams BT, Webb-Peploe MM, Crowther A, Coltart DJ. Thallium-201 myocardial imaging in assessment of results of aortocoronary bypass surgery. Br Heart J 1979;42:455–462.

40. Vlietstra RE, Kronmal RA, Oberman A, Frye RL, Killip T III. Effect of cigarette smoking on survival of patients with angiographically documented coronary artery disease. Report from the CASS Registry. JAMA 1986;255:1023–1027.

41. Hermanson B, Omenn GS, Kronmal RA, Gersh BJ and participants in the Coronary Artery Surgery Study. Beneficial six-year outcome of smoking cessation in older men and women with coronary artery disease. Results from the CASS Registry. N Engl J Med 1988;319:1365–1369.

42. CASS Principal Investigators. Coronary artery surgery study (CASS): a randomized trial of coronary artery bypass surgery. Quality of life in patients randomly assigned to treatment groups. Circulation 1983;68:951–960.

43. Warner MA, Offord KP, Warner ME, Lennon RL, Conover MA, Jansson-Schumacher U. Role of preoperative cessation of smoking and other factors in postoperative pulmonary complications: a blinded prospective study of coronary artery bypass patients. Mayo Clin Proc 1989;64:609–616.

44. National Cholesterol Education Program. Report of the National Cholesterol Education Program Expert Panel on detection, evaluation, and treatment of high blood cholesterol in adults. Arch Intern Med 1988;148:38–69.

45. Watt P, Becker DM, Salaita K, Pearson TA. Hypercholesterolemia in patients undergoing coronary bypass surgery: are they aware, under treatment, and under control? Heart Lung 1988;17:205–208.

46. Campeau L, Enjalbert M, Lesperance J, et al. The relation of risk factors to the development of atherosclerosis in saphenous-vein bypass grafts and the progression of disease in the native circulation. N Engl J Med 1984;311:1329–1332.

47. Stewart WJ, Goormastic M, Healy BP, et al. Clinical outcome ten years after coronary bypass effects of cholesterol and triglycerides in 4913 patients. J Am Coll Cardiol 1988;11:7A.

48. Neitzel GF, Barboriak JJ, Pintar K, et al. Atherosclerosis in aortocoronary bypass grafts. Morphologic study and risk factor analysis 6–12 years after surgery. Atherosclerosis 1986;6:594–600.

49. Blankenhorn DH, Nessim SA, Johnson RL, Sanmarco ME, Azen SP, Cashin-Hemphill L. Beneficial effects of combined colestipol-niacin therapy on coronary atherosclerosis and coronary venous bypass grafts. JAMA 1987;257:3233–3240.

50. Salomon NW, Page US, Okies JE, Stephens J, Krause AH, Bigelow JC. Diabetes mellitus and coronary artery bypass: short-term risk and long-term prognosis. J Thoracic Cardiovasc Surg 1983;85:264–271.

51. Horneffer PJ, Gardner TJ, Manolio TA, et al. The effects of age on outcome after coronary bypass surgery. Circulation 1987;76(suppl V):V6–V12.

52. Edmunds LH Jr, Stephenson LW, Edie RN, Ratcliffe MB. Open heart surgery in octogenarians. N Engl J Med 1988;319:131–136.

53. Loop FD, Golding FR, Macmillan JP, Cosgrove DM, Lytle BW, Sheldon WC. Coronary artery surgery in women compared with men: analyses of risk and long-term results. J Am Coll Cardiol 1983;1:383–390.

54. Davis KB. Coronary artery bypass graft surgery in women. In: Eaker ED, Packard B, Wenger NK, Clarkson TB, Tyroler HA (eds): Coronary heart disease in women. New York: Haymarket Doyma Inc., 1987:247–250.

55. Eaker ED, Kronmal R, Kennedy JW, Davis K. Comparison of the long-term, postsurgical survival of women and men in the Coronary Artery Surgery Study (CASS). Am Heart J 1989;117:71–81.

56. Johnson WD, Kayser KL, Pedraza PM. Angina pectoris and coronary bypass sur-

gery: patterns of prevalence and recurrence in 3105 consecutive patients followed up to 11 years. Am Heart J 1984;108:1190–1197.

57. Maynard C, Fisher LD, Passamani ER, Pullum T. Blacks in the Coronary Artery Surgery Study: risk factors and coronary artery disease. Circulation 1986;74:64–71.

58. Maynard C, Fisher LD, Passamani ER, Pullum T. Blacks in the Coronary Artery Surgery Study (CASS): race and clinical decision-making. Am J Public Health 1986;76:1446–1448.

59. Jenkins CD, Stanton BA, Savageau JA, et al. Coronary artery bypass surgery: physical, psychological, social and economic outcomes six months later. JAMA 1983;250:782–788.

60. Magni G, Unger HP, Valfre C, et al. Psychosocial outcome one year after heart surgery. A prospective study. Arch Intern Med 1987;147:473–477.

61. Williams MA, Maresh CM, Esterbrooks DJ, Harbrecht JJ, Sketch MH. Early exercise training in patients older than age 65 years compared with that in younger patients after acute myocardial infarction or coronary artery bypass grafting. Am J Cardiol 1985;55:263–266.

62. Kornfeld DS, Heller SS, Frank KA, Wilson SN, Malm JR. Psychological and behavioral responses after coronary artery bypass surgery. Circulation 1982;66(suppl III):24–28.

63. Papadopoulos C, Shelley SI, Piccolo M, Beaumont C, Barnett L. Sexual activity after coronary bypass surgery. Chest 1986;90:681–685.

64. Davidson DM. Family and sexual adjustments after cardiac events. Qual Life Cardiovasc Care 1989;5:66–71,77–79.

65. Davidson DM. Return to work after cardiac events: a review. J Cardiac Rehabil 1983;3:60–67.

66. Johnson WD, Kayser KL, Pedraza PM, Shore RT. Employment patterns in males before and after myocardial revascularization surgery. A study of 2229 consecutive male patients followed for as long as 10 years. Circulation 1982;65:1086–1093.

67. Zyzanski SJ, Rouse BA, Stanton BA, Jenkins CD. Employment changes among patients following coronary bypass surgery: social, medical, and psychological correlates. Publ Health Rep 1982;97:558–565.

68. Hammermeister KE, DeRouen TA, English MT, Dodge HT. Effect of surgical vs. medical therapy on return to work in patients with coronary artery disease. Am J Cardiol 1989;44:105–111.

69. Logue B, King SD III, Douglas JS. A practical approach to coronary artery disease with special reference to coronary artery bypass surgery. Curr Probl Cardiol 1976;1:5–10.

70. Davidson DM. Recovery after cardiac events. In: Spittell JA (ed): Clinical medicine, vol 6, chapter 20. New York: JB Lippincott, 1983.

71. Barnes GK, Ray MJ, Oberman A, Kouchoukos MT. Changes in working status of patients following coronary bypass surgery. JAMA 1977;238:1259–1263.

72. Almeida D, Bradford JM, Wenger NK, King SB, Hurst JW. Return to work after coronary bypass surgery. Circulation 1983;68(suppl II):II205–II213.

73. Gohlke H, Schnellbacher K, Samek L, Sturzenhofecker P, Roskamm H. Long-term improvement of exercise tolerance and vocational rehabilitation after bypass surgery: a five-year follow-up. J Cardiac Rehabil 1982;2:531–540.

74. Niles NW II, VanderSalm TJ, Cutler BS. Return to work after coronary bypass operation. J Thorac Cardiovasc Surg 1980;79:916–921.

Section VI

Dysrhythmias and Sudden Cardiac Death

19

sudden cardiac death

Each day, approximately 1000 residents of Canada and the United States die suddenly from cardiac causes (1). Lown has noted that sudden cardiac death

> was recognized at the dawn of recorded history and even depicted in Egyptian relief sculpture . . . approximately 4500 years ago. Sudden cardiac death has left no age untouched. Sparing neither saint nor sinner, it has burdened man with a sense of uncertainty and fragility (2).

A majority of sudden cardiac death (SCD) cases occur out of the hospital and in emergency rooms (3), with higher percentages in blacks, men, and younger persons. Between 1980 and 1985, age-adjusted SCD rates for women and men in the United States declined 15 to 20%, with similar reductions in deaths occurring within hospitals and without (1). In the first three decades of life, a variety of causes are present (3–5). These include hypertrophic cardiomyopathy (6), congenital coronary-artery aneurysms and other anomalies (7), myocarditis (8), valvular diseases (9), sickle cell trait (10), and cocaine abuse (11, 12). Sudden death in young athletes often comes to the public's attention, and screening programs have been proposed to detect risk for SCD.

While echocardiography would be the logical choice for detecting hypertrophic and dilated cardiomyopathies and valvular diseases (13), it is not presently considered to be cost-effective (14). Recommendations are available regarding eligibility for athletic competition in persons with known cardiac disease (15).

In middle-aged persons and elders, most SCD victims have extensive coronary atherosclerosis (6); other causes include congestive heart failure, valvular heart disease, and primary electrophysiologic abnormalities (16). Alcohol and exercise have also been associated with SCD episodes.

The underlying dysrhythmia accounting for most cases of SCD is ventricular fibrillation, which results from myocardial electrical instability. Psychological stressors of various types may lower the threshold for ventricular fibrillation through neurohumoral or neural pathway mechanisms (16).

These topics are discussed in further detail in this chapter.

CORONARY ARTERY DISEASE AND SCD

In the Framingham Study, investigators defined sudden death as any death occurring within one hour of onset of symptoms without other probable cause of death suggested by medical history. After 26 years of surveillance of their original cohort, 6.2% of their male subjects and 1.7% of women participants had died suddenly. A majority of the men had known CAD at the time of death, but less than one-third of the women did (17). After four more years of follow-up, another 23 women and 14 men had died suddenly. In subjects who had experienced a CAD event in the three decades, the relative risk of SCD was 6.7. A history of myocardial infarction (MI) imposed greater risk than development of angina; asymptomatic MIs were as dangerous as infarctions accompanied by symptoms. In persons with known CAD, factors reflecting cumulative myocardial damage and dysfunction were the most important predictors of SCD. The investigators also noted that, in persons with CAD, the proportion of deaths that were sudden did not decline over the three decades (18).

The Finnish Social Insurance Institution (SII) Coronary Heart Disease Study population includes 3589 men initially aged 40 to 59 years who have been followed prospectively for more than 11 years. Of 234 CAD deaths occurring during that interval, 150 were considered sudden. The severity of CAD at baseline was the most effective predictor of SCD (19).

Hinkle and colleagues followed 301 men for more than 20 years; 65 of 148 deaths were sudden. Factors from the baseline evaluation predictive of SCD were blood pressure, conduction abnormalities, smoking level, chronic airway disease, and sedentary leisure habits (20).

In their surveillance of 7591 Hawaiian-Japanese men initially free of evidence of CAD, investigators found that predictors of SCD included blood pressure, serum cholesterol, serum glucose, smoking, history of parental MI, and ECG evidence of left ventricular hypertrophy.

These same factors predicted other manifestations of CAD (21).

Several prospective studies have examined the occurrence of SCD after baseline exercise tests in their asymptomatic enrollees. Although those with a normal test had a lower incidence of SCD, the large majority of subjects who subsequently died suddenly had normal responses to exercise testing at baseline. Such observations raise questions about the mechanisms of sudden death in persons with undetectable atherosclerosis, including the likelihood of silent ischemia (22).

Epstein and colleagues have pointed out that coronary resistance does not increase appreciably until the coronary lumen diameter has been reduced below 50% of its original size, making detection through exercise testing very unlikely. In persons with 25 to 50% obstruction, for example, thrombus or spasm could develop suddenly. In the absence of collateral circulation, the risk of MI and SCD is greatly increased. In contrast, in persons with gradual development of coronary luminal obstruction to 75% or more of the diameter, collateral circulation may develop in some. Development of angina is also more likely under the second scenario. If acute coronary occlusion appears in such a patient, unstable angina is more common than acute MI or SCD (22).

Exercise testing is also of limited value in predicting SCD in persons with established CAD, because of its limited sensitivity and specificity (23). After a first cardiac arrest, the recurrence rate may be as high as 30% during the first year (24). Cox survival analysis has been employed to identify three major variables as independent predictors of recurrent cardiac arrest. These include persistence of inducible ventricular dysrhythmias, a left ventricular ejection fraction of 30% or less, and the absence of coronary artery bypass surgery (25).

CAD Risk Indicators and SCD

Cigarette smoking and hypertension increased SCD risk in Finnish SII Study men and women (19) and in Framingham Study male subjects (17). Investigators in the Medical Research Council (UK) trial of treatment of mild hypertension found significantly higher risks in smoking participants; relative risk for MI or SCD was 1.7 in men and 3.5 in women who smoked (26). A case-control study by Mayo Clinic investigators included 15 women younger than 60 years who died suddenly during the years 1960 through 1974. The relative risk incurred by "ever smoking" was 8.6 (27).

Hallstrom and co-workers studied 310 survivors of out-of-hospital cardiac arrest who had been habitual cigarette smokers at the time of their event. During a mean follow-up of 47 months, the incidence of recurrent arrest was 18% in those who had quit smoking versus 27% in those who persisted in smoking (28). In an Irish investigation of men who had survived a first attack of unstable angina or MI, follow-up after the first two years revealed similar SCD rates in those who continued to smoke and those who quit, although overall mortality was much higher in smokers (29).

After 102 months of the Oslo Study Diet and Antismoking Trial, reductions in serum cholesterol in the intervention group subjects were accompanied by marked decreases in SCD and sudden unexplained death. After the first five years, intervention subjects were smoking considerably less; after formal completion of the trial, per capita daily cigarette consumption tended to increase toward that of the control group (30). High levels of serum cholesterol were also associated with a higher incidence of SCD in the Framingham men (17) and in Finnish men and women in the SII Study (19).

There are several mechanisms by which CAD risk indicators may unfavorably influence SCD rates. Cigarette smoking causes release of epinephrine and free fatty acids, increases heart rate, blood pressure, and platelet adhesiveness, and lowers the ventricular fibrillation threshold (31, 32). Diuretic-induced hypokalemia during treatment of hypertension may be associated with increased SCD rates. While awaiting definitive data, many practitioners have reduced doses in those patients for whom diuretics are indicated (33).

ALCOHOL CONSUMPTION

Evidence for a direct effect of heavy alcohol consumption on SCD is largely indirect, although ventricular dysrhythmias are more common and more easily induced in alcoholics. In a Soviet series of 50 autopsies, 30 persons (all chronic alcoholics) had died suddenly. Compared with control subjects, those with SCD had greater degrees of myocardial fibrosis and necrosis (34).

Considerable evidence linking alcohol and SCD comes from Swedish studies. In 50-year-old men followed for 10 years, registration with the Temperance Board was associated with an increased SCD risk (35). Men who chose not to enroll in the Göteborg Primary Prevention Trial were more often registered for alcohol problems and had a significant excess of SCD (36). In a longitudinal study of 50-year old men in Uppsala, half of all men dying suddenly were registered with the Temperance Board (37).

In the Finnish SII Study, SCD incidence was much less in abstaining middle-aged men, regardless of the presence of CAD and smoking status. The reduced risk was most pronounced in the age 60 to 64 group (38). In the Mayo Clinic study of women, alcoholics represented 40% of SCD cases, compared with 6.7% of women with

MI and 3.3% of controls (27). New Zealand investigators interviewed spouses of SCD victims, noting that heavy alcohol consumers had a higher percentage of cardiac events as SCD (39). However, not all studies have found a positive relation between SCD and alcohol. In the Kaiser Permanente experience to 1981, "instantaneous" sudden cardiac death was no more likely in current drinkers than in those who reported no alcohol intake during the preceding year (40). Investigators in the Seattle, Washington area interviewed spouses of 152 SCD cases (without prior heart disease) and controls. After adjustment for hypertension, smoking, and physical activity, they found that light (less than 1 drink/day) to moderate (1 to 3 drinks daily) consumption was associated with a reduced rate of primary cardiac arrest (41).

EXERCISE

Exercise-related cardiac arrest is typically a primary dysrhythmic event not due to acute MI (42). Epidemiologically, SCD occurs with a disproportionately higher frequency during vigorous activity. This appears to be true regardless of the level of habitual activity and the degree of CAD; however, the overall risk of primary cardiac arrest in habitually vigorous men is only approximately 40% of that in men who are sedentary (43). It is likely that this improved risk reflects a higher ventricular fibrillation threshold that results from frequent vigorous activity. Exercise decreases sympathetic tone and increases parasympathetic tone, factors that are associated with a reduced incidence of ventricular fibrillation during myocardial ischemia (2).

PSYCHOSOCIAL CONSIDERATIONS

Anxiety manifestations of emotional stress can markedly exacerbate ventricular dysrhythmias, but they may be successfully treated with β-adrenergic blockade (44). Coronary-prone (type A) behavior was an independent predictor of SCD in the Recurrent Coronary Prevention Project; investigators proposed that increased sympathetic responses to environmental stimuli may account for this observation (45).

Depression and cognitive impairment can also adversely affect outcome in persons with dysrhythmias, as documented by a study of 88 persons undergoing electrophysiologic studies. The investigators suggested that cognitive and emotional impairment may lessen one's ability to comply with lifesaving therapy, maintain a stable physiologic milieu, and continue an adaptive emotional life (46). Antidepressive treatment in patients with chronic dysrhythmias can significantly reduce ventricular ectopy (47). Bereavement may increase the risk of SCD; in one study, women who died suddenly were six times more likely to have experienced the death of a significant other during the preceding six months (48).

The day and time of occurrence of SCD may also implicate biobehavioral mechanisms. Mondays (49) and mid-late morning are times disproportionately represented in sudden cardiac death statistics.

In some cases, psychosocial variables are associated with SCD by mechanisms that are currently unclear. For example, Laotian-Hmong refugees who migrate to Thailand and the United States are at relatively high risk for sudden death during sleep (50). Munger has noted similar patterns in other diverse Asian populations; their risk seems to accompany them during migration (51).

Studies in England (52) and New Zealand (53) revealed an inverse relation of SCD incidence with social class and education. Within North America, a man's risk of SCD is inversely related to his own educational level (54), as well as that of his wife (55).

CONDUCTION DISORDERS

Bharati and Lev have classified conduction system abnormalities in their large series of persons who died suddenly. Abnormalities were found in the sinoatrial (S-A) node, the atrial preferential pathways, the approaches to the atrioventricular (A-V) node as well as the A-V node itself, the bundle of His, and the bundle branches. Hemorrhage, granulomatous or fatty infiltration, and fibrosis were noted in S-A and A-V nodes of persons who had died suddenly. In many cases of sudden infant death, the A-V node did not have its normal orientation to the central fibrous body. In younger persons, they noted increased sclerosis of the summit of the ventricular septum, especially the right side. In older subjects, sclerosis of the left side of the cardiac skeleton involved the A-V node and the bundles (56).

Chronic alcoholism can cause a variety of conduction disorders, including a prolonged P-R interval, Mobitz I and II blocks, right and left bundle branch blocks, and complete heart block. Acute alcohol ingestion can prolong atrial conduction and decrease ventricular refractory periods in nonalcoholics with cardiac disease (57).

DYSRHYTHMIAS

Although most people dying of sudden cardiac arrest have CAD and associated left ventricular dysfunction, unexpected cardiac arrest is usually a primary electrical event not associated with new MI. When treated immediately, ventricular fibrillation is reversible. In the smaller percentage of patients who have asystole or electromechanical dissociation when resuscitation begins, survival is rare (58).

The hypothesis that ventricular dysrhythmias are a risk indicator for SCD has been examined in many studies. Most have used the Lown grading system for VPCs (59), as shown in Table 19.1

Surawicz surveyed published studies, concluding that ventricular dysrhythmias, including short runs of ventricular tachycardia, do not increase SCD risk in persons without heart disease or in those with heart disease and normal myocardial function. In MI survivors, however, susceptibility to sudden death as a result of ventricular ectopy depends upon myocardial function. He reports an overall incidence of 3 to 5% in all MI patients, but a four-fold higher rate is found in persons with severely impaired ventricular function (60).

While ventricular dysrhythmias are most closely associated with cardiac arrest and SCD, a minority of patients may have nonventricular dysrhythmias as the sole precipitating rhythm for ventricular fibrillation. One team of investigators noted two cases each of sinus arrest and rapid, hypotensive A-V nodal reentrant tachycardia, which were the immediate precursors

Table 19.1. Lown Classification for Ventricular Dysrhythmias

Grade	Observation
0	No ventricular premature complexes (VPCs)
1	Occasional, isolated VPCs
2	VPC frequency > 1/min or > 30/hr
3	Multiform VPCs
4	Repetitive VPCs
	a. Pairs (couplets)
	b. Salvos (3 or more consecutive
5	Early VPCs (R or T phenomenon)

of ventricular fibrillation. Appropriate therapy prevented recurrence in each patient (61).

Detection

Ambulatory electrocardiographic monitoring has become standard for assessment of dysrhythmias. In screening asymptomatic persons, ambulatory monitoring is considered insufficiently sensitive and specific for accurate categorization by SCD risk (62). Further, 30 to 50% of patients with recurrent sustained ventricular tachycardia or those resuscitated after cardiac arrest have infrequent ectopy, reducing the benefit of monitoring (63). However, it is particularly useful in identifying patients after MI who are at risk for SCD. Several cases of SCD have occurred while monitoring was underway, documenting the predominance of ventricular fibrillation as the preterminal rhythm (64, 65). Monitoring can now provide information on silent ischemia as well as on dysrhythmias, which may be useful for determining drug doses for the evening hours. Investigators have noted increased ventricular ectopy during REM sleep; lobile non-REM sleep generally reduces the frequency of ventricular dysrhythmias (66).

Survivors of cardiac arrest frequently undergo electrophysiologic studies during which ventricular tachycardia is deliberately introduced and terminated. Intravenous medications are introduced, followed by repeat induction of the dysrhythmias, allowing testing of the effectiveness of various pharmacologic preparations. When ventricular tachycardia is successfully suppressed, recurrent dysrhythmic events are fewer over a five-year surveillance period (67).

Treatment

Basing drug therapy on the results of electrophysiologic ventricular fibrillation induction studies, the risk of recurrent SCD has been reduced to 5 to 10% per year (68). The automatic implantable cardiac defibrillator has reduced the risk of SCD even further (69, 70).

In persons who have not experienced cardiac arrest and do not display life-threatening dysrhythmias on other testing, nonpharmacologic therapy may contribute to a reduction of ventricular ectopy and risk. Avoidance of nicotine and caffeine, as well as biofeedback and relaxation techniques, may be of help to some patients (66).

Drug treatment of dysrhythmias increased substantially from 1970 to 1986 (71). However, recent studies such as the Cardiac Arrhythmia Suppression Trial (CAST) have led to the abandonment of routine treatment of dysrhythmias, particularly when the patient is asymptomatic (72). Despite the worse prognosis for dysrhythmic patients with poor left ventricular function, they are particularly susceptible to the "pro-dysrhythmia" effects that have been noted with most pharmacologic agents (73). The regulatory implications of CAST for North American and European medical communities have been recently discussed (74, 75).

The treatment effectiveness of β-adrenergic blocking agents after MI was discussed in Chapter 17. When begun beyond the first 24 hours after the infarct, mortality reductions approximating 25% have been noted during follow-up extending up to six years (76).

REFERENCES

1. Gillum RF. Sudden coronary death in the United States, 1980–1985. Circulation 1989;79:756–765.

2. Lown B. Sudden cardiac death: the major challenge confronting contemporary cardiology. Am J Cardiol 1979;43:313–328.

3. Gillum RF. Geographic variation in sudden coronary death. Am Heart J 1990; 119:380–389.

4. Lambert EC, Menon VA, Wagner HR, Vlad P. Sudden unexpected death from cardiovascular disease in children: a cooperative international study. Am J Cardiol 1974;34:89–96.

5. Topaz O, Edwards JE. Pathologic features of sudden death in children, adolescents, and young adults. Chest 1985;87:476–482.

6. Maron BJ, Epstein SE, Roberts WC. Causes of sudden death in competitive athletes. J Am Coll Cardiol 1986;7:204–214.

7. Gorgels AP, Braat SH, Becker AF, et al. Multiple aneurysms of the coronary arteries as the cause of sudden death in childhood. Am J Cardiol 1986;57:1193–1194.

8. Phillips M, Robinowitz M, Higgins JR, Boran KJ, Reed T, Virmani R. Sudden cardiac death in Air Force recruits. A 20-year review. JAMA 1986;256:2696–2699.

9. Maron BJ. Right ventricular cardiomyopathy: another cause of sudden death in the young. N Engl J Med 1988;318:178–180.

10. Kark JA, Posey DM, Schumacher HR, Ruehle CJ. Sickle-cell trait as a risk factor for sudden death in physical training. N Engl J Med 1987;317:781–787.

11. Isner JM, Estes NA III, Thompson PD, et al. Acute cardiac events temporally related to cocaine abuse. N Engl J Med 1986;315:1438–1443.

12. Isner JM, Chokshi SK. Cocaine and vasospasm. N Engl J Med 1989;321:1604–1606.

13. Epstein SE, Maron BJ. Sudden death and the competitive athlete: perspectives on preparticipation screening studies. J Am Coll Cardiol 1986;7:220–230.

14. Lewis JF, Maron BJ, Diggs JA, Spencer JE, Mehrotra PP, Curry CL. Preparticipation echocardiographic screening for cardiovascular disease in a large, predominantly black population of college athletes. Am J Cardiol 1989;64:1029–1033.

15. Mitchell JE, Maron BJ, Epstein SE. Cardiovascular abnormalities in the athlete: recommendations regarding eligibility for competition. J Am Coll Cardiol 1985;6:1189–1232.

16. Lown B. Sudden cardiac death: biobehavioral perspective. Circulation 1987;76:(Suppl I):I86–I96.

17. Schatzkin A, Cupples LA, Heeren T, Morelock S, Kannel WB. Sudden death in the Framingham Heart Study. Am J Epidemiol 1984;120:888–899.

18. Kannel WB, Cupples LA, D'Agostino RB. Sudden death risk in overt coronary heart disease: the Framingham Study. Am Heart J 1987;113:799–804.

19. Suhonen O, Reunanen A, Knekt P, Aromaa A. Risk factors for sudden and nonsudden coronary death. Acta Med Scand 1988;223:19–25.

20. Hinkle LE Jr, Thaler HT, Merke DP, Renier-Berg D, Morton NE. The risk factors for arrhythmia death in a sample of men followed for 20 years. Am J Epidemiol 1988;127:500–515.

21. Kagan A, Yano K, Reed DM, MacLean CJ. Predictors of sudden cardiac death among Hawaiian-Japanese men. Am J Epidemiol 1989;130:268–277.

22. Epstein SE, Quyyumi AA, Bonow RO. Sudden cardiac death without warning. N Engl J Med 1989;321:320–324.

23. McHenry PL. Role of exercise testing in predicting sudden death. J Am Coll Cardiol 1985;5:9B–12B.

24. Myerburg RJ, Kessler KM, Estes D, et al. Long-term survival after prehospital cardiac arrest: analysis of outcome during an 8-year study. Circulation 1984;70:538–546.

25. Wilber DJ, Garan H, Finkelstein D, et al. Out-of-hospital cardiac arrest. Use of electrophysiologic testing in the prediction of long-term outcome. N Engl J Med 1988;318:19–24.

26. Medical Research Council Working Party on Mild Hypertension. Coronary heart disease in the Medical Research Council trial of treatment of mild hypertension. Br Heart J 1988;59:364–378.

27. Beard CM, Griffin MR, Offord KP, Edwards WD. Risk factors for sudden unexpected death in young women in Rochester, MN, 1960 through 1974. Mayo Clinic Proc 1986;61:186–191.

28. Hallstrom AP, Cobb LA, Ray R. Smoking as a risk factor for recurrence of sudden cardiac arrest. N Engl J Med 1986;314:271–275.

29. Daly IF, Hickey N, Graham IM, Mulcahy R. Predictors of sudden death up to 18 years after a first attack of unstable angina or myocardial infarction. Br Heart J 1987;58:567–571.

30. Hjermann I, Holme I, Leren P. Oslo Study Diet and Antismoking Trial. Results after 102 months. Am J Med 1986;80(suppl 2A):7–11.

31. Cryer PE, Haymond MW, Santiago JV, Shah SD. Norepinephrine and epinephrine release and adrenergic mediation of smoking-associated hemodynamic and metabolic events. N Engl J Med 1976;295:573–577.

32. Bellet S, DeGuzman NT, Kostis JB, Roman L, Fleischmann D. The effect of inhalation of cigarette smoke on ventricular fibrillation threshold in normal dogs and dogs with acute myocardial infarction. Am Heart J 1972;83:67–76.

33. Moser M. Suppositions and speculations—their possible effects on treatment decisions in the management of hypertension. Am Heart J 1989;118:1362–1369.

34. Velisheva LS, Goldina BG, Boguslavsky VI. Sudden death in alcohol-induced cardiomyopathy. In: Proceedings of the First US-USSR Symposium on Sudden Death. Bethesda, MD: National Institutes of Health, 1978. NIH Publ no., 78–1470.

35. Wilhelmsen L, Wedel H, Tibblin G. Multivariate analysis of risk factors for coronary heart disease. Circulation 1973;48:950–958.

36. Rosengren A, Wilhelmsen L, Wedel H. Separate and combined effects of smoking and alcohol abuse in middle-aged men. Acta Med Scand 1988;223:111–118.

37. Lithell H, Aberg H, Selinus I, Hedstrand H. Alcohol intemperance and sudden death. Brit Med J 1987;294:1456–1458.

38. Suhonen O, Aromaa A, Reunanen A, Knekt P. Alcohol consumption and sudden coronary death in middle-aged Finnish men. Acta Med Scand 1987;221:335–341.

39. Fraser GE, Upsdell M. Alcohol and other discriminants between cases of sudden death and myocardial infarction. Am J Epidemiol 1981;114:462–476.

40. Klatsky AL, Friedman GD, Siegelaub AB. Alcohol use and cardiovascular disease: the Kaiser-Permanente experience. Circulation 1981;64:(suppl III):32–41.

41. Siscovick DS, Weiss NS, Fox N. Moderate alcohol consumption and primary cardiac arrest. Am J Epidemiol 1986;123:499–503.

42. Cobb LA, Weaver WD. Exercise: a risk for sudden death in patients with coronary heart disease. J Am Coll Cardiol 1986;7:215–219.

43. Siscovick DS, Weiss NS, Fletcher RH, Lasky T. The incidence of primary cardiac arrest during vigorous exercise. N Engl J Med 1984; 311:874–877.

44. Brodsky MA, Sato DA, Iseri LT, Wolff LJ, Allen BJ. Ventricular tachyarrhythmia associated with psychologic stress. JAMA 1987; 257:2064–2067.

45. Brackett CD, Powell LH. Psychosocial and physiological predictors of sudden cardiac death after healing of acute myocardial infarction. Am J Cardiol 1988;61:979–983.

46. Kennedy GJ, Hofer MA, Cohen D, Schindledecker R, Fisher JD. Significance of depression and cognitive impairment in patients undergoing programmed stimulation of cardiac arrhythmias. Psychosom Med 1987; 49:410–421.

47. Giardina E, Bigger JT, Glassman AH, Perel JM, Kantor SJ. The electrocardiographic and antiarrhythmic effects of imipramine hydrochloride at therapeutic plasma concentrations. Circulation 1979;60:1045–1052.

48. Cottington EM, Mathews KA, Talbott E, Kuller LH. Environmental effects preceding sudden death in women. Psychosom Med 1980;42:567–574.

49. Rabkin SW, Mathewson FA, Tate RB. Chronobiology of cardiac sudden deaths in men. JAMA 1980;244:1357–1358.

50. Kirschner RN, Eckner FA, Baron RC. The cardiac pathology of sudden unexplained nocturnal death in Southeast Asian refugees. JAMA 1986;256:2700–2705.

51. Munger RG. Sudden death in sleep of Laotian-Hmong refugees in Thailand: a case-control study. Am J Public Health 1987; 77:1187–1190.

52. Myers A, Dewar HA. Circumstances attending 100 sudden deaths from coronary artery disease with coroner's necropsies. Br Heart J 1975;37:1133–1143.

53. Fraser GE. Sudden death in Auckland. Aust NZ J Med 1978;8:490–499.

54. Ruberman W, Weinblatt E, Goldberg JD, Chaudhary BS. Education, psychosocial stress and sudden cardiac death. J Chron Dis 1983;36:151–160.

55. Strogatz DS, Siscovick DS, Weiss NS, Rennert G. Wife's level of education and husband's risk of primary cardiac arrest. Am J Public Health 1988;78:1491–1493.

56. Bharati S, Lev M. Cardiac disease in sudden death. Arch Intern Med 1984;144:1811–1812.

57. Davidson DM. Cardiovascular effects of alcohol. West J Med 1989;151:430–439.

58. Ruskin JN. Automatic external defibrillators and sudden cardiac death. N Engl J Med 1988;319:713–715.

59. Lown B, Wolf M. Approaches to sudden death from coronary heart disease. Circulation 1971;44:130–142.

60. Surawicz B. Prognosis of ventricular arrhythmias in relation to sudden cardiac death: therapeutic implications. J Am Coll Cardiol 1987;10:435–437.

61. Hays LJ, Lerman BB, DiMarco JP. Nonventricular arrhythmias as precursors of ventricular fibrillation in patients with out-of-hospital cardiac arrest. Am Heart J 1989; 118:53–57.

62. Armstrong WF, McHenry PL. Ambulatory electrocardiographic monitoring: can we predict sudden death? J Am Coll Cardiol 1985;5:13B–16B.

63. Josephson ME. Antiarrhythmic agents and the danger of proarrhythmic events. Ann Intern Med 1989;111:101–103.

64. Gradman AH, Bell PA, DeBusk RF. Sudden death during ambulator monitoring. Circulation 1977;55:210–211.

65. Hohnloser S, Weiss M, Zeiher A, Wollschlager H, Hust MH, Just H. Sudden cardiac death recorded during ambulatory electrocardiographic monitoring. Clin Cardiol 1984;7:517–523.

66. Verrier RL, DeSilva RA, Lown B. Psychologic factors in cardiac arrhythmias and sudden death. In: Krantz DS, Baum A, Singer JE (eds): Handbook of psychology and health. Hillsdale, NJ: Lawrence Erlbaum, Publishers, 1983:125–154.

67. Lo YS, Nguyen KP. Electrophysiologic study in the management of cardiac arrest survivors: a critical review. Am Heart J 1987;114:596–606.

68. Lampert S, Lown B, Graboys TB, Podrid PJ, Blatt C. Determinants of survival in patients with malignant ventricular arrhythmia associated with coronary artery disease. Am J Cardiol 1988;61:791–797.

69. Lehmann MH, Steinman RT, Schuger CD, Jackson K. The automatic implantable cardioverter defibrillator as antiarrhythmic treatment modality of choice for survivors of cardiac arrest unrelated to acute myocardial infarction. Am J Cardiol 1988; 62:803–805.

70. Weaver WD, Hill D, Fahrenbruch CE. Use of the automatic external defibrillator in the management of out-of-hospital cardiac arrest. N Engl J Med 1988;319:661–666.

71. Hine LK, Gross TP, Kennedy DL. Outpatient antiarrhythmic drug use from 1970 to 1986. Arch Intern Med 1989;149:1524–1527.

72. Podrid PJ, Marcus FI. Lessons to be learned from the Cardiac Arrhythmia Suppression Trial. Am J Cardiol 1989;64:1189–1191.

73. Pratt CM, Eaton T, Francis M, et al. The inverse relationship between baseline left ventricular ejection fraction and outcome of antiarrhythmic therapy: a dangerous imbalance in the risk-benefit ratio. Am Heart J 1989; 1128:433–440.

74. Pratt CM, Brater DC, Harrell FE, et al. Clinical and regulatory implications of the Cardiac Arrhythmia Suppression Trial. Am J Cardiol 1990;65:101–103.

75. Akhtar M, Breithardt G, Camm AJ, et al. CAST and beyond. Implications of the Cardiac Arrhythmia Suppression Trial. Circulation 1990;81:1123–1127.

76. Yusuf S, Peto R, Collins R, Sleight P. Beta blockade during and after myocardial infarction: an overview of the randomized trials. Prog Cardiovasc Dis 1985;27:335–371.

Section VII

Cerebrovascular Disease

20

stroke

The World Health Organization has defined a stroke as a syndrome composed of "rapidly developed clinical signs of focal (or global) disturbance of cerebral function, lasting more than 24 hours or leading to death, with no apparent cause other than of vascular origin" (1). The National Survey of Stroke in the United States specified that "vascular origins are limited to: (a) thrombotic or embolic occlusion of a cerebral artery resulting in infarction, or (b) spontaneous rupture of a vessel resulting in intracerebral or subarachnoid hemorrhage." From their definition of stroke, the investigators excluded vascular occlusion or rupture due to traumatic, neoplastic, or infectious processes (2). In addition to thrombosis and embolism, ischemic stroke may result from hypoxia. Symptoms of an ischemic stroke often include only progressive weakness or paralysis, while a hemorrhagic stroke usually is characterized by headache and increased intracranial pressure and may include loss of consciousness and death.

Duration of such signs and symptoms distinguishes a stroke from a transient ischemic attack (TIA). In the latter syndrome, evidence of cerebrovascular blood flow insufficiency is no longer present 24 hours after its onset.

Normally, cerebral blood flow (CBF) is autoregulated, providing constancy of flow despite fluctuations in cerebral perfusion pressure (mean arterial pressure minus intracranial pressure) within a range of 60 to 150 mm Hg. Below the lower limit, CBF becomes insufficient. Even below this level, however, vasodilation can be further increased with hypercapnia or pharmacologic therapy. The oxygen requirements of the brain can be met by further increasing oxygen extraction from the blood, since in the cerebral circulation, extraction is not always near maximal as it is in the coronary artery circulation. Above 150 mm Hg mean arterial pressure, vasoconstriction results in increased CBF, but the increased intraluminal pressure may lead to brain edema.

Autoregulation is mainly accomplished by smaller, resistance vessels, while the influence of the sympathetic nervous system is largely on larger, cerebral vessels. In the face of chronic hypertension, the lower and upper limits of autoregulation shift upward. However, the ability of resistance vessels to maximally dilate is inhibited by structural changes within the arterial wall. Treatment can restore the CBF autoregulatory mechanism in the absence of irreversible structural changes in

the arteries, although the relative influences of various antihypertensive agents is
not currently known (3).

STROKE EPIDEMIOLOGY

The incidence of stroke in most economically developed countries ranges from
150 to 250 new cases annually per 100,000
population of all ages (1), of which 10 to
20% are hemorrhagic. While methods of ascertainment differ in various studies, reports from Europe (4), Australia (5), Japan
(6), Hawaii (7), and the North American
continent (8, 9) provide similar incidence
rates.

The Ni-Hon-San Study of men of
Japanese ancestry living in Japan, Hawaii,
and the San Francisco Bay area documented markedly higher stroke rates in
those living in Japan during the 1965 to
1972 period (10). However, during the
1980s, mortality from stroke has been
halved in Japan (11). Reed has suggested
that low CAD rates and high stroke incidence in Japan may be due not to atherosclerotic disease in major cerebral arteries,
but to lesions in the small intracerebral arteries (12).

In middle-aged whites in the US,
stroke mortality decreased by one-third
over a 20-year period (13). Although survival following stroke has improved, stroke
incidence in the US has decreased even
more dramatically (14). These gains may
be attributed in part to enhanced detection
and treatment of hypertension and dyslipidemias, as well as to reductions in the
prevalence of smoking (15), as will be discussed later.

The probability of surviving for six
months after a hemorrhagic stroke in the
US is approximately 30%, whereas approximately 60% of individuals experiencing
ischemic strokes are alive six months
thereafter. Five-year survival for persons

with hemorrhagic and ischemic strokes is
20% to 30%, respectively (16).

Racial and ethnic differences in
stroke incidence may be noted within a
given country. For example, stroke mortality in black men in the United States was
nearly double the rate in white men from
1979 to 1982 (17). In 1983, the years of potential life lost before age 65 years due to
cerebrovascular disease were nearly three
times higher for black women and men
than for their white counterparts (18). The
inverse relation of stroke and socioeconomic status may account for some observed differences among racial and ethnic
groups (12).

Age plays an important role in stroke
mortality; rates more than triple with each
succeeding decade (5). In most countries,
men have an overall excess of cerebrovascular deaths compared with women. For
ischemic stroke, the male excess is approximately 45%. For intracerebral hemorrhage, rates are similar for the two genders,
while subarachnoid hemorrhage is nearly
twice as common in women (19). In the US
National Survey of Stroke during 1975–
1976, the age-adjusted incidence rate for
hemorrhagic stroke was 53% higher in
women (8).

In persons under the age of 45 who
have experienced a focal cerebral or retinal
event, male and female rates are equal. In
the youngest subjects, women's rates may
exceed those of men. As was discussed in
Chapter 11, this may be attributed in part
to the vascular complications of oral contraceptives (20), smoking, and their combination (21), as well as the influence of
pregnancy (22). Other medical conditions,
such as mitral valve prolapse, may further
add to this concentration of strokes in
young women (23).

Occupation may influence stroke
rates. In Japan, farmers have the highest
stroke rates, where miners occupy that po-

sition in England and Wales. Professional persons in both countries have considerably lower rates (24). Of course, occupation may reflect lower economic conditions and access to medical care, along with the tendency of persons in lower social classes to have higher levels of disease risk indicators.

Family history of stroke is probably an independent predictor for first-degree relatives. The relative risk in one California study was 2.3 for women aged 50 to 79 years after controlling for other cardiovascular risk indicators. In that population sample, however, men did not appear to be at increased risk of stroke, although a family history of stroke did give them a relative risk of 3.3 for coronary artery disease events (25). A case-control study in the UK revealed that a family history of stroke or MI was associated with increased risk of stroke in women (26).

The existence of chronic atrial fibrillation is recognized as a risk indicator of cerebral embolism and infarction, largely as a result of the migration of intracardiac thrombi (27). Transesophageal echocardiography is the method of choice for detection of these lesions. In elderly participants in the Framingham Study, a moderate degree of mitral annular calcification doubled the risk for stroke (28). Likewise, left atrial size correlated with stroke risk, which doubled with every 10 mm increase in left atrial diameter (29).

RISK INDICATORS

Ischemic Stroke

Indicators of ischemic stroke risk are similar to those for coronary artery disease (CAD). In fact, preexisting CAD serves as a marker for increased stroke risk (25). Conversely, some authors recommend coronary angiography more readily in persons

with documented extracranial atherosclerosis, since the leading cause of death in patients who have a history of stroke or TIA is myocardial infarction rather than recurrent stroke or other neurological disease (30).

LIPIDS AND LIPOPROTEINS

Serum total cholesterol and stroke mentality were examined in more than 350,000 men without history of MI, who were not being treated for diabetes. During six years' surveillance of men who had been screened for the Multiple Risk Factor Intervention Trial (MRFIT), a positive association was noted between ischemic stroke and total cholesterol. In contrast, men with total cholesterol levels under 160 mg/dl had a threefold greater risk for intracranial hemorrhage. The authors suggest that very low serum cholesterol levels may weaken the endothelium of intracerebral arteries. In the face of hypertension, arterionecrosis may ensue, leading to the rupture of microaneurysms and cerebral hemorrhage. They conclude that, despite the risk of hemorrhagic stroke at low total cholesterol levels, the public health impact is far greater for persons with elevated cholesterol and their consequent risk for CAD and ischemic stroke (31).

Meyer et al. studied cerebral blood flow in elderly volunteers and age-matched patients with TIA symptoms. Significantly higher total cholesterol and triglyceride levels were noted in the TIA patients, and cerebral blood flow in the TIA patients was inversely related to lipid levels (32). In another study, an increased risk of brain infarction in persons with familial hypercholesterolemia was noted (33). Acheson and Williams demonstrated an inverse relation between stroke and consumption of fresh green vegetables and fresh fruit, but they did not draw firm conclusions about the mechanism (34).

SMOKING

In a case-control study encompassing nearly one-quarter of the New Zealand population, men and women who smoked cigarettes were noted to have a threefold increase in the risk of stroke compared with nonsmokers. Smokers who were also hypertensive had an almost 20-fold risk compared to those with neither condition. The authors attributed roughly 37% of stroke events to smoking and a similar percentage to hypertension (35).

In the Honolulu Heart Study of 8006 men of Japanese ancestry, those who continued to smoke through 12 years of surveillance had twice the risk of ischemic stroke as those who had never smoked (36). In the Nurses' Health Study, which was initially composed of more than 100,000 women aged 30 to 55 years, subjects smoking 1 to 14 cigarettes per day had a relative risk of stroke of 2.2; those smoking 25 or more cigarettes daily had a relative risk of 3.7, compared with nonsmoking participants (37). Investigators in the Framingham Study also confirmed the independent predictive value of smoking on stroke incidence (38).

HYPERTENSION

The effects of hypertension and left ventricular hypertrophy on stroke incidence was clearly seen during the 30-year surveillance of participants in the Framingham Study (39). Investigators also suggested that isolated systolic hypertension predisposes to stroke, independent of arterial rigidity (40). In men aged 35 to 57 years, who were MRFIT screenees, the incidence of stroke mortality was three times higher in those with isolated systolic hypertension as in those with systolic and diastolic blood pressures less than 160 mm Hg and 90 mm Hg, respectively (41).

In the Hypertension Detection and Follow-up Program in the US, five-year stroke incidence in the stepped-care group was 34% lower than in the community-treated referred-care group. These reductions were experienced by all race-gender groups, at all ages and diastolic blood pressure strata, and among those with and without long-standing hypertension (42). A pooled analysis of nine long-term, randomized, clinical trials revealed a 38% reduction in stroke mortality among participants in the intervention groups (43). Bonita and Beaglehole have analyzed these and other studies and concluded that, despite these notable results, approximately three-fourths of the observed reduction in stroke mortality in economically developed countries is due to factors other than high blood pressure reduction (44). They note reports that stroke mortality is increasing in eastern European countries, suggesting further examination of other stroke risk indicators as well (45).

During the past two decades, stroke mortality has also decreased in Australia, but rates continue to exceed those in the United States for both women and men. Higher blood pressures and a greater prevalence of hypertension are consistent with a 40 to 55% greater mortality in Australia from 1968 to 1977. Investigators also note a higher consumption of alcohol in Australia, which may account for some differences in hypertension levels (46).

As noted in Chapter 4, guidelines for the detection, evaluation, and treatment of high blood pressure have been promulgated by the National High Blood Pressure Education Program in the United States (47).

ALCOHOL

During the past three decades, the relation of alcohol abuse and stroke has been firmly established. The direct association has been noted in Finland (48), the United Kingdom (49), Yugoslavia (50), Japan (51), Hawaii (52), and the North American continent, particularly in persons below the age of 50 (53, 54).

In a case-control study from England, light drinkers (10 to 90 g per week) had only half the stroke rate of nondrinkers. In contrast, men consuming 300 g or more weekly had a relative stroke risk of 4.2 compared with nondrinkers (49). Investigators have suggested that alterations in cerebral blood flow and its autoregulation, secondary to altered cerebral metabolism and vasospasm of cerebral vascular smooth muscle, occur with habitual alcohol intake (55). These effects, combined with alcohol-related disturbances of blood pressure, coagulation, and cardiac rhythm, place the heavy drinker at greater risk of stroke (56).

DIABETES

Persons with glucose intolerance or frank diabetes mellitus have a relative risk of 2 to 4 for stroke. Although diabetes is associated with other risk indicators, such as hypertension, it exerts an independent effect on stroke incidence, as measured in the United Kingdom and the United States (57). In Göteborg, Sweden, stroke patients aged 65 to 75 years had a 22% prevalence of diabetes, compared with 6% from the general population of 70-year-old residents of that city (58).

PHYSICAL INACTIVITY AND OBESITY

In the Framingham Study, an inverse relation between obesity and stroke risk in the elderly was noted. In younger Japanese-Hawaiian men, however, the two variables were directly related (59). Investigators in a case-control study of stroke in the Netherlands suggest that vigorous physical activity may reduce the risk of stroke (60).

SOCIOLOGIC FACTORS

British investigators reported two cases of stroke in young women, titling their report "Conjugal Disharmony." Neither had been taking oral contraceptives, nor had either any other conventional risk indicators for stroke. After some probing, both women admitted to a strangulation attempt by their husbands, resulting in traumatic internal carotid artery occlusion (61).

Hemorrhagic Stroke

Modifiable risk indicators for hemorrhagic stroke are similar to those for ischemic stroke (62), but hypertension, smoking, and coagulation abnormalities, including those induced by alcohol (63), play a particularly important part.

Investigators from the Honolulu Heart Study noted that consumption of alcohol greater than 30 ml daily doubled the risk of hemorrhagic stroke (64). Hillbom noted the precipitation of hemorrhagic and ischemic strokes during intoxication, rather than withdrawal. In other studies, he and his colleagues observed that the incidence of alcohol-related strokes correlated with the relative alcohol consumption in Finnish men and women, but alcohol-unrelated strokes are approximately equal in the two genders (48). Chronic use of alcohol is also associated with a variety of clotting and platelet abnormalities (56).

In a study of physicians in the United States, participants were randomized to every-other-day doses either 325 mg aspirin or placebo. Hemorrhagic strokes were doubled in the aspirin group, although the incidence of fatal and nonfatal MI was sufficiently lower to warrant termination of that component of the trial (65).

In the aforementioned Honolulu Heart Study, the risk of hemorrhagic stroke was four-fold in continuing smokers compared with those who were nonsmokers during the first 12 years of follow-up (36). In the Nurses' Health Study, women smoking 25 or more cigarettes daily had a relative risk of subarachnoid hemorrhage of 9.8 compared to those who had never smoked (37).

DIAGNOSTIC ASSESSMENT

Investigators in two large studies have documented an increased risk of stroke in persons with asymptomatic carotid bruits. In the Evans County, Georgia Study of blacks and whites, aged 45 years and older, men with asymptomatic bruits were 7.5 times more likely to have a new stroke; women displayed a threefold risk (66). In the Framingham Study, strokes were twice as common in men and women with asymptomatic bruits (67).

However, in both studies, correlation of the bruits and the affected hemisphere was poor. It is clear that bruits indicate generalized atherosclerotic disease, since myocardial infarction rates are also higher in persons with such signs.

In 1988, Feussner and Matcher published their criteria for carotid studies. Their recommendations depend heavily upon the presence and location of symptoms and are summarized below.

When neck bruits are asymptomatic, no diagnostic testing is indicated, even before vascular reconstruction or coronary artery bypass surgery. Instead, patients can be educated about symptoms indicative of TIAs.

If TIA symptoms exist in the distribution of the carotid circulation, a surgical candidate should have noninvasive testing, preferably duplex ultrasonography. This procedure combines pulsed-echo or B-mode ultrasonography with pulsed Doppler, and has 85% sensitivity and 90% specificity in detecting high-grade stenoses. If such a positive result is obtained, carotid angiography is indicated. If persons with a previous minor stroke develop TIA symptoms, they may proceed directly to angiography.

When signs are nonlateralizing, such as syncope, dizziness, vertigo, diplopia, and tonic clonic motor activity, neurologic consultation is indicated. If the consultant determines that symptoms may arise from the carotid circulation, noninvasive testing is recommended. If not, diagnostic testing is not indicated. The authors indicate that this last set of recommendations is conservative, but they point out the high rate of false positives that may result from indiscriminate noninvasive testing, as well as the unnecessary carotid angiography and endarterectomy procedures that may ensue (68).

PREVENTION OF STROKE AND ITS RECURRENCE

Therapeutic regimens proposed for the primary prevention of stroke have included hypertension treatment, platelet antiaggregants, anticoagulation, fibrinolytic therapy, and surgery. While thrombolytic therapy holds promise as the treatment for acute stroke, dipyridamole, sulfinpyrazone, anticoagulation, carotid endarterectomy, and extracranial-to-intracranial bypass operations have not been demonstrated to contribute significantly to the primary prevention of stroke (69, 70). In contrast, successful treatment of hypertension, aspirin, and ticlopidine have been documented to significantly reduce primary stroke incidence.

Hypertension Treatment

The beneficial effects of treatment of hypertension have been noted in several randomized controlled studies (71–75) as noted in Table 20.1.

Further analysis of the Medical Research Council (MRC) trial data suggested that diuretic treatment was equally effec-

Table 20.1.   Reduction in Stroke Incidence with Antihypertensive Therapy

Study	Intervention	% Stroke Reduction	Reference
VA Cooperative (USA)	Diuretic	76	(71)
Australian Therapeutic	Diuretic	45	(72)
European Working Party	Diuretic, methyldopa prn	43	(73)
MRC[a] Working Party (UK)	Diuretic	67	(74)
	β-blocker	24	
HDFP[b] (USA)	Stepped care versus referred	34	(75)

[a]MRC = Medical Research Council.
[b]HDFP = Hypertension Detection and Follow-up Program.

tive in stroke reduction in smokers and nonsmokers of both genders. In contrast, propranolol was effective only in nonsmokers. The effects were greatest in persons with the highest initial blood pressures, leading the MRC Working Party to recommend that routine prescription of drugs for all persons with mild hypertension should be avoided (76).

Platelet Antiaggregants

As noted earlier, the Physicians' Health Study in the United States found increased stroke rates among their participants (all male) taking aspirin. The relative risk for ischemic stroke was 1.11, but it was 2.14 for hemorrhagic stroke (65). A smaller study in British physicians produced even higher stroke rates in the aspirin-treated (500 mg daily) group. The principal investigators of the two studies issued a joint letter, comparing these rates (Table 20.2). They concluded that the prescription of aspirin for primary prevention should remain a matter of judgment, in which the physicians balance the risk of aspirin against the "clearly established reduction in the incidence of a first myocardial infarction" (77).

Several studies have confirmed that 1300 mg aspirin daily will reduce stroke incidence after TIA by 25 to 30%, while sulfinpyrazone and dipyridamole offer no advantage over aspirin therapy alone (69). In the United Kingdom Transient Ischemic Attack (UK-TIA) Aspirin Trial, 2435 persons thought to have had a TIA or minor ischemic stroke were allocated to aspirin 1200 mg daily, aspirin 300 mg daily, or placebo regimens. After a four-year follow-up, stroke incidence was significantly reduced in both groups receiving aspirin, with no appreciable advantage of the higher dose (78).

The use of antithrombolitic agents to prevent stroke resulting from other cardio-

Table 20.2.   Nonfatal Stroke Rates in Aspirin Studies in Physicians in United Kingdom and United States

	Nonfatal strokes/1000 men	
	Aspirin	No Aspirin
Disabling and nondisabling		
United Kingdom (UK)	17.8	15.8
United States (US)	7.2	6.3
Disabling strokes only		
UK	10.5	4.1
US	1.5	1.1
Nondisabling strokes		
UK	7.3	11.7
US	5.7	5.3

vascular conditions has recently been reviewed by a panel from the American College of Chest Physicians (79).

Modification of Other Risk Indicators

Much less has been written about the
effects of dyslipidemias, smoking, diabetes
control, and obesity after stroke or documentation of TIA. Leonberg and Elliot
provided individual risk-indicator assessment and treatment in 88 survivors of a
first stroke. They noted that most prior
studies showed an anticipated five-year
mortality of 35 to 65% and a recurrence
rate of 20 to 40%. In their patients, five-
year mortality was 17%, with a 16% incidence of stroke recurrence (80).

REFERENCES

1. Aho K, Harmsen P, Hatano S, Mar-
quardsen J, Smirnov VE, Strasser T. Cerebrovascular disease in the community: results of a
WHO collaborative study. Bull WHO
1980;58:113–130.

2. Walker AE, Robins M, Weinfeld FD.
The National Survey of Stroke. Clinical findings. Stroke 1981;12(suppl I):I13–I44.

3. Paulson OB, Waldemar G, Schmidt JF,
Strandgaard S. Cerebral circulation under normal and pathologic conditions. Am J Cardiol
1989;63:2C–5C.

4. Harmsen P, Berglund G, Larsson O,
Tibblin G, Wilhelmson L. Stroke registration
in Goteborg, Sweden, 1970–1975. Acta Med
Scand 1979;206:337–344.

5. Dobson AJ, Gibberd RW, Wheeler DJ,
Leeder SR. Age-specific trends in mortality
from ischemic heart disease and cerebrovascular disease in Australia. Am J Epidemiol
1981;113:404–412.

6. Tamashiro H, Enomoto N, Minowa M,
et al. Geographical distributions of cerebrocar-
diovascular diseases in Japan: 1969–1974. Soc
Sci Med 1981;15D:173–186.

7. Kagan AG, Popper JS, Rhoads GG.
Factors related to stroke incidence in Hawaii

Japanese men. The Honolulu Heart Study.
Stroke 1981;11:14–21.

8. Robins M, Baum HM. The National
Survey of Stroke. Incidence. Stroke
1981;12(suppl I):I45–I57.

9. American Heart Association. 1990
Heart and stroke facts. Dallas, TX: American
Heart Association, 1989.

10. Worth RM, Kato H, Rhoads GG,
Kagan A, Syme SL. Epidemiologic studies of
coronary heart disease and stroke in Japanese
men living in Japan, Hawaii and California:
mortality. Am J Epidemiology 1975;102:481–
490.

11. Uemura K. International trends in
cardiovascular diseases in the elderly. Eur
Heart J 1988;9(suppl D):1–8.

12. Reed DM. The paradox of high risk of
stroke in populations with low risk of coronary
heart disease. Am J Epidemiol 1990;131:579–
588.

13. Wing S, Casper M, Davis WB, Pellum
A, Riggan W, Tyroler HA. Stroke mortality
maps. United States whites aged 35–74 years,
1962–1982. Stroke 1988;19:1507–1513.

14. Wolf PA. Cigarettes, alcohol, and
stroke. N Engl J Med 1986;315:1087–1089.

15. Klag MG, Whelton PK, Seidler AJ.
Decline in US stroke mortality. Demographic
trends and antihypertensive treatment. Stroke
1989;20:14–21.

16. Baum HM, Robins M. The National
Survey of Stroke. Survival and prevalence.
Stroke 1981;12(suppl I):I59–I68.

17. Savage DD, McGee DL, Oster G. Reduction of hypertension-associated heart disease and stroke among black Americans: past
experience and new perspectives on targeting
resources. Milbank Quarterly 1987;65:(suppl
2):297–321.

18. Anonymous. Premature mortality due
to cerebrovascular disease—United States,
1983. MMWR 1987;36(20),316–317.

19. Haberman S, Capildeo R, Rose FC.
Sex differences in the incidence of cerebrovascular disease. J Epidemiol Comm Health
1981;35:45–50.

20. Collaborative Group for the Study of
Stroke in Young Women. Oral contraception
and increased risk of cerebral ischemia or
thrombosis. N Engl J Med 1973;288:871–878.

21. Petitti DB, Wingerd J. Use of oral contraceptives, cigarette smoking, and risk of subarachnoid hemorrhage. Lancet 1978;2:234–235.

22. Jennett WB, Cross JN. Influence of pregnancy and oral contraception on the incidence of strokes in women of childbearing age. Lancet 1967;1:1019–1023.

23. Donaldson JO. Stroke. Clin Obstet Gynecol 1981;24:828–835.

24. Kagamimori S. Occupational life tables for cerebrovascular disease and ischemic heart disease in Japan compared with England and Wales. Jpn Circul J 1981;45:195–201.

25. Khaw KT, Barrett-Connor E. Family history of stroke as an independent predictor of ischemic heart disease in men and stroke in women. Am J Epidemiol 1986;123:59–66.

26. Thompson SG, Greenberg G, Meade TW. Risk factors for stroke and myocardial infarction in women in the United Kingdom as assessed in general practice: a case-control study. Br Heart J 1989;61:403–409.

27. Dyken ML, Wolf PA, Barnett HG, et al. Risk factors for stroke. Stroke 1987;18:9–15.

28. Benjamin EJ, Levy D, D'Agostino RB, et al. Mitral annular calcification and the risk of stroke in a free living elderly cohort. Circulation 1989;80(suppl II):II-403.

29. Benjamin EJ, Levy D, Plehn JF, Belanger AJ, D'Agostino RB, Wolf PA. Left atrial size: an independent risk factor for stroke. The Framingham Study. Circulation 1989;80(suppl II):II-615.

30. Graor RA, Hetzer NR. Management of coexistent carotid artery and coronary artery disease. Curr Concepts Cardiovasc Dis 1988;23:19–23.

31. Iso H, Jacobs DR Jr, Wentworth D, Neaton JD, Cohen JD for the MRFIT Research Group. Serum cholesterol levels and six-year mortality from stroke in 350,977 men screened for the Multiple Risk Factor Intervention Trial. N Engl J Med 1989;320:904–910.

32. Meyer JS, Rogers RL, Mortel KF, Judd BW. Hyperlipidemia is a risk factor for decreased cerebral perfusion and stroke. Arch Neurol 1987;44:418–422.

33. Kaste M, Koivisto P. Risk of brain infarction in familial hypercholesterolemia. Stroke 1988;19:1097–1100.

34. Acheson RM, Williams DR. Does consumption of fruit and vegetables protect against stroke? Lancet 1983;1:1191–1193.

35. Bonita R, Scragg R, Stewart A, Jackson R, Beaglehole R. Cigarette smoking and risk of premature stroke in men and women. Brit Med J 1986;293:6–8.

36. Abbott RD, Yin Y, Reed DM, Yano K. Risk of stroke in male cigarette smokers. N Engl J Med 1986;315:717–720.

37. Colditz GA, Bonita R, Stampfer MJ, et al. Cigarette smoking and risk of stroke in middle-aged women. N Engl J Med 1988;318:937–941.

38. Wolf PA, D'Agostino RB, Kannel KB, et al. Cigarette smoking as a risk factor for stroke: the Framingham Study. JAMA 1988;259:1025–1029.

39. Stokes J III, Kannel WB, Wolf PA, D'agostino RB, Cupples LA. Blood pressure as a risk factor for cardiovascular disease. Hypertension 1989;13(suppl I):I13–I18.

40. Kannel WB, Wolf PA, McGee DL, Dawber TR, McNamara P, Castelli WP. Systolic blood pressure, arterial rigidity, and risk of stroke. The Framingham Study. JAMA 1981;245:1225–1229.

41. Rutan GH, Kuller LH, Neaton JD, Wentworth DN, McDonald RH, Smith WM. Mortality associated with diastolic hypertension and isolated systolic hypertension among men screened for the Multiple Risk Factor Intervention Trial. Circulation 1988;77:504–514.

42. Hypertension Detection and Follow-Up Program Cooperative Group. Five-year findings of the Hypertension Detection and Follow-Up Program. III. Reduction in stroke incidence among persons with high blood pressure. JAMA 1982;247:633–638.

43. MacMahon SW, Cutler JA, Furberg CD, Payne GH. The effects of drug treatment for hypertension on morbidity and mortality from cardiovascular disease: a review of randomized controlled trials. Prog Cardiovasc Dis 1986;29:99–118.

44. Bonita R, Beaglehole R. Increased treatment of hypertension does not explain the decline of stroke mortality in the United States, 1970–1980. Hypertension 1989;13(suppl I):I69–I73.

45. Uemura K, Pisa Z. Recent trends in cardiovascular disease mortality in 27 industrialized countries. World Health Stat Q 1985;38:142–156.

46. MacMahon SW, Leeder SR. Blood pressure levels and mortality from cerebrovascular disease in Australia and the United States. Am J Epidemiol 1984;120:865–875.

47. Joint National Committee. The 1988 report of the Joint National Committee on the Detection, Evaluation, and Treatment of High Blood Pressure. Arch Intern Med 1988; 148:1023–1038.

48. Hilbom ME. What supports the role of alcohol as a risk factor for stroke? Acta Med Scand 1987;717(suppl):93–106.

49. Gill JS, Zezulka AV, Shipley MJ, Gill SK, Beevers DG. Stroke and alcohol consumption. N Engl J Med 1986;315:717–720.

50. Kozararevic D, McGee D, Vojvodic N, et al. Frequency of alcohol consumption and morbidity and mortality. Lancet 1980;1:613–616.

51. Kono S, Ikeda M, Tokudome S, Nishizumi M, Kuratsune M. Smoking and mortalities from cancer, coronary heart disease and stroke in male Japanese physicians. J Cancer Res Clin Oncol 1985;110:161–164.

52. Blackwelder WC, Yano K, Rhoads GG, Kagan A, Gordon T, Palech Y. Alcohol and mortality: the Honolulu Heart Study. Am J Med 1980;68:164–169.

53. Hilbom M, Kaste M, Ravi V. Can ethanol intoxication affect hemocoagulation to increase the risk of brain infarction in young adults? Neurology 1983;33:381–384.

54. Taylor JR, Coombs-Orme T. Alcohol and strokes in young adults. Am J Psychiatry 1985;142:116–118.

55. Rogers RL, Meyer JS, Shaw TG, Mortel KF. Reductions in regional cerebral blood flow associated with chronic consumption of alcohol. J Am Geriatr Soc 1983;31:540–543.

56. Gorelick PB. Alcohol and stroke. Stroke 1987;18:268–271.

57. Wade DT, Hewer RL, Skilbeck CE, David RM. Stroke. London: Chapman and Hall, 1985.

58. Himmelmann A, Hansson L, Svensson A, Harmsen P, Holmgren C, Svanborg A. Predictors of stroke in the elderly. Acta Med Scand 1988;224:439–443.

59. Rhoads GG, Kagan A. The relation of coronary disease, stroke, and mortality to weight in youth and middle age. Lancet 1983;1:492–495.

60. Herman B, Leyten AC, Van Luijk JH, Frenken CW, Op de Coul AA, Schulte BP. An evaluation of risk factors for stroke in a Dutch community. Stroke 1982;13:334–339.

61. Milligan N, Anderson M. Conjugal disharmony: a hitherto unrecognised cause of strokes. Br Med J 1980;9:421–422.

62. Davidson DM. Cardiovascular effects of alcohol. West J Med 1989;151:430–439.

63. Weisberg LA. Alcoholic intracranial hemorrhage. Stroke 1988;29:1565–1569.

64. Donahue RP, Abbott RD, Reed DM, Yano K. Alcohol and hemorrhagic stroke. The Honolulu Heart Program. JAMA 1986; 255:2311–2314.

65. Steering Committee of the Physicians' Health Study Research Group. Final report on the aspirin component of the ongoing Physicians' Health Study. N Engl J Med 1989; 321:129–135.

66. Heyman A, Wilkinson WE, Heyden S, et al. Risk of stroke in asymptomatic persons with cervical arterial bruits. N Engl J Med 1980;302:838–841.

67. Wolf PA, Kannel WB, Sorlie P, McNamara P. Asymptomatic carotid bruit and risk of stroke. The Framingham Study. JAMA 1981;245:1442–1445.

68. Feussner JR, Matchar DB. When and how to study the carotid arteries. Ann Intern Med 1988;109:805–818.

69. Grotta JC. Current medical and surgical therapy for cerebrovascular disease. N Engl J Med 1987;317:1505–1516.

70. Hass WK, Easton JD, Adams HP Jr, et al. A randomized trial comparing ticlopidine hydrochloride with aspirin for the prevention of stroke in high-risk patients. N Engl J Med 1989;321:501–507.

71. Freis ED. The Veterans Administration Cooperative Study on Antihypertensive Agents. Implications for stroke prevention. Stroke 1974;5:76–77.

72. Management Committee. The Australian Therapeutic Trial in Mild Hypertension. Lancet 1980;1:1261–1267.

73. Amery A, Brixko P, Clement D, et al. Mortality and morbidity results from the Eu-

ropean Working Party on High Blood Pressure in the Elderly Trial. Lancet 1985;1:1349–1354.

74. Medical Research Council Working Party. MRC Trial of Treatment of Mild Hypertension: principal results. Br Med J 1985; 291:97–102.

75. Hypertension Detection and Follow-up Program Cooperative Group. Persistence of reduction in blood pressure and mortality of participants in the Hypertension Detection and Follow-up Program. JAMA 1988;259:2113–2122.

76. Medical Research Council Working Party. Stroke and coronary heart disease in mild hypertension: risk factors and the value of treatment. Br Med J 1988;296:1565–1570.

77. Hennekens CH, Peto R, Hutchison GB, Doll R. An overview of the British and American aspirin studies. N Engl J Med 1988;318:923–924.

78. UK-TIA Study Group. United Kingdom transient ischaemic attack (UK-TIA) aspirin trial: interim results. Br Med J 1988;296:316–320.

79. Sherman DG, Dyken ML, Fisher M, Harrison MJ, Hart RG. Antithrombotic therapy for cerebrovascular disorders. Chest 1989;95(suppl):140S–155S.

80. Leonberg SC, Elliott FA. Prevention of recurrent stroke. Stroke 1981;12:731–735.

index

Page numbers in bold denote chapter headings.